Respiratory
Pharmacology and
Pharmacotherapy

Series Editors:

Dr. David Raeburn
Discovery Biology
Rhône-Poulenc Rorer Ltd
Dagenham Research Centre
Dagenham
Essex RM10 7XS
England

Dr. Mark A. Giembycz
Department of Thoracic Medicine
National Heart and Lung Institute
Imperial College of Science, Technology and Medicine
London SW3 6LY
England

Rhinitis: Immunopathology and Pharmacotherapy

Edited by
D. Raeburn
M. A. Giembycz

Birkhäuser Verlag
Basel · Boston · Berlin

Editors:

Dr. David Raeburn
Discovery Biology
Rhône-Poulenc Rorer Ltd
Dagenham Research Centre
Dagenham
Essex RM10 7XS
England

Dr. Mark A. Giembycz
Department of Thoracic Medicine
National Heart and Lung Institute
Imperial College of Science, Technology and Medicine
London SW3 6LY
England

Library of Congress Cataloging-in-Publication Data

Rhinitis: immunopathology and pharmacotherapy / edited by D. Raeburn, M.A. Giembycz
p. cm. – (Respiratory pharmacology and pharmacotherapy)
Includes bibliographical references and index.
ISBN-13: 978-3-0348-9937-6 e-ISBN-13: 978-3-0348-9181-3
DOI: 10.1007/978-3-0348-9181-3

1. Rhinitis – Pathophysiology. 2. Rhinitis – Immunological aspects. 3. Rhinitis – Chemotherapy. I. Raeburn, D. (David), 1953- II. Giembycz, M. A. (Mark A.), 1961- . III. Series.
[DNLM: 1. Rhinitis – immunology. 2. Rhinitis – drug therapy. 3. Rhinitis – physiopathology. WV 335 R47264 1997]
RF361.R48 1997
616.2' 12 – dc21
DNLM/DLC
for Library of Congress

Deutsche Bibliothek Cataloging-in-Publication Data

Rhinitis: immunopathology and pharmacotherapy / ed by D. Raeburn ; M. A. Giembycz. – Basel ; Boston : Berlin : Birkhäuser, 1997
(Respiratory pharmacology and pharmacotherapy)
ISBN-13: 978-3-0348-9937-6
NE: Raeburn, David [Hrsg.]

The publisher and editors cannot assume any legal responsibility for information on drug dosage and administration contained in this publication. The respective user must check its accuracy by consulting other sources of reference in each individual case.

Softcover reprint of the hardcover 1st edition 1997
Printed on acid-free paper produced from chlorine-free pulp. TCF ∞
Cover design: Markus Etterich

9 8 7 6 5 4 3 2 1

Contents

Contributors

Morgan Andersson, Department of Otorhinolaryngology, University Hospital, S-221 85 Lund, Sweden

Jean Bousquet, Clinique des Maladies Respiratoires, Hôpital Arnaud de Villeneuve, Centre Hospitalier Universitaire, 34295 Montpellier Cedex 5, France

Moisés A. Calderón, Department of Respiratory Medicine and Allergy, St. Bartholomew's Hospital, London EC1A 7BE, UK

Ker-Sang Chen, Procter & Gamble Pharmaceutical Research Division, Health Care Research Center, Procter & Gamble Company, Mason, Ohio 45040-8006, USA

James A. Cook, Department of Otolaryngology, Leicester Royal Infirmary, Leicester, UK

S. Criscione, Department of Experimental Medicine, University of Aquila, 67100 Aquila, Italy

Robert J. Davies, Department of Respiratory Medicine and Allergy, St. Bartholomew's Hospital, London EC1A 7BE, UK

Pascal Demoly, Clinique des Maladies Respiratoires, Hôpital Arnaud de Villeneuve, Centre Hospitalier Universitaire, 34295 Montpellier Cedex 5, France

Jonas Erjefält, Department of Physiology and Neuroscience, University Hospital, S-221 85 Lund, Sweden

Lennart Greiff, Department of Otorhinolaryngology, University Hospital, S-221 85 Lund, Sweden

Jane Krasnick, Division of Allergy-Immunology and the Ernest S. Bazley Asthma and Allergic Diseases Center of the Department of Medicine of Northwestern Memorial Hospital and Northwestern University Medical School, Chicago, Illinois 60611-3008, USA

Valerie J. Lund, Institute of Laryngology and Otology, University College London, London WC1X 8DA, UK

François-B. Michel, Clinique des Maladies Respiratoires, Hôpital Arnaud de Villeneuve, Centre Hospitalier Universitaire, 34295 Montpellier Cedex 5, France

Roy Patterson, Division of Allergy-Immunology and the Ernest S. Bazley Asthma and Allergic Diseases Center of the Department of Medicine of Northwestern Memorial Hospital and Northwestern University Medical School, Chicago, Illinois 60611-3008, USA

Carl G. A. Persson, Department of Clinical Pharmacology, University Hospital, S-221 85 Lund, Sweden

E. Porro, Department of Experimental Medicine, University of Aquila, 67100 Aquila, Italy

Glenis K. Scadding, Royal National Throat, Nose and Ear Hospital, London WC1X 8DA, UK

Christer Svensson, Department of Otorhinolaryngology, University Hospital, S-221 85 Lund, Sweden
John Widdicombe, Department of Physiology, St. George's Hospital Medical School, London SW17 0RE, UK

Rhinitis: Immunopathology
and Pharmacotherapy
ed. by D. Raeburn and M. A. Giembycz

CHAPTER 1
Anatomy and Physiology of the Nasal Cavity and Paranasal Sinuses

Valerie J. Lund

Institute of Laryngology and Otology, University College London, London, UK

1. Introduction

In considering the anatomy and physiology of the nose, this chapter must inevitably pay some attention to the adjacent paranasal sinuses, forming as they do an integral functional structure and subject to the same pathophysiological processes.

2. Nasal Cavity

2.1. Gross Anatomy

The nasal cavity extends from the nostrils to the posterior choanae, where it becomes continuous with the nasopharynx [1]. Vertically it extends from the palate to the cribriform plate, narrowing into the olfactory cleft. The nasal cavity is divided in two by a septum, and its configuration and dimensions show considerable ethnic variation. Each half has a floor, a roof, a lateral wall and a medial (septal) wall. The *floor* is composed anteriorly of the palatine process of the maxilla and posteriorly by the horizontal process of the palatine bone. The *roof* is narrow from side to side, and its highest part relates to the cribriform plate of the ethmoid. This area is covered by olfactory epithelium which spreads down a little distance onto the upper lateral and medial walls of the nasal cavity. The rest of the nasal cavity (with the exception of the nasal vestibule) is lined by respiratory mucous membrane which is intimately adherent to the underlying periosteum and perichondrium and is continuous with that of the paranasal sinuses, nasolacrimal duct and nasopharynx.

The *nasal septum* is composed of a small anterior membranous portion, cartilage and several bones; the perpendicular plate of the ethmoid, the vomer and two bony crests of the maxilla and palatine. The cartilaginous portion is composed of a quadrilateral cartilage with a contribution from the lower and upper lateral alar cartilages forming the anterior nasal septum. It is bound firmly by collagenous fibres to the nasal bones and to the perpendicular plate of the ethmoid and vomer, and sits inferiorly in the nasal crest of the palatine process of the maxilla. The perpendicular plate forms the superior and anterior bony septum, is continuous above with the cribriform plate and crista galli and abuts a variable amount of the nasal bones. The vomer forms the posterior and inferior nasal septum and articulates by its two alae with the rostrum of the sphenoid, inferiorly with the nasal crest formed by the maxillae and palatine bones and anteriorly with the perpendicular plate of the ethmoid and the quadrilateral cartilage. The posterior edge of the vomer forms the posterior free edge of the septum. Deflections can occur at any of these articulations.

The lateral wall is divided up by a number of baffles, or *turbinates*, which are the remnants of more complicated structures in lower mammals, in whom they increase surface area for olfaction and air conditioning (Figure 1). The wall adjacent to the turbinates is termed a meatus. Thus the *inferior meatus* is that part of the lateral wall of the nose lateral to the inferior turbinate. It is the largest meatus, extending almost the entire length of the nasal cavity. The meatus is highest at the junction of the anterior and middle third with the nasolacrimal duct opening just anterior to this highest point.

The *inferior turbinate* is a separate bone with an irregular surface, perforated and grooved by vascular channels to which the mucoperiosteum is firmly attached (Figure 2). The bone articulates with the inferior margin of the maxillary hiatus and with the ethmoid, palatine and lacrimal bones, completing the medial wall of the nasolacrimal duct. The turbinate possesses an impressive submucosal cavernous plexus with large sinusoids under autonomic control which provides the major contribution to nasal resistance.

The *middle meatus* is that portion of the lateral nasal wall lying lateral to the *middle turbinate*. It receives drainage from the frontal, maxillary and

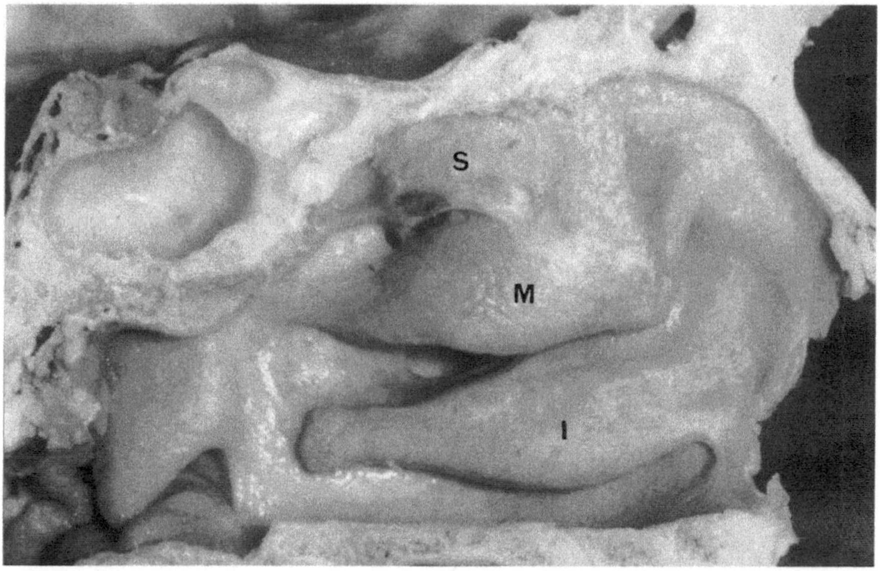

Figure 1. Photograph of sagittal section showing lateral wall of nasal cavity, with three main turbinates (I: inferior, M: middle and S: superior) and sphenoid sinus cavity posteriorly.

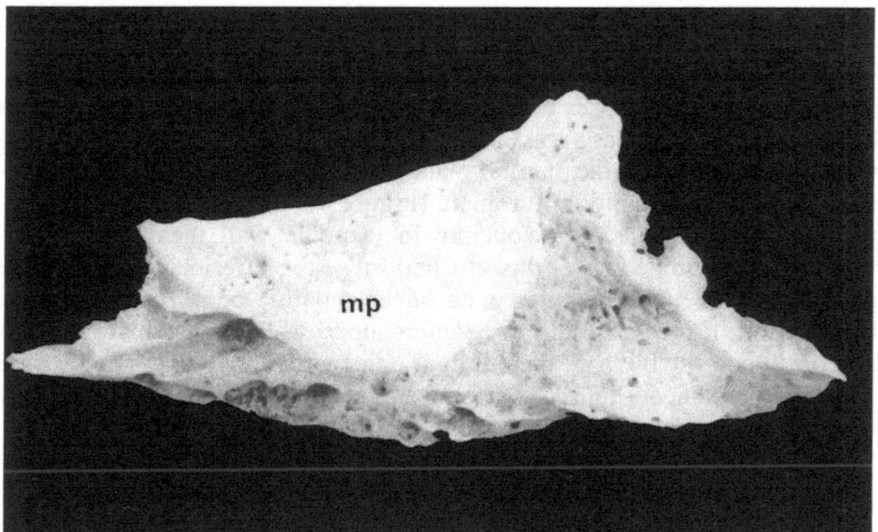

Figure 2. Photograph of inferior turbinate bone, showing maxillary process (MP) which articulates with maxillary hiatus and irregularities in the bone due to vascular structures.

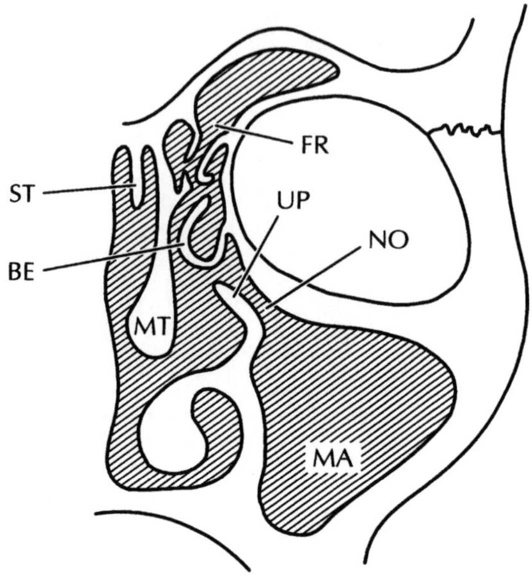

Figure 3. Diagram of coronal view of anterior middle meatus showing relationship of maxillary, anterior ethmoid and frontal sinuses draining into the ostiomeatal complex. ST: superior turbinate; MT: middle turbinate; MA: maxillary sinus (antrum); NO: natural ostium of maxillary sinus; UP: uncinate process; BE: bulla ethmoidalis (anterior ethmoid cell); FR: frontal recess.

anterior ethmoidal sinuses (Figure 3). The configuration of the structures of the middle meatus are complex and variable. If the topographical anatomy is considered in the sagittal plane, a number of structures are apparent covered by the middle turbinate (Figure 4). In a disarticulated skull, the maxillary bone has a large opening in its medial wall, the maxillary hiatus. In the articulated skull this is filled in by the inferior turbinate bone (inferiorly), the perpendicular plate of the palatine bone (posteriorly), a tiny portion of the lacrimal bone (anterosuperiorly), the uncinate process anteriorly and the bulla of the ethmoid (superiorly). The uncinate process is a crescent-shaped bone of variable size, and the bulla is a bony bulge made by one or more of the anterior ethmoidal sinuses.

A portion of the maxillary hiatus is nevertheless left open by these osseous attachments which in life is filled by the mucous membrane of the middle meatus and the maxillary sinus and the intervening connective tissue forming the membranous portion of the lateral wall. This membranous area can be defined as lying anterior or posterior to the uncinate process, constituting the anterior and posterior fontanelles respectively. These may break down in acute maxillary sinusitis to form extra or accessory ostia.

Between the posterior edge of the uncinate process and the anterior surface of the ethmoidal bulla lies the hiatus semilunaris, a two-dimensional

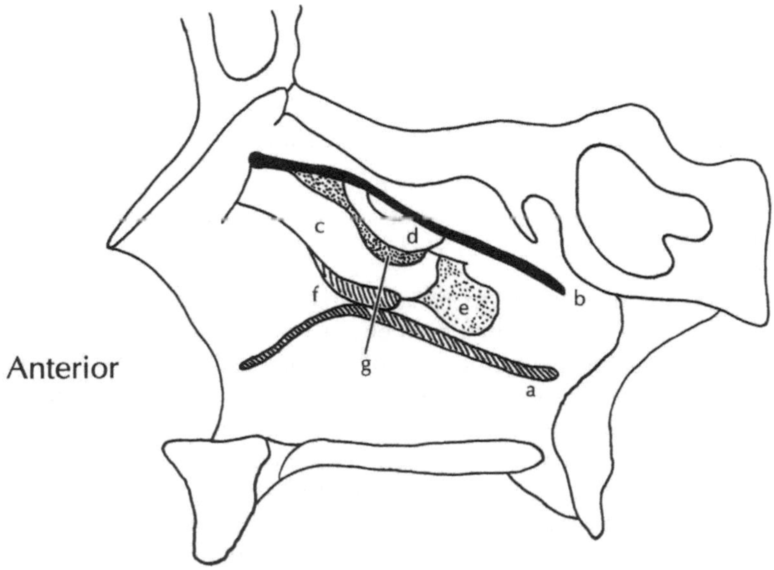

Figure 4. Diagram showing lateral wall of nasal cavity after removal of turbinates. a: position of inferior turbinate; b: position of middle turbinate; c: uncinate process; d: bulla ethmoidalis; e: posterior fontanelle; f: anterior fontanelle; g: hiatus semilunaris.

space leading into the ethmoidal infundibulum. This funnel connects the middle meatus with the natural ostium of the maxillary sinus, which therefore cannot usually be seen until the uncinate process has been removed.

The opening into the frontal sinus is found in the most anterosuperior portion of the middle meatus. The term "frontonasal duct" has been generally abandoned in favour of "frontal recess", as no true duct exists either histologically or topographically in the majority of cases. The natural ostium of the frontal sinus is somewhat variable in its configuration but most frequently is an hourglass narrowing opening directly into the recess. Rarely, a longer narrowed region is found.

There is a considerable range of anatomic variation in this area, which has been implicated in the development of sinus infection [2]. This includes pneumatisation of the middle turbinate, enlargement of the ethmoidal bulla, a paradoxically bent middle turbinate, everted uncinate process, the presence of Haller cells (anterior ethmoidal cell which pneumatise the floor of the orbit), Onodi cells (posterior ethmoidal cells which pneumatise lateral to the sphenoid sinus) or a septal deflection. The incidence with which these occur in a "normal" population may appear to be less frequent than in those individuals with chronic rhinosinusitis, but on closer inspection it is clear that it is narrowing of the ostiomeatal complex (see p 17) rather than the existence of the variant which is the important factor [3].

The *superior meatus* is again defined by its relationship to the superior turbinate. The posterior ethmoidal cells open into this region. A *supreme turbinate* is discernible above the superior meatus in 60–67% of subjects [4, 5]. The *sphenoethmoidal recess* lies medial to the superior turbinate and is the location of the ostium of the spenoid sinus.

2.2. Histology

The mucous membrane of the nasal cavity is predominantly respiratory with a small area of olfactory epithelium onto the cribriform plate and spreading down over a variable area of septum and lateral wall. Areas of squamous metaplasia are often found on the lateral wall, particularly in areas subject to greatest air flow such as the anterior inferior turbinate.

Respiratory epithelium is composed of ciliated and non-ciliated pseudostratified columnar cells, basal pluripotential stem cells and goblet cells (Figure 5). The columnar cells are 25 µm in height and 7 µm wide, tapering to 2–4 µm at the basement membrane. Each cell bears 300–400 microvilli, irrespective of the presence of cilia. These microvilli are fingerlike cytoplasmic extensions, 2 µm in length and 0.1 µm in diameter. Their

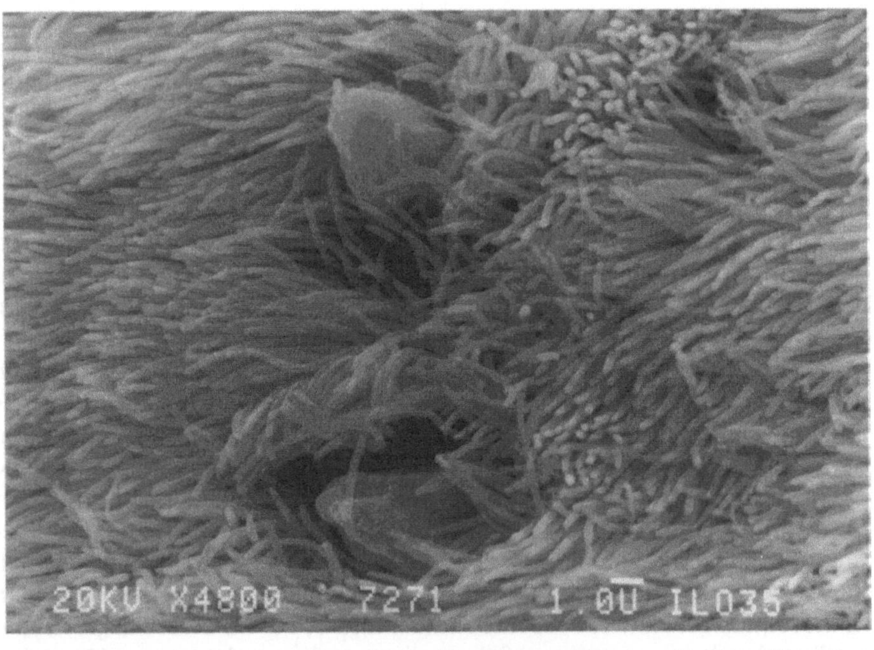

Figure 5. Scanning electronmicrograph of showing ciliated respiratory epithelium with packets of mucus indicating the position of underlying goblet cells.

function is to increase surface area and thus prevent drying. Where cilia are present, there are 50–100 per cell, though the number varies with their position in the nose and with age. The cilia are composed of the classical axonema of nine peripheral doublets and two central single microtubules. Each peripheral pair (A and B) connects to the next doublet and to the central microtubule with hexin links. The A microtubule bears an outer and inner dynein arm, composed of Adenosine triphosphatase (ATPase), which can attach to the B microtubule, leading to axonemal displacement and cilial beating.

Seromucinous glands are found in the submucosa and are more important in mucus production in the nasal cavity than are the goblet cells, which are more numerous in the sinuses. On the septum the number of goblet cells increases from anterior to posterior and from superior to inferior [6]. By contrast, the glands decrease from anterior to posterior and from superior to inferior and also decrease with age. The neonatal septum is 450 mm^2 in area, with 17–18 glands/mm^2, compared with the adult septum of 1700 mm^2 and 8.5 glands/mm^2.

The olfactory epithelium is composed of receptor cells, supporting cells with microvilli and basal stem cells conferring on olfactory epithelium the capacity for regeneration. Each receptor cell has approximately 17 cilia, but these differ from their respiratory counterparts in their radial arrangement, greater length and poorly developed ultrastructure. Dynein arms are not present, preventing linking between the microtubules and conventional beating. The sensory endings have a characteristic knoblike vesicular structure from which olfactory fibres join the axonal bundle. There is a sharp transition zone between the olfactory and respiratory epithelium, though the relative area of each varies with age and reflects the decrease in olfactory acuity. Secretion for the olfactory epithelium is provided by Bowman's glands.

2.3. Blood Supply

The external and internal carotid arteries are responsible for the rich blood supply to the nose. The sphenopalatine artery (branch of the maxillary artery and thus external carotid) supplies the posteroinferior septum. The greater palatine artery (also a branch of the maxillary) supplies the anteroinferior portion. The superior labial branch of the facial artery contributes anteriorly, in particular to *Kiesselbach's plexus*, composed of unusually long capillary loops, situated in Little's area on the anterior septum and a common source of epistaxis. The internal carotid supplies the septum superiorly via the anterior and posterior ethmoidal arteries and also contributes to Kiesselbach's plexus.

The external and internal carotid arteries also supply the lateral wall. The sphenopalatine artery brings the majority of the supply to the turbinates and meatuses. It enters through the sphenopalatine foramen, which lies just inferior to the horizontal attachment of the middle turbinate and may be damaged in excessive enlargement of a middle meatal antrostomy. Its branches to the respective turbinates and meatuses enter posteriorly. On the conchae the vessels are partially embedded in deep grooves. In the inferior meatus the sphenopalatine branch dips below the level of the palate to re-emerge anteriorly, leaving the central portion of the meatus relatively avascular [7]. An area anteriorly is supplied by a branch from the facial artery, and part of the lateral wall adjacent to the palate receives blood from the greater palatine artery. The internal carotid contribution is via the ethmoidal arteries which supply the superior lateral wall. There is considerable overlap between the internal and external carotid systems on each side and between the right and left sides, which may complicate attempts at arterial ligation in the management of epistaxis [8].

A sinusoid system is found in the nasal submucosa which is under autonomic control and which has been well described in relation to the turbinates but is also present on the septum adjacent to the inferior turbinate and on the most anterior septum. This anterior septal tubercle or intumescence was first described by Morgagni [9] and may be related to control of airflow into the olfactory cleft. A similar structure is seen on the posterior septum in two-thirds of individuals. The cavernous plexuses are most prominent in the lamina propria of the inferior and middle turbinates. The veins of the plexus are between 0.1 and 0.5 mm wide and anastomose with each other. In addition, numerous arteriovenous anastomoses are found in the deep mucosa and around the glands [10].

The cavernous venous system of the nasal cavity drains via the sphenopalatine vessels into the pterygoid plexus posteriorly and into the facial and ophthalmic veins anteriorly. Superiorly the ethmoidal veins communicate with the superior ophthalmic system, and there may be direct intracranial connections through the foramen caecum into the superior sagittal sinus.

2.4. Nerve Supply

The maxillary division of the trigeminal nerve provides the sensory supply to the majority of the nasal septum. The nasopalatine nerve supplies the bulk of the bony septum, entering the nasal cavity via the sphenopalatine foramen. The anterosuperior part of the septum is supplied by the anterior ethmoidal branch of the nasociliary nerve, and a smaller anteroinferior portion receives a branch from the anterior superior alveolar nerve. The postero-inferior septum also receives a small supply from the nerve to the pterygoid canal and a posterior inferior nasal branch of the anterior palatine nerve. The sensory nerves are accompanied by postganglionic sympathetic fibres to blood vessels, and postganglionic parasympathetic secretomotor fibres pass to glands with the branches from the pterygopalatine ganglion.

The olfactory epithelium covers the inferior surface of the cribriform plate spreading down to cover a variable area on the upper septum and adjacent lateral wall, over the medial surface of the superior concha. The area is encroached upon by respiratory epithelium with increasing age, though in an adult covers an area of approximately 2–5 cm^2. The nerve fibres arising from the olfactory receptors are slim (0.2 µm in diameter) and non-myelinated. They join up into approximately 20 bundles which traverse the cribriform plate to reach the olfactory bulbs. Each bundle carries a tubular sheath of dura and pia-arachnoid, which may be sheared in head injuries, destroying olfaction and potentially producing cerebrospinal fluid leakage. The fibres synapse in the glomeruli of the olfactory bulbs, which in turn connect with the olfactory tract. The olfactory tract passes on the inferior surface of the frontal lobe to the olfactory trigone from which diverging bundles, the medial and lateral olfactory striae, connect with the hypothalamus, amygdala and hippocampus. These complex connections link smell with taste, feeding and reproductive behaviour.

Apart from the olfactory supply on the superior concha, the lateral wall receives ordinary sensation from the anterior ethmoidal nerve anterosuperiorly and from branches of the pterygopalatine ganglion and anterior palatine nerves posteriorly. There is a small area of infraorbital supply anteriorly and an area of overlap between the ethmoidal and maxillary nerves. The anterior superior alveolar nerve sends a small branch to the anterior inferior meatus, which may be damaged in inferior meatal surgery, affecting dental sensation [11, 12].

2.5. Lymphatic Drainage

The septum and lateral nasal wall drain with the external nose to the submandibular nodes anteriorly and to the lateral pharyngeal, retropharyngeal and upper deep cervical nodes posteriorly.

3. The Paranasal Sinuses

3.1. The Ethmoid Bone and Sinuses

This complex bone is composed of five parts: two ethmoidal labyrinths suspended on either side of a perpendicular plate which forms the upper portion of the bony nasal septum, with an intervening cribriform plate and a superior midline extension, the crista galli. The bone is roughly cruciate in form. All components of the bone are subject to individual variation. The perpendicular plate is quadrilateral in shape and articulates anteriorly with the nasal spine of the frontal bone and nasal bones and posteriorly with the sphenoid and vomer. The cribriform plate divides the nasal cavity from the anterior cranial cavity. The fenestrations in the plate give the area its name, which the olfactory filaments, ethmoidal vessels and nerves and dural prolongations traverse. The roof of the ethmoidal labyrinths is predominantly

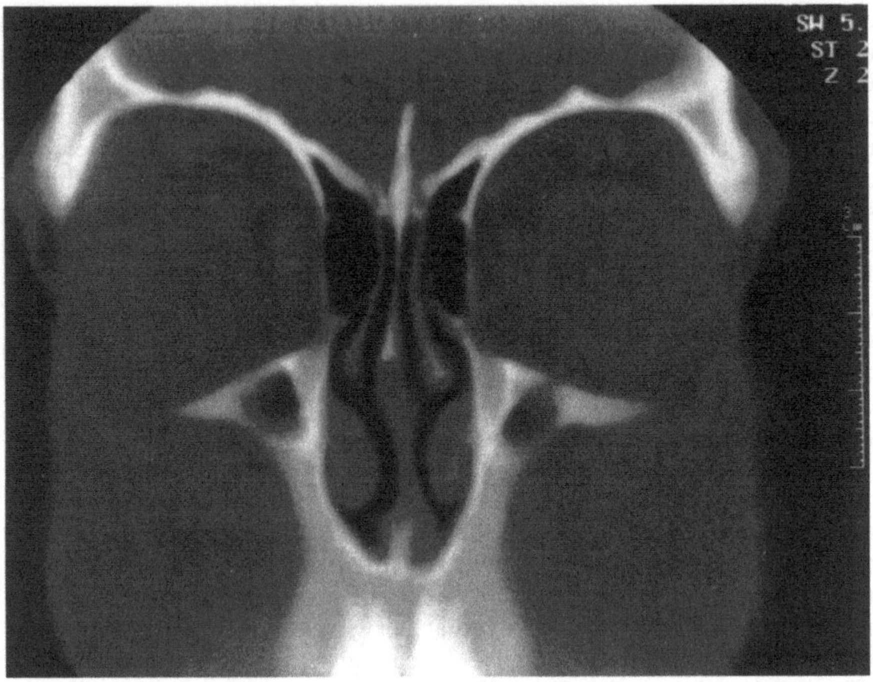

Figure 6. Coronal computerised tomography (CT) scan showing anterior vertical attachment of middle turbinate to skull base.

completed by the frontal bone. The point at which the frontal and ethmoid bones meet is at a variable height above the cribriform niche (1 – 17 mm) [13], and the ethmoid roof themselves are often asymmetric with the right more often lower than the left [14].

The *middle turbinate* is crucial to understanding the anatomy of the ethmoid complex by virtue of its three main attachments. The anterior third attaches vertically to the skull base at the lateral border of the cribriform niche with the frontal bone as it forms the roof of the ethmoids (Figure 6). The posterior third attaches horizontally to the lamina papyracea and medial wall of the maxilla (Figure 7). Between these two portions of the turbinate, there is an obliquely disposed plate of bone, the *basal lamella* of the middle turbinate, attaching laterally to the lamina papyracea. The basal lamella divides the ethmoidal labyrinth into an anterior and posterior group of cells, and thus there are no true middle ethmoidal cells.

The ethmoidal labyrinth is a collection of cells and clefts. The lateral walls constitute the orbital plates or lamina papyracea (Figure 8). The lamina is extremely thin and may be dehiscent, particularly in the very young or old. The anterior cells are generally smaller and more numerous (2 – 8) than the posterior group (1 – 5), which are closed off posteromedially

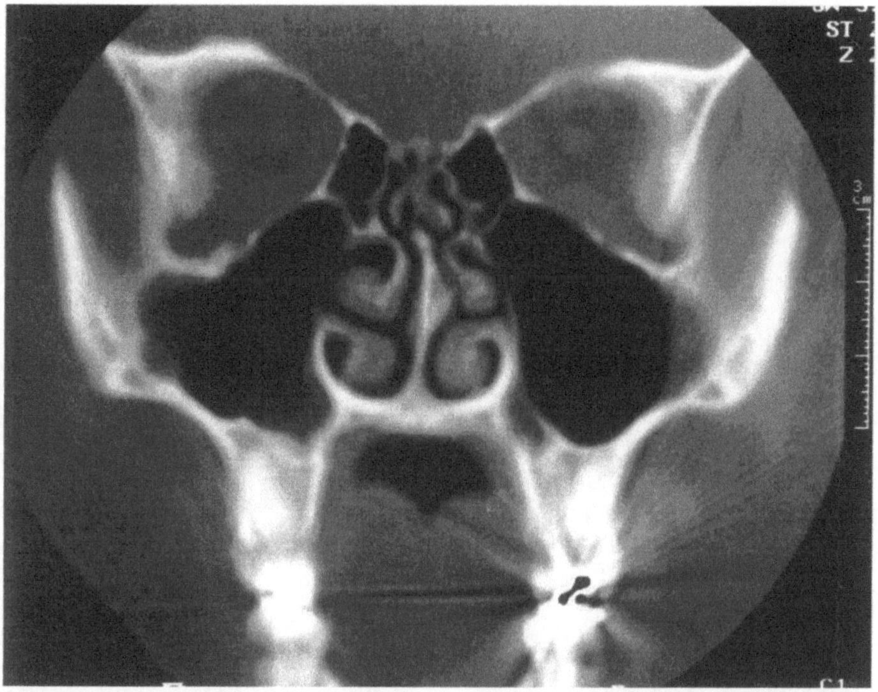

Figure 7. Coronal CT scan showing posterior lateral attachment of middle turbinate to the maxilla.

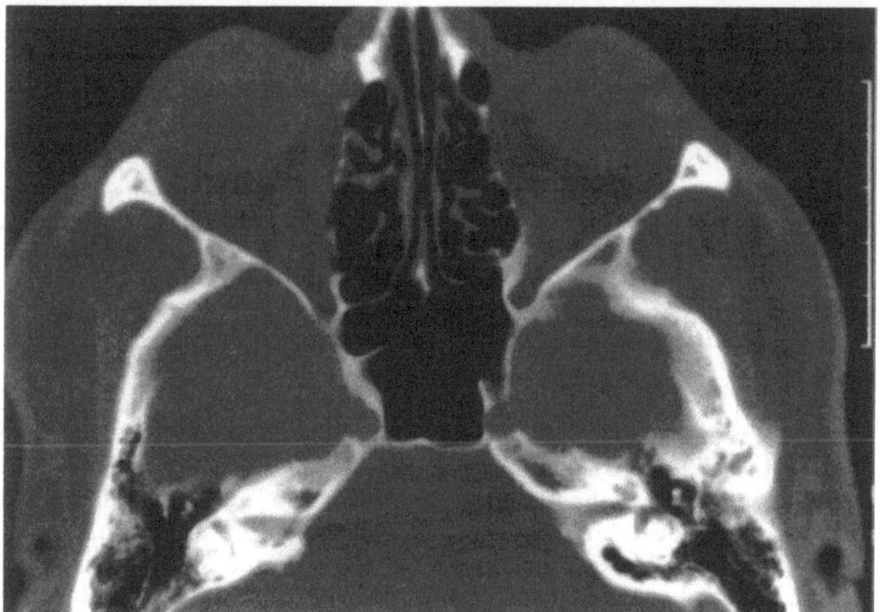

Figure 8. Axial CT scan showing the ethmoid labyrinths separated from the orbits by the lamina papyracea.

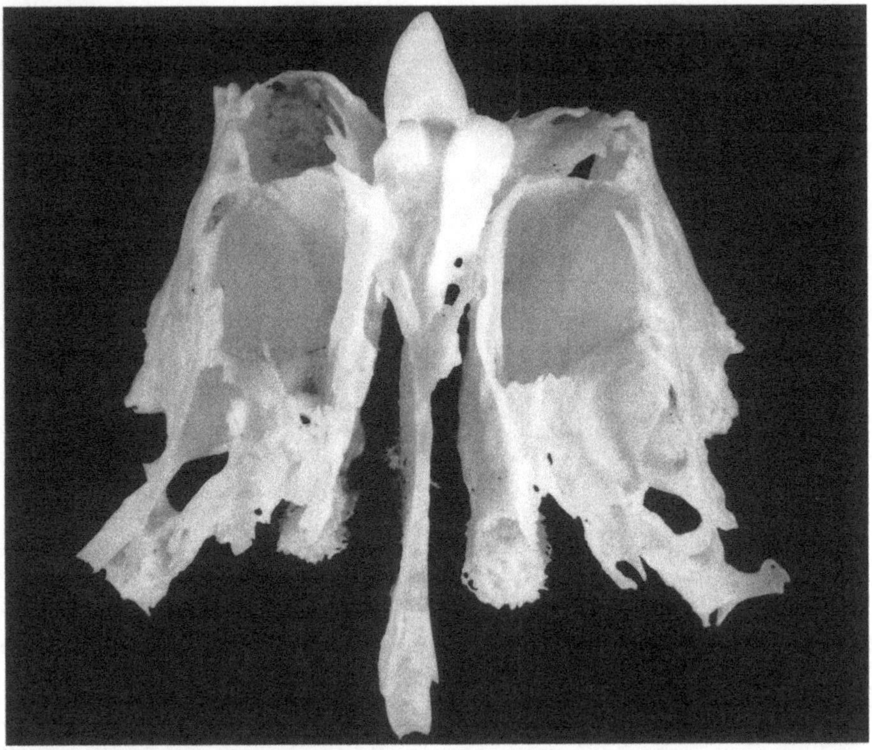

Figure 9. Photograph of disarticulated ethmoid bone showing view into large posterior ethmoid cells, closed in life by the sphenoid bone.

by the sphenoid bone (Figure 9). The ethmoid sinuses thus have an intimate relationship with the orbit, and the optic nerve may be particularly vulnerable in the posterior cells.

3.2. The Maxillary Sinus

The maxilla is the second largest facial bone, forming the majority of the roof of the mouth, the lateral wall and floor of the nasal cavity and the floor of the orbit (Figure 10). The body is usually described as a quadrilateral pyramid, and contains the maxillary sinus. The roof of the maxillary sinus forms most of the orbital floor. It is traversed by the infraorbital canal, which may be dehiscent. Inferiorly the floor of the sinus is generally thicker, but can be encroached upon by the roots of teeth – for instance the second premolar and three molar teeth. The medial wall contains a large defect, the maxillary hiatus, which is completed in life by a number of bones and mucous membrane leaving only the natural maxillary ostium

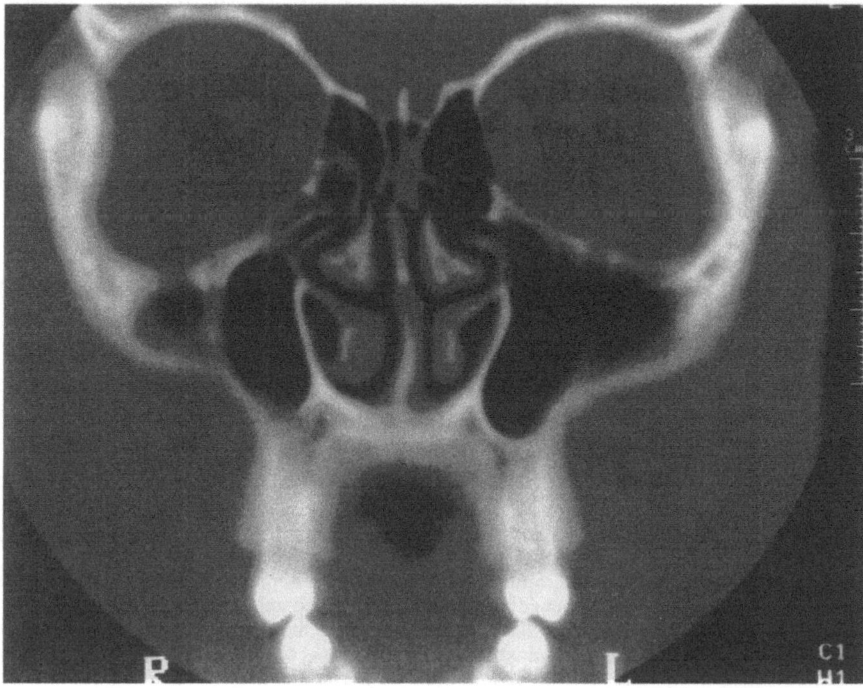

Figure 10. Coronal CT scan showing relationship of maxillary sinus to orbit and dentition.

which is localised at the base of the ethmoidal infundibulum. The maxillary sinuses are relatively symmetrical and only rarely absent.

3.3. The Frontal Sinuses

The frontal bone forms the forehead, the orbital roof and the roof of the ethmoidal sinuses. The frontal sinuses are unique in shape and size to each individual and are absent in 1% of the British population. When present, the sinus is usually "L" shaped, composed of a horizontal and a vertical compartment, but in addition diverticula, supernumerary sinuses and incomplete septa are frequently encountered. An intersinus septum is usually present, but this may be paramedian and is partially dehiscent in 9%. The sinus drains into the frontal recess though accessory channels which are found in 10% of the population [15], and there may be accessory connections of the ethmoidal system.

3.4. The Sphenoid Sinuses

The sphenoid bone is the largest in the skull base, dividing the anterior and middle cranial fossa. It is composed of a body (pneumatised to a variable

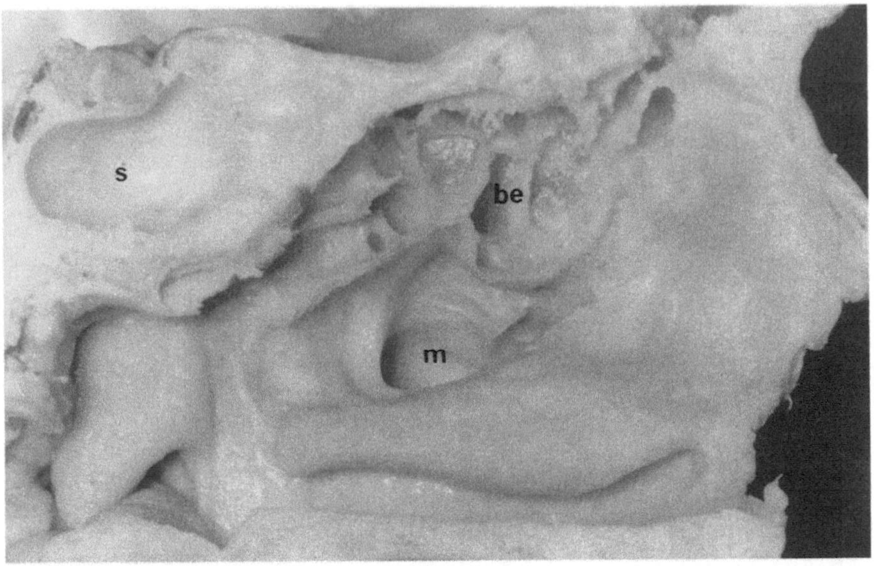

Figure 11. Photograph of lateral wall of nasal cavity after removal of inferior, middle and superior turbinates, showing opened ethmoid labyrinth and relationship to sphenoid sinus posteriorly. A large accessory maxillary ostium is seen in the posterior fontanelle. be: bulla ethmoidalis; s: sphenoid sinus; m: maxillary sinus through accessory ostium.

degree), two wings (greater and lesser) and two inferior plates (lateral and medial pterygoid plates). The lateral surface of the body is grooved by the carotid artery on each side as it traverses the cavernous sinus. Halfway up on either side of the face lie the ostia of the sinuses. These are large on a macerated skull (5–8 mm in diameter) but are substantially closed by mucous membrane in life. The sinuses open into the sphenoethmoidal recess (Figure 11). The sinus cavities are also variable in size an shape, and pneumatisation can be very extensive. By contrast, the sinus may be completely absent in 1% of the population [16]. Although the most posterior ethmoidal cell is closed by the sphenoidal concha, the sphenoid sinus may only be entered safely through the most inferior and medial portion of the posterior ethmoidal cell. Alternatively, it may be readily approached directly via its natural ostium in the sphenoethmoidal recess.

The optic nerve and internal carotid artery produce prominences of variable size in the lateral and posterior walls of the sinus, with an intervening cleft which can be deep. The bone overlying these structures can be extremely thin or dehiscent (internal carotid: 25%; optic nerve: 6% of the normal population).

3.5. *Histology*

All the paranasal sinuses are lined by thin ciliated columnar respiratory epithelium. The density of goblet cells is highest in the maxillary sinus, with a mean of 9700/mm^2. The respiratory epithelium of the ethmoid, sphenoid and frontal sinuses has a relatively smaller number of goblet cells (6500, 6200 and 5900/mm^2 respectively) [6]. Tubuloalveolar seromucinous glands are found throughout the mucosa, being more numerous in the ethmoids, least numerous in the sphenoid and concentrated in the maxillary sinus around the ostium.

3.6. *Blood, Nerves and Lymphatic Drainage*

The vascular supply of the ethmoid labyrinth is derived from the sphenopalatine and ethmoidal (anterior and posterior) arteries and drains by corresponding veins. The ethmoid sinuses are innervated by the anterior and posterior ethmoidal nerves and orbital branches of pterygopalatine ganglion. Lymphatic drainage of all the sinuses is relatively poor. From the ethmoids drainage is to the submandibular nodes anteriorly and retropharyngeal nodes posteriorly.

Small branches of the facial, maxillary, infraorbital and greater palatine arteries and veins supply the maxilla. Venous drainage is to the anterior facial vein and pterygoid plexus. The maxillary division of the trigeminal nerve supplies sensation via the infraorbital, superior alveolar (anterior, middle and posterior) and greater palatine nerves. Near the midpoint of the infraorbital canal, a small branch, the anterior superior alveolar nerve arises, passes in its own canal anterior to the inferior turbinate and reaches the nasal septum in front of the incisive foramen. It supplies the anterior wall of the maxillary sinus, the pulps of the canines and incisors, the anteroinferior quadrant of the lateral nasal wall, the floor of the nose and a small portion of the anterior nasal septum.

The posterior superior alveolar nerves arise from the maxillary nerve in the pterygopalatine fossa and enter the maxilla through the posterior wall to supply the adjacent mucosa and molar teeth. The middle superior alveolar nerve, when present, arises from the infraorbital nerve in its canal and supplies the lateral wall of the sinus and upper premolar teeth. The posterior medial wall of the sinus is supplied by the greater palatine nerve and the roof by perforating branches from the infraorbital nerve. Lymphatic drainage is predominantly into the pterygopalatine fossa and to the submandibular nodes.

The supraorbital and anterior ethmoidal arteries supply the frontal sinuses. Venous drainage includes accompanying veins, diploic veins draining into the sagittal and sphenoparietal sinuses and an anastomotic vein in the supraorbital notch connecting the supraorbital and superior ophthalmic vessels. The nerve supply derives from the supraorbital nerve, and the lymphatic drainage is to the submandibular gland.

The sphenoid sinuses are supplied by the posterior ethmoidal vessels and nerves, with additional supply from the orbital branches of the pterygopalatine ganglion. Lymphatic drainage is again to the retropharyngeal nodes.

4. Nasal Physiology

The nose, as the principal portal of the respiratory tract, serves an important protective function at a macroscopic and microscopic level. The functions of the paranasal sinuses, however, remain obscure and the subject of much speculation. Air entering the respiratory tract must be filtered, warmed and humidified, and noxious agents removed. The other main function (olfaction) has been ostensibly reduced in humans though the significance of the most primitive of senses has almost certainly been underestimated and underinvestigated.

4.1. Air Conditioning

The complex arrangement of turbinates with their vascular sinusoid system and glandular elements of the mucosa permits air to be humidified and warmed for optimum delivery to the lower respiratory tract. When air reaches the nasopharynx, it is normally 31 °C and 95% saturated. A number of nasopulmonary reflexes exist which may enhance this activity, and certainly its importance can be best appreciated in patients deprived of nasal airflow, as following total laryngectomy.

4.2. Mucociliary Clearance

The respiratory epithelium continuously produces secretions, both from the seromucinous glands and from the goblet cells, which form a blanket throughout the nasal cavity and sinuses [17]. The blanket forms two distinct layers, a liquid sol layer in which the cilia beat, on top of which is a thicker gel layer into which the “claws” of the cilia can engage, progressively dragging the mucous blanket along with each effective cilial stroke. The blanket changes in the nasal cavity every 20–30 min, and has an average speed of 6 mm/min. Under normal circumstances the cilia of the lower septum and inferior turbinate beat at 12–15 Hz, a frequency which may be measured photometrically. The direction of flow is posteriorly towards the nasopharynx and thence to the oropharynx and hypopharynx, where secretions may be swallowed. This has a most important protective function, removing any particulate material which becomes trapped in the mucus. Thus larger allergens such as grass pollens (30 μm in diameter) are filtered by the nose and prevented from reaching the lungs but may still provoke allergic reactions in the nasal cavity.

The mucus produced mainly by the goblet cells in the sinuses is similarly carried to their respective ostia. These patterns are pre-determined and will vary in a cyclical fashion, with certain parts of a sinus draining better at some times than others. Thus mucus from the floor of the maxillary sinus is carried a considerable distance against gravity to the natural ostium, reflecting the embryological development of the sinus from the region of the infundibulum (Figure 12). Similarly the frontal sinus, which may be regarded as embryologically an anterior ethmoidal cell, has fascinating mucociliary pathways which may even carry mucus back into the sinus from the frontal sinus (Figure 13). The maxillary, anterior ethmoids and frontal sinus all drain, as previously stated, into the middle meatus, an area frequently referred to as the "ostiomeatal complex" in recognition of its functional importance in the aetiology of sinus infection [18]. Although in health only 5% of sinonasal secretions come from the sinuses, any obstruction to outflow in the ostiomeatal complex will inevitably lead to problems within the dependent sinuses, and much surgery for sinusitis now focuses on this area, facilitated by the visualisation afforded by rigid endoscopes and computerised tomography. The importance of anatomic variants in the

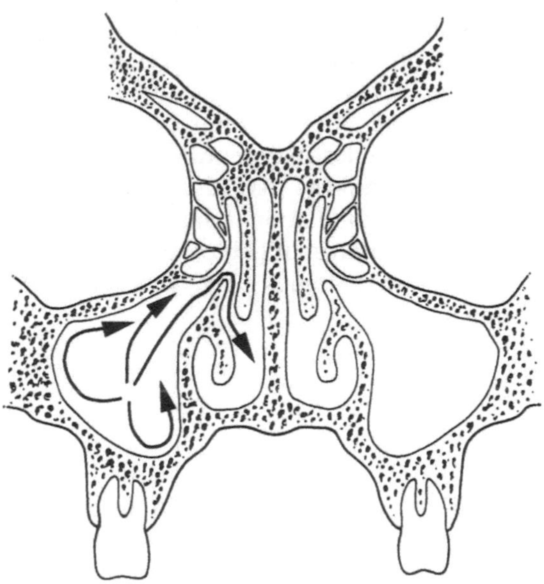

Figure 12. Diagram of showing mucociliary clearance from maxillary sinus into infundibulum and thence through hiatus semilunaris into middle meatus.

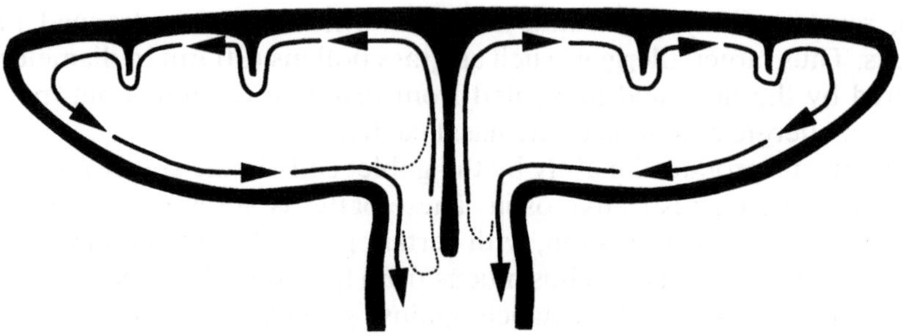

Figure 13. Diagram showing mucociliary clearance within the frontal sinuses.

development of infection will be determined by the degree of obstruction to outflow which they produce, and it is often a combination of this with allergy, decreased mucociliary clearance and/or subtle immune deficiencies which determines progression from acute to chronic rhinosinusitis.

Nasal secretion is, therefore, a complex mixture from goblet cells, seromucinous glands, lacrimal glands, material transported across the epithelial surfaces and condensed water whose composition varies in response to internal and external factors. Glycoproteins, lactoferrin, albumin, lysozymes and all major immunoglobulins are present. Immunoglobulin (Ig) A forms up to 50% of the total protein content and together with IgG may be secreted on a cyclical diurnal basis. The equally complex profile of electrolytes, cytokines and other mediators such as histamine, 5-hydroxytryptamine, bradykinin and substance P will be discussed in succeeding chapters.

The main nervous control of nasal secretion is autonomic, with parasympathetic stimulation increasing secretion, in particular mediated by the nerve to the pterygoid canal. Although this system is mainly cholinergic, the presence of vasoactive intestinal peptide (VIP) amongst others, suggests non-cholinergic mechanisms may also be important. Conversely, in general terms, sympathetic stimulation reduces secretion from the seromucinous glands, whereas the control of goblet cell secretion remains obscure, and transudation across membranes may be mainly of significance in response to inflammation.

4.3. Airflow

In the first few months following birth, nasal breathing is obligatory to facilitate suckling, and this has important life-threatening consequences when nasal obstruction occurs, as in bilateral choanal atresia. Nasal breathing remains the optimal route for the majority of adults, who only resort to an oral or oronasal route under demanding situations (such as exercise), thus subserving the protective functions of the nose. Normally airflow passes through the cavities by the least turbulent routes in quiet inspiration. Air passes almost vertically up through the anterior nares at a rate of 2–3 m/s. The flow converges to become laminar and horizontal and achieves a velocity of 12–18 m/s at the narrowest point, the valve area. Most of the air continues through the lower two-thirds of the cavity with approximately 10% of inspired air reaching the olfactory area under these circumstances, but this may double with sniffing. There is, however, considerable turbulence of expiratory air within the nasal cavity, sweeping inspired air out of the olfactory niche.

Airflow is controlled in a number of ways, with the nose providing up to 60% of total airway resistance in normal respiration. The nasal cavity should be regarded in three areas when considering resistance to flow: the vestibule, the valve region and the lateral nasal wall. The vestibule contributes approximately one-third of resistance and acts as the flow-limiting segment on inspiration. It is normally stented by the alar cartilages, though it will collapse to a greater or lesser extent if flow exceeds 30 l/min.

The valve region is generally regarded as being located at the anterior end of the inferior turbinate just within the first few millimetres of the bony pyriform aperture [19]. However, evidence from acoustic rhinometry studies suggests that its position may alter slightly with decongestion [20]. Here changes in the size of the turbinate generally as a result of engorgement of the sinusoid system will produce the greatest effects on airflow. Posterior to this area, the turbinates contribute relatively little. The autonomic control of the capacitance vessels in the venous erectile tissue largely relates to stimulation of the sympathetic adrenergic supply, resulting in vasoconstriction and increased flow. There appears to be a continuous level of sympathetic tone which when removed, as in cervical sympathectomy, results in an increase in nasal resistance and congestion.

Parasympathetic stimulation largely affects glandular secretion and has little impact on the erectile tissue. A curious manifestation of this may be observed in "honeymoon" rhinitis [21]. A number of other physiologic circumstances will alter nasal resistance.

The existence of a *nasal cycle* of spontaneous reciprocating congestion and decongestion has been known since the end of the nineteenth century. It is found in at least 80% of adults, and although it is not known at what age it begins, it has been found in children as young as 3 years old. It largely goes unnoticed, as the total resistance remains unchanged, and a number of patterns are recognised. The duration of the cycle varies from 2–7 h (usually 3–4 h) and is found throughout the day. The effect of posture is interesting in that the cycle can be overridden by lying down on one side when the dependent side becomes the more congested. This reflex is in response to pressure on the side of the body and can also be provoked when standing upright. The most sensitive areas to pressure are the axilla and the lateral chest wall, but it is hard to see what protective function such a reflex affords [22]. The fact that the nasal cycle persists, albeit with reduced magnitude, after nasal airflow ceases (such as after total laryngectomy) confirms a central control with local modulation [23].

Nasal airway resistance does alter with age in that it is at a maximum in infancy, declining to a minimum by adolescence. Little change occurs thereafter until middle age, attributed to slight atrophy of the tissues, though there does not appear to be any correlation with age or sex.

Exercise also has an impact on nasal resistance, causing a reduction due to increased sympathetic tone and vasoconstriction of the erectile tissues. This occurs, rapidly, though it is generally unnoticed, and the normal situation is restored within 15–30 min after activity ceases, when a rebound congestion may be noticed. Similarly any situation resulting in an increase in PCO_2, such as rebreathing expired air, leads to vasoconstriction and a fall in resistance within in a few breaths and vice versa with hyperventilation.

Changes in skin temperature and that of inspired air also lead to alterations in nasal mucosal blood flow as part of the thermoregulatory mechanisms which facilitate heat conservation or loss. Breathing cold air causes nasal congestion and an increase in nasal resistance. In contrast, the application of a cold stimulus to the skin causes nasal vasoconstriction but no change in resistance to airflow, as no change in the venous erectile tissue occurs. More intense thermal, chemical or physical stimulation produces sneezing in addition to congestion and secretion. This reflex is mediated via the trigeminal nerve, the respiratory muscles and the autonomic nervous system. In its most exaggerated form, such as falling into extremely cold water, closure of the laryngeal sphincter and apnoea can occur.

Emotional disturbance may influence the nasal airway. Stress increases sympathetic stimulation, decreasing resistance in anticipation of "flight". In contrast, the subjective sensation of airflow can be altered by certain chemicals such as menthol, which can stimulate thermal receptors in nasal mucosa, making the airway feel clearer even though no real change in resistance has occurred [24].

4.4. Olfaction

The gradual devolution of our olfactory acuity in comparison with other mammals should not obscure its importance. The surface area of olfactory epithelium is relatively small in humans, and only the vestiges of ancillary olfactory structures such as the vomeronasal organ remain [25]. However, olfaction continues to have a primary role in the regulation of food intake and reproductive behaviour and has an important protective function in the detection of noxious and toxic substances. A complex interaction exists between the olfactory system and other cranial nerves (V, VII, IX, X). Of these, the trigeminal response may contribute up to 30% of odour perception in some situations, and it is trigeminal irritation which is largely responsible for detection of ammonia.

Many theories exist about the nature of olfactory detection, transduction and recognition. Recent studies suggest that odour molecules are carried to receptors on the cilia of olfactory neurones by a binding globulin found in nasal mucus. The cilial receptors are glycoproteins which may have the capacity to selectively bind to different odour molecules. The binding activates a stimulatory GTP-binding protein, which activates adenyl cyclase and provokes a cascade of events resulting in ion conductance changes in the cell membrane and depolarisation.

It seems that olfactory cells are broadly "tuned", so that whilst each neurone may respond to many odours, no two neurones are identical. Odour recognition thus depends upon unique combinations of neuronal response. Thence, electrical stimulation passes along the primary olfactory neurone, through the cribriform plate to synapse in the olfactory bulbs. Second-order neurones form the lateral olfactory tracts which project to the olfactory cortex in the temporal lobe. However, a plethora of other connections exist with the hypothalamus, amygdala and hippocampus that are responsible for the complex interactions of smell, taste, feeding behaviour, reproduction and memory.

References

1. Lang J. Clinical Anatomy of the nose, nasal cavity and paranasal sinuses. Stuttgart: Georg Thieme Verlag, 1989.
2. Zinreich SJ, Kennedy DW, Gayler BW. CT of nasal cavity, paranasal sinuses: an evaluation of anatomy in endoscopic sinus surgery. Clear Images 1988; 2: 2–10.
3. Lloyd GAS, Lund VJ, Scadding GK. Computerised tomography in the pre-operative evaluation of functional endoscopic sinus surgery. J Laryngol Otol 1991; 105: 181–185.
4. Schaeffer JP. The nose, paranasal sinuses, Nasolacrimal passageways and olfactory organ in man. Philadelphia: Blakiston, 1920.
5. Van Alyea OE. Ethmoid labyrinth. Archiv Otolaryngol 1939; 29: 881–902.
6. Tos M, Morgensen C. Mucus production in the nasal sinuses. Acta Otolaryngol 86: (suppl 360) 1979; 131–134.
7. Lund VJ. Inferior meatal antrostomy: fundamental considerations of design and function. J Laryngol Otol 102: (suppl 15) 1988: 1–18.
8. Shaheen OH. Epistaxis. In: Mackay IS, Bull TR, editors. Scott-Brown's otolaryngology, 5th ed, vol 4. London: Butterworths, 1987: 272–282.
9. Zuckerkandl E. Normale and pathologische Anatomie der Nasenhöhle und interpneumatischen Anhage. Leipzig: W. Braumuller, 1893.
10. Cauna N. The fine structure of the arteriovenous anastomosis and its nerve supply in the human nasal respiratory mucosa. Anat Rec 1970; 168: 9–22.
11. Wood Jones F. The anterior superior alveolar nerve and vessels. J Anatomy 1939; 73: 583–591.
12. Heasman P. Clinical anatomy of the superior alveolar nerves. Br J Oral Maxillo-facial Surg 1984; 6: 439–447.
13. Kainz J, Stammberger H. The roof of the anterior ethmoid: a place of least resistance in the skull base. Am J Rhinol 1989; 4: 191–99.
14. Dessi P, Moulin G, Triglia JM, Zanaret M, Cannoni M. Difference in the height of the right and left ethmoid roofs: a possible risk factor for ethmoid surgery. J Laryngol Otol 1995; 108: 261–262.
15. Lund VJ. Anatomical considerations in the aetiology of fronto-ethmoidal mucocoeles. Rhinology 1987; 25: 83–88.

16. Grunwald L. Anatomie und Entwicklungsgeschichte. In: Denker H, Kahler O. Handbuch der Hals-Nasen-Ohrenheilkunde. Band 1; Die Krankheiten der Luftwege und Mundhöhle. Berlin: Springer, 1925.
17. Proetz AW. Essays on the applied physiology of the nose, 2nd ed. St. Louis: Annals Publishing, 1953.
18. Stammberger H. Functional endoscopic sinus surgery: the Messerklinger technique. Philadelphia: BC Dekker, 1991.
19. Haight JSJ, Cole P. The site and function of the nasal valve. Laryngoscope 1983; 93: 49–55.
20. Lenders H, Pirsig W. Diagnostic value of acoustic rhinometry: patients with allergic and vasomotor rhinitis compared with normal controls. Rhinology 1990; 28: 5–16.
21. Watson Williams E. Endocrines and the nose. J Laryngol Otol 1952; 66: 29–35.
22. Burrows A, Eccles R. Reciprocal changes in nasal resistance to airflow caused by pressure applied to the axilla. Acta Otolaryngol 1985; 99: 154–59.
23. Fisher E, Lund VJ, Ming L. The nasal cycle after deprivation of airflow: a study of laryngectomy patients using acoustic rhinometry. Acta Otolaryngol 1994; 114: 443–446.
24. Eccles R. Neurological and pharmacological considerations. In: Proctor DF, Andersen I, editions. The nose: upper airway physiology and the atmospheric environment. Amsterdam: Elsevier Biomedical, 1982: 191–214.
25. Johnson A, Josephson R, Hawke M. Clinical and histological evidence for the presence of the vomeronasal organ in adult humans. J Otolaryngol 1985; 14: 71–79.

Rhinitis: Immunopathology
and Pharmacotherapy
ed. by D. Raeburn and M.A. Giembycz

CHAPTER 2
Pathophysiology of the Nose in Rhinitis

John Widdicombe

Department of Physiology, St. George's Hospital Medical School, London, UK

1. Introduction

The nose has structural and functional features that make its response to disease unique in the body. It is the only thoroughfare air-filled tube surrounded by bone and cartilage, so that any changes in mucosal thickness will be reflected in luminal calibre. The tracheobronchial tree, similar in many respects, can expand and contract in response to changes in surrounding tissue compliance, or to smooth muscle contraction. For the nose, the surrounding tissue has zero compliance, and there is no smooth muscle, apart from that in blood vessels, which can change airway calibre. The closest analogy to the nose is the eustachian tube, but here the lumen is essentially a cul-de-sac, unlike the nose. The upper airway sinuses are also cul-de-sacs, with rigid bony surrounds to a vascular and glandular mucosa.

The nose has features in common with many other air-containing tubes. It has a copious system of submucosal seromucous glands [1, 2], and a vascular bed which can determine liquid extravasation into the interstitium and exudation into the lumen [3, 4]. However, the nasal mucosa additionally has a conspicuous system of capacitance vessels which can distend with blood and block the nose or constrict down and open the nasal air passages [5, 6]. The nose also has unusual secretory structures such as the anterolateral submucosal glands that secrete a watery fluid into the front of a nose [7] and Bowman's glands at the back of the nose that have an unknown secretory function, probably in relation to smell. Some species have a specialised structure (the vomeronasal gland) at the front of the nose which, at least in rats, is associated with sexual awareness [8]. It is vestigial in humans.

The classification of rhinitis is controversial [9–11]. Some categories are straightforward, such as infectious rhinitis, which is caused either by viruses or by bacteria, with a few additional other specific forms of infection. Allergic rhinitis is also fairly easy to define and to diagnose based on the response to specific allergens, and may be either seasonal or perennial. Nonallergic types of rhinitis, however are more difficult to classify. Apart from infectious rhinitis, a large residuum of types of rhinitis remains, much of which is usually thought to be "vasomotor rhinitis", sometimes referred to as "hyperreactive rhinitis", as well as number of nasal diseases which are difficult to classify. Of course, more than one type of rhinitis may coexist.

Classification is usually based on case history, on the occurrence of nasal blockage, sneezing and sense of irritation, and a running nose which could be a combination of glandular secretion and plasma exudation [2, 3]. These signs and symptoms are common to all the pathological forms of rhinitis and do not themselves lead to accurate definitions. Investigative tests, such as tests for reactions to allergens, challenge with drugs and histopathological analysis, are seldom done except in some hospital clinics.

In all forms of rhinitis underlying mechanisms lead to certain signs and symptoms:

- Blockage. This is probably caused mainly by the distension of the vascular capacitance vessels which will thicken the mucosa and block the airway lumen. The extent to which the thickening of the mucosa is associated with oedema is usually not well analysed. A third component of nasal blockage could be the accumulation of secretions in the lumen, but this is unlikely to be a major factor in most conditions since the secretions can be cleared by sniffing or by blowing the nose. In theory the relative contributions of vascular congestion and oedema could be analysed by appropriate use of drugs, but in practice one would expect most drugs that act on the vascular bed and cause decongestion also to decrease tissue oedema, although the time course of latter change might be slower.
- Secretions. Nasal secretions are the combination of outputs from the copious seromucous glands, secretion from the anterolateral nasal glands and exudate of plasma-like liquid from the blood vessels and through the epithelium [1–4]. The relative contributions of these three factors are difficult to determine in most conditions. Antisecretory drugs such as atropine, if effective, should point to the role of glandular secretions, since plasma exudate should not be affected. Anti-inflammatory drugs might be expected to have equal actions on glandular secretions and on plasma exudate.

- Nervous influences. The involvement of mucosal nerves, probably mainly from C-fibre and Aδ-fibre receptors, is certainly established when there is either sneezing or the sensation of nasal irritation, which can only be mediated by sensory nerves [12–14]. However, such symptoms point to further mechanisms, since activation of these sensory receptors will cause a local neurogenic inflammation [14–16], with axon reflex vasodilatation and glandular secretion. There will also be central nervous reflex changes both in breathing and back to the airway mucosa with further vasodilatation and secretion. The role of sensory neuropeptides, such as substance P (SP), neurokinin (NK) A, and calcitonin gene-related peptide (CGRP), has recently aroused much interest [14–16].
- Hyperresponsiveness. The hyperresponsiveness of the nose to various challenges, such as allergens, histamines or chemical irritants, can be found in all rhinitic conditions and is not diagnostic of any particular one [17–18]. Which mechanism in the nose is hyperresponsive is usually harder to define. It could be vascular beds, glandular tissues or the sensory nerves, or some combination of the three.

It can be seen that each of these signs of rhinitis involves several target tissues, and the pathophysiology of each of these will now be described.

2. Pathophysiological Mechanisms

2.1. Vasculature

Both vascular tone and permeability are changed in rhinitis, especially the allergic form, and both contribute to mucosal thickening and nasal blockage.

The nasal vasculature has several features that distinguish it from mucosal circulations elsewhere (Figure 1). The rich subepithelial capillary network consists of fenestrated vessels, with the fenestrations pointing towards the epithelium and lumen [6, 19]. Presumably these fenestrations are related to water loss into the airways in association with air conditioning and temperature control. No particular role for them in rhinitis has been described. Deeper in the mucosa the nose has a copious system of capacitance vessels, also called blood sinuses [5, 6, 20]. The distension and collapse of this system is probably the main cause of nasal blockage and its reverse. The control of the sinuses, however, is little unterstood. One concept is that they are filled by blood flowing through arteriovenous anastomoses (AVAs), the dilation of which would cause nasal congestion (Figure 1) [21], but there is some evidence against this [5, 6]. The sinuses have thick muscular walls, and probably the main mechanism determining their distension is contraction or relaxation of this muscle. There may also be venous sphincters at the points of emptying of the sinuses, and

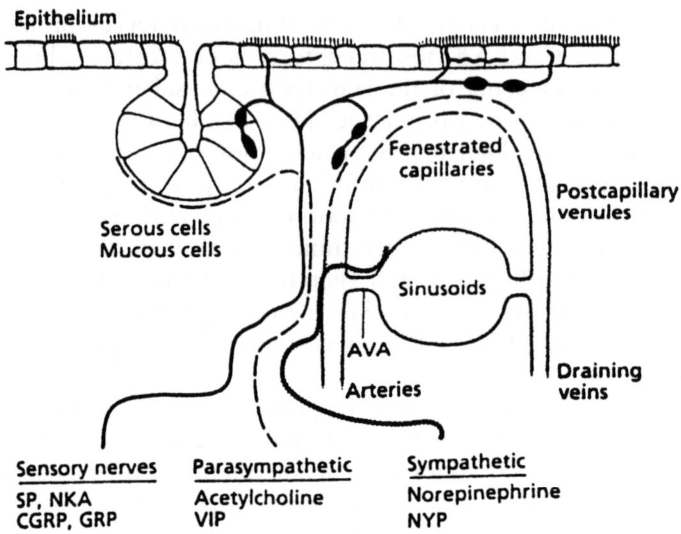

Figure 1. Schematic representation of human nasal mucosa. Arterial vessels carry blood to AVAs, which regulate blood flow into venous sinusoids, and a superficial plexus of periglandular and subepithelial fenestrated capillaries. Sensory, parasympathetic and sympathetic neurons innervate the vessels and glands, while sensory neurons also innervate the epithelium. Sensory neurons have neurosecretory varicosities, which release tachykinins, CGRP and other peptides during the axonal response. Reprinted with permission from [49].

constrictions of these could distend the vascular bed [21]. Whatever the mechanisms of sinus control, the control can be functionally distinguished from that of the main resistance vessels of the nose [22].

In rhinitis several processes will change vascular congestion and permeability. The vessels are under nervous control, dominantly sympathetic and "vasoconstrictor" but with a parasympathetic dilator component (Figure 1) [5, 23, 24]. Nasal reflexes set up in rhinitis can cause a reflex vascular congestion due at least in part due to a cholinergic dilatation [25]. The role of sensory nerves in neurogenic inflammation will be mentioned later.

However, the dominant mechanism controlling vascular tone and volume rhinitis is probably the release of mediators [5, 24]. The list of active agents is long and includes histamine, 5-hydroxytryptamine (5-HT), prostaglandins (PG) D_2 and E, neuropeptides such as vasoactive intestinal polypeptide (VIP), SP and CGRP, and bradykinin. All these agents cause arteriolar dilatation and all (except CGRP) increase postcapillary venular permeability. Vasoconstrictor mediators are less common, but may include leukotrienes and possibly platelet activating factor (PAF) [26]. The actions of some of these mediators are shown in Figure 2. Full descriptions of their actions can be read elsewhere [5, 6, 24, 25, 27].

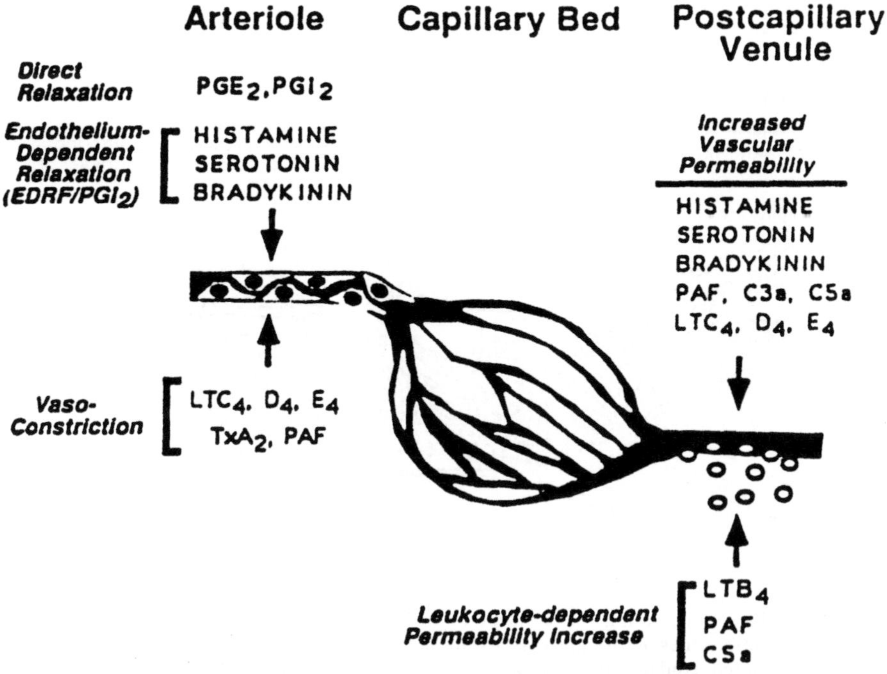

Figure 2. Effects of mediators on the microcirculation. Vasodilation and vasoconstriction prominently affect the arterioles and precapillary sphincters, which together constitute the resistance vessels within the mucosa. Changes in vascular permeability and leukocyte adherence and migration occur largely in the postcapillary venules. Some agents, such as PAF, induce increased vascular permeability by a mechanism that depends at least partly on neutrophil adhesion and release of secondary mediators. Vasodilation induced by some compounds such as histamine, bradykinin and serotonin results, at least in part, from receptor-mediated release of endothelial-derived relaxing factor (EDRF) and PGI_2 from endothelial cells. Not shown are effects on the venous sinusoids, the capacitance vessels of the nasal mucosa, which undergo vasodilation and constriction in response to mediators as well. This illustration also does not include indirect effects of neural mediators on the microvasculature, e.g. vasoconstriction and increased vascular permeability produced by antidromic release of tachykinins. Reprinted with permission from [24].

The increase in postcapillary venular permeability is important in rhinitis because it leads both to mucosal oedema and thickening and also to an exudate of plasma-like liquid into the airway lumen (Figure 3) [3, 4]. The increased permeability occurs because of the opening of gaps between the endothelial cells in the vessels. The increase in interstitial liquid pressure would in turn open gaps between the epithelial cells, allowing liquid to enter the lumen. This liquid is rich in plasma proteins of all molecular weights, as well as various plasma-derived mediators. It could contribute an important defensive mechanism by lining the epithelium with liquid containing protective agents [3, 4].

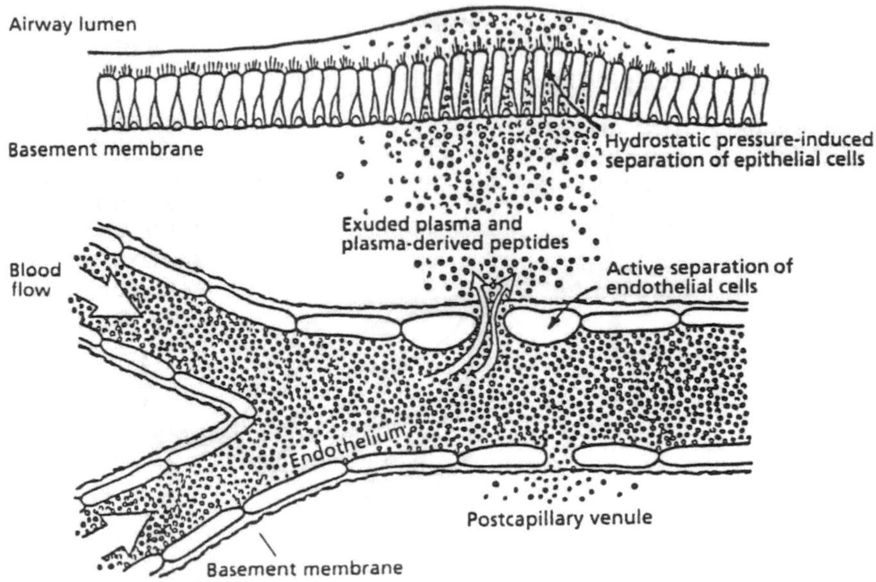

Figure 3. Scheme illustrating the concept of inflammatory stimulus-induced exudation of plasma macromolecules across the vessel wall and the mucosal barrier. Note that the luminal entry of unfiltered exudate can occur across a normal epithelium. Reprinted with permission from [3].

The relative importance of different mediators in causing vascular congestion in rhinitis is not very clear. Antihistamines tend to be ineffective on nasal congestion, as are drugs acting on the production of prostaglandins [27]. The most effective vascular-acting agents are the α_1-adrenoceptor agonists [28], which bypass the inflammatory systems and act directly on the vascular smooth muscle, causing it to contract.

2.2. Secretion

Most of the nasal secretions in rhinitis come from submucosal seromucous glands [1, 2, 29], although added to their secretion will be that of epithelial cells and possibly exudate of plasma-like liquid from the submucosal interstitium (Figure 4) [3, 4].

The submucosal glands have a predominantly cholinergic innervation, which is secretomotor and blocked by atropinic drugs [29]. The effectiveness of these drugs in limiting the secretions in rhinitis is partial, however, suggesting that other agents are at work. The cholinergic cotransmitter VIP also causes glandular secretion, as do some of the adrenergic transmitters such as noradrenaline and possibly neuropeptide Y [30, 31].

A large number of inflammatory and immunological mediators can stimulate secretion, and few seem to inhibit it [1, 2, 29, 30]. These media-

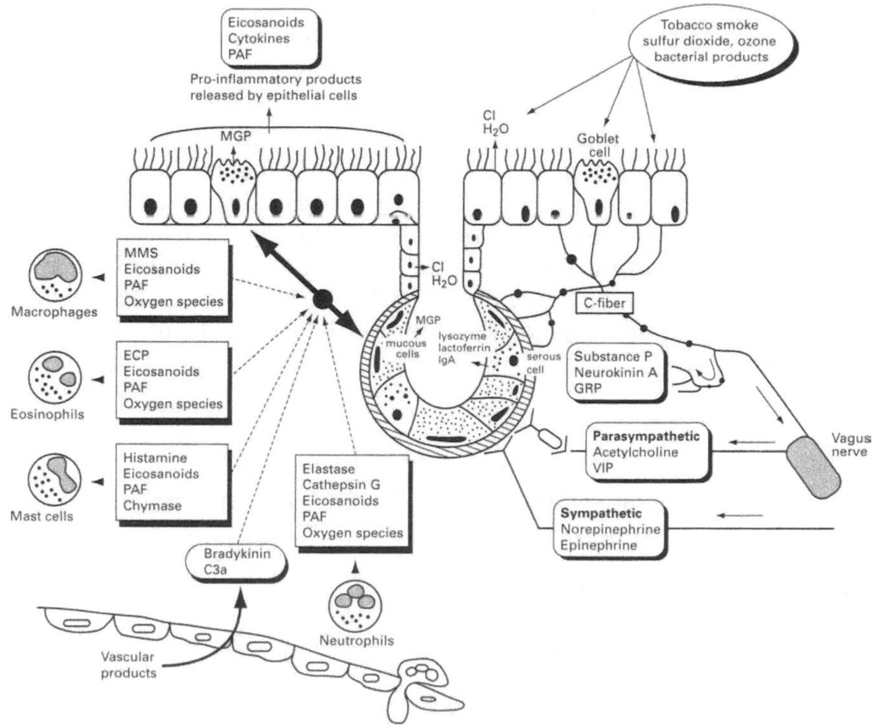

Figure 4. Mechanisms by which control of mucous production in the airways may occur. Reprinted with permission from [30].

tors include prostaglandins, leukotrienes and their derivatives, PAF, and probably various enzymes and mediators derived from migratory cells. Endothelins are also powerful secretor drugs, although their role in rhinitis is uncertain [30].

The copious supply of submucosal glands in the nose makes the contribution of epithelial secretory processes from goblet cells and via ion-transport mechanisms quantitatively far less important. In any event, the secretory activities of the epithelium have been little studied in the nose, compared with the tracheobronchial tree. As already indicated, any vascular extravasation of plasma-like liquid into the submucosa will open gaps between the epithelial cells with exudation into the lumen. Quantitative estimations of the volume of such an exudate in the lower airways suggests that it is small compared with that of glandular secretion [32], but it may be qualitatively important in view of the chemical constituents brought into the lumen as part of a defence reaction.

2.3. *Reflexes*

Activation of sensory nerves in the nasal mucosa in rhinitis by various mediators will set up axon reflexes (see later) and central nervous reflexes (Figure 5) [12–16]. The latter can be demonstrated by causing provocation on one side of the nasal cavity, for example by histamine, and recording changes on the other side [14, 25]. These include glandular secretion, which is largely atropine-sensitive and presumably cholinergic, and vasodilatation and increase in mucosal thickness; the last is only partially blocked by atropine and is probably mainly due to VIP [25]. The main involvement of nasal nerves in rhinitis, however, is probably their role in neurogenic inflammation.

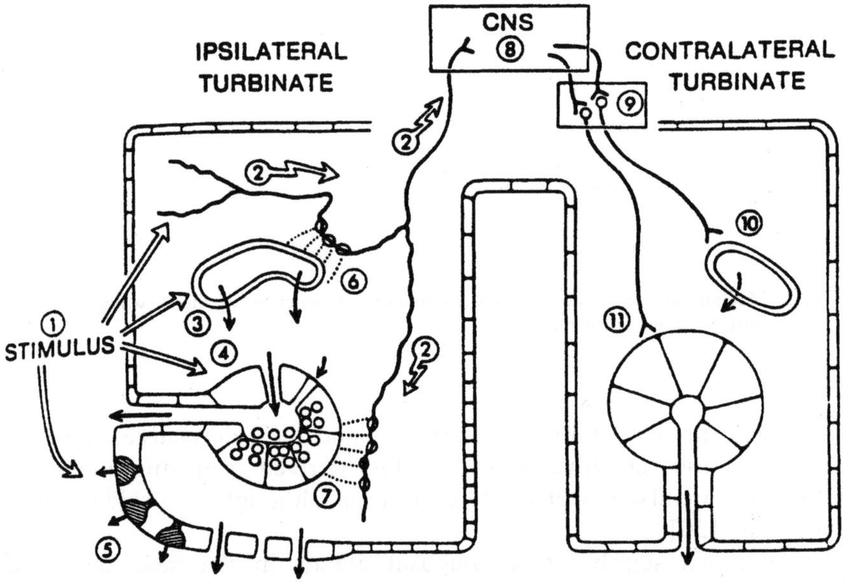

Figure 5. Schematic representation of the nose with two turbinates. The ipsilateral turbinate can be stimulated by (1) factors that act upon nociceptive sensory nerves (2), vessels (3), glands (4), or epithelial cells (5). Depolarization of the entire sensory neuron (2) leads to the release of neuropeptides such as SP, NKA, CGRP and others from neurosecretory vesicles by the axon-response mechanism, as well as stimulation of the central nervous system. Neuropeptides released by the axon-response mechanism can act upon vessels (6) to induce vasodilation (SP, CGRP) and vascular permeability (SP), and may also induce glandular secretion (7) (SP, GRP). In the central nervous system, specific populations of nociceptive and other sensory nerves produce sensations of pain and itch, and induce central reflexes such as sneeze (8). One of the most important consequences of sensory-nerve stimulation is the initiation of bilateral parasympathetic reflexes via the sphenopalatine ganglion (9). For simplicity, only the contralateral parasympathetic reflex is shown. Postganglionic fibres innervate vessels and release acetylcholine and VIP, which can induce vasodilation (10) and glandular secretion (11). Reprinted with permission from [49].

2.4. *Neurogenic Inflammation*

Abundant evidence in experimental animals points to this process being important in rhinitis [14–16], although it has never been established in humans either for rhinitis or asthma. It consists of activation of sensory nerves, probably C-fibre receptors, by various inflammatory mediators or irritants. The nerves may not only set up central nervous reflexes but, more important in this context, conduct a spread of impulses along the sensory receptor terminals with release of neuropeptides to cause local axon reflex responses (Figure 5). Such responses are abolished if the nerves are caused to degenerate by large doses of capsaicin, or to be rendered nonfunctional through local anaesthetics [14].

Apart from inhaled irritants such as cigarette smoke, ammonia or capsaicin, sensory receptors are stimulated by many local mediators [12, 14]. These include bradykinin and histamine, and thus in allergen-induced rhinitis the sensory nerves will be activated, releasing in particular SP, NKA and CGRP. These act on local blood vessels to cause dilatation and vascular congestion, including swelling of the capacitance vessels or sinuses; SP and NKA will open gaps in the post-capillary venules to produce extravasation of plasma, oedema and luminal exudate.

Neurogenic inflammation in the lower airways also includes the secretion of submucosal glands [29] and the action of neuropeptides on the epithelium itself, which may increase its permeability [15]. These two processes probably also apply to the nasal mucosa, but this is not yet established.

The existence of neurogenic inflammation in the nose has been demonstrated in experimental animals by retrograde stimulation of the trigeminal nerve, which contains sensory fibres from the nose [14]. The vascular responses are associated with release of CGRP-like peptide into the nasal venous blood. The responses can be mimicked by administration of SP or CGRP, and in humans nasal SP causes vasodilatation, mucus secretion and autonomic nervous responses [14].

2.5. *Hyperresponsiveness*

In objective terms nasal hyperresponsiveness is usually determined by the reduction in threshold dose of a provoking agent on nasal airflow resistance (Figure 6C), due presumably to local or reflex vascular changes in the mucosa [17, 18]. However, hyperresponsiveness can also be demonstrated for the number of sneezes and the volume of secretion from the nose induced by challenge (Figure 6A and B) [33–35].

Although hyperresponsiveness is usually nonspecific, the choice of challenge agents is important when considering mechanisms. Thus hista-

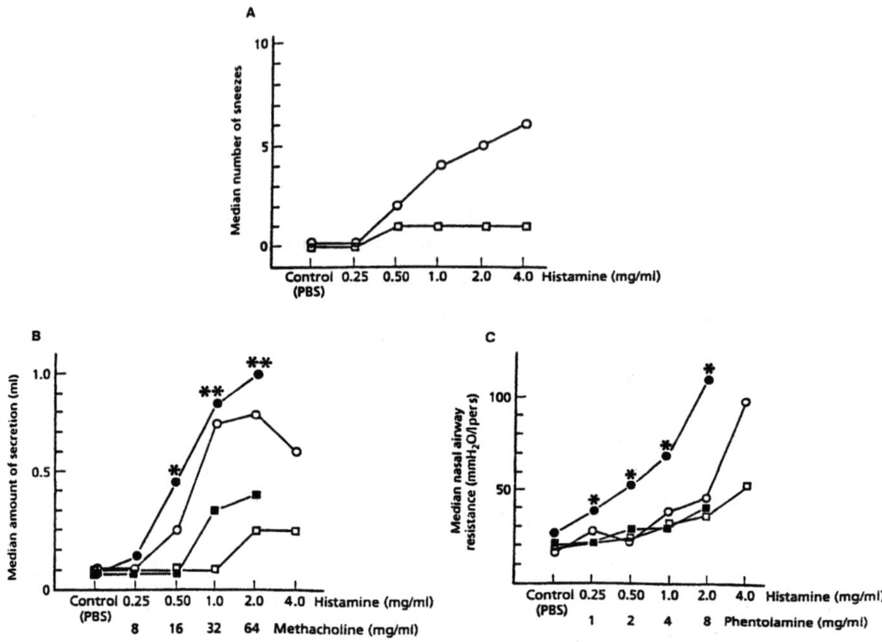

Figure 6. A: Relationship between the concentration of histamine used for nasal challenge and the median number of sneezes induced in patients with perennial allergic rhinitis (circles) and in normal controls (squares). B: Relationship between the concentration of histamine (open symbols) and methacholine (closed symbols) and the median amount of secretion. $*P < 0.05$, $**P < 0.01$ for patients compared with controls. C: Relationship between the concentrations of histamine (open symbols) and phentolamine (closed symbols) and the median nasal airway resistance. $*P < 0.05$ for patients compared with controls. Reprinted with permission from [17].

mine causes intense itching and some sneezing, which establishes that it is stimulating sensory nerves (Figures 6A, 7). The increased nasal discharge and airflow resistance could be due in part to a central nervous reflex (Figure 7), since they occur on the contralateral side when histamine is restricted to one side of the nose (Figure 5), but the histamine will also have a local action that could be hyperresponsive. Methacholine predominantly causes glandular secretion [17], and the hyperresponsiveness to this agent seen in rhinitis is presumably a local effect on the glands.

Hyperresponsiveness to allergen in allergic rhinitis is definitive and usually measured as nasal airflow resistance changes. The mediators involved in this hyperresponsiveness are uncertain, although PAF has been suggested [36], and eosinophils may play an important part [37]. However, there seems to be little correlation between the numbers of eosinophils in the nasal mucosa and the degree of hyperresponsiveness. Epithelial damage, leading to more ready penetration of active agents and exposure

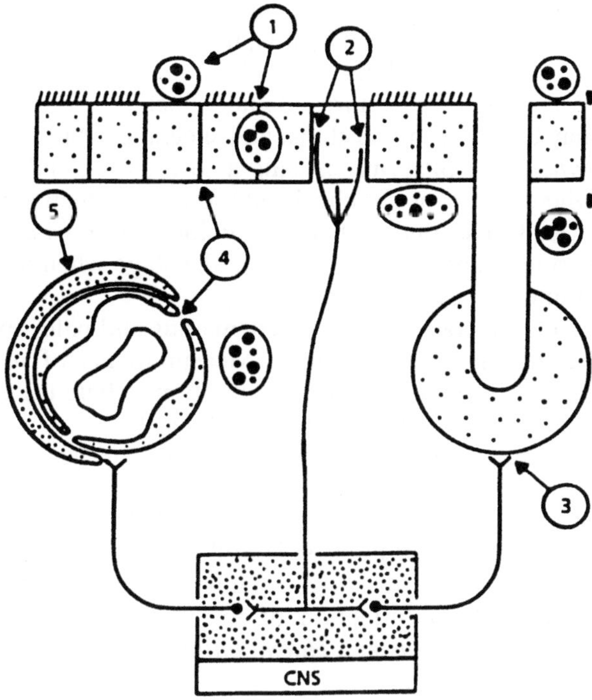

Figure 7. A schematic outline of the nasal allergic reaction with some potential sites of changes that might be responsible for an increase in responsiveness at allergen challenge. (1) A changed distribution of mediator cells towards a more superficial site. (2) An increased excitability of nerve endings. (3) An increase in reactivity of the glands. (4, 5) Changes in the barrier function of the epithelium and endothelium. (6) An increased number of eosinophils. Reprinted with permission from [17].

of mucosal and epithelial nerves, could play a part in hyperresponsiveness (Figure 7).

3. Pathological Conditions

3.1. Infectious Rhinitis

This is far and away the most common form of rhinitis, but in terms of pathophysiological mechanisms it has been studied much less than allergic and vasomotor rhinitis [38]. Nasal infections, including the common cold, certainly affect most city dwellers at least once a year; but because the pathology only lasts for a few days, it has either proved more intransigent to study or less important, compared with the chronic nasal diseases.

Infectious rhinitis is most commonly caused by rhinoviruses, but other agents include coronovirus, influenza virus, respiratory syncytial virus and adenoviruses [39, 40]. Although the clinical features due to different viral infections may vary, common features include blockage of the nose, nasal secretion that may be either thin or thick, and sneezing. Many of the infections spread down to the pharynx, causing a sore throat, and even to the lower airways where they cause tracheal and bronchial infections. The viral infections often lead to secondary bacterial colonisation, when the secretions become purulent, and this may occur at the stage when the infection is passing down into the lower airways.

Pathologically the mucosa is usually oedematous and pale, and the epithelium may be damaged or destroyed. Measurements of mucociliary transport show that it is deranged even in conditions where the epithelium has not been visually damaged or destroyed [38–40].

When there is bacterial infection in the nose, either by itself or superimposed on viral infection, although the overall pathological picture is similar to that of viral infection, the mucosa tends to be reddened rather than pale, and the secretions are thick and purulent rather than watery. With acute bacterial rhinitis the invading organisms are almost invariably aerobic; anaerobic bacterial infection of the nose is rare for obvious reasons. *Staphylococcus aureus* and *Haemophilus influenzae* are common bacterial invaders of the nose.

3.2. Seasonal Allergic Rhinitis

Seasonal allergic rhinitis, sometimes called atopic rhinitis or more commonly hay fever, is associated with inflammation due to specific allergens such as pollen, house-dust mite, dander from animals and products of various moulds [38, 41]. The last three may not always be seasonal and therefore may cause perennial allergic rhinitis. Seasonal allergic rhinitis is by far the most common chronic respiratory disease in humans: probably up to 20% of humans in the western world have it, and it is twice as common as asthma and over twice as common as vasomotor rhinitis.

The allergen first penetrates the nasal epithelium. It is likely that, as for the lower airways, there are specific areas such as bronchus-associated lymphoid tissue (BALT) where penetration of the allergen may be facilitated (see below), but presumably penetration is easier in conditions where the epithelium has already been damaged, such as established hay fever [38, 42]. The quantitation of allergen cleared on the one hand by adhesion to mucous with mucociliary transport and on the other by penetration through the epithelium does not seem to have been greatly studied, but could be important. The allergens eventually bind to cells such as mast cells, although the intermediate process involves other cells that may carry the allergen and lead to the production of immunoglobulin (Ig)E. IgE is bound both to mast cells and to various other migratory cells such as basophils, monocytes and eosinophils, and to some epithelial fixed cells. The combination of the IgE on various migratory cells with allergen leads to the release of a range of bioactive substances such as histamine, bradykinin, leukotrienes, enzymes and cytokines. These mediators then set up various pathophysiological responses. These include vasodilatation and engorgement of capacitance vessels; increased capillary vascular pressure and opening of interendothelial gaps in postcapillary venules leading to oedema and plasma exudation into the airway lumen; secretion by submucosal glands and epithelial goblet cells; and stimulation of sensory nerves that will cause irritation, sneezing and various reflex responses.

3.2.1. Migratory cells: There has been exhaustive study of the populations of migratory cells in various forms of rhinitis ([43] and see other chapters in this book), and only a brief summary will be given here. Mast cells have traditionally been regarded as the leading actor in allergic rhinitis, although it is now increasingly evident that many other migratory and fixed cells are also involved [38]. The mast cell membrane IgE reacts with antigen both to release preformed mediators from intracellular granules and also to cause synthesis of mediators such as cytokines with their subsequent release. In patients with allergic rhinitis more mast cells (of the mucosal type) are found in and under the epithelium; presumably they have migrated from deeper sites (Figure 8) [44, 45], and are well situated to respond to inhaled allergens. After challenge with allergen mast cell mediators including bradykinin, histamine, PG D2 and enzymes such as tryptase can be found in nasal lavage liquid [44]. These released mediators presumably set up the pathophysiological changes that follow allergen challenge. The relative importance of the many types of mediators released from mast cells in allergic rhinitis has not been established, although histamine seems to be important. This conclusion is based on the fact that histamine is found in abundance in nasal washings after challenge with allergen and that antihistamines can relieve many if not all of the symptoms of allergic rhinitis [27].

Blood eosinophilia usually occurs in allergic rhinitis and the eosinophils may have different secretory characteristics from those found normally [46].

In seasonal allergic rhinitis there is an increased number of eosinophils in the nasal mucosa and in nasal washings, especially after exposure to allergen [46]. The eosinophil seems to be in activated state, and different structural types of eosinophils have been identified. In response to a nasal challenge with an allergen, eosinophils appear in nasal secretions about 30 min after challenge and are present for up to 48 h

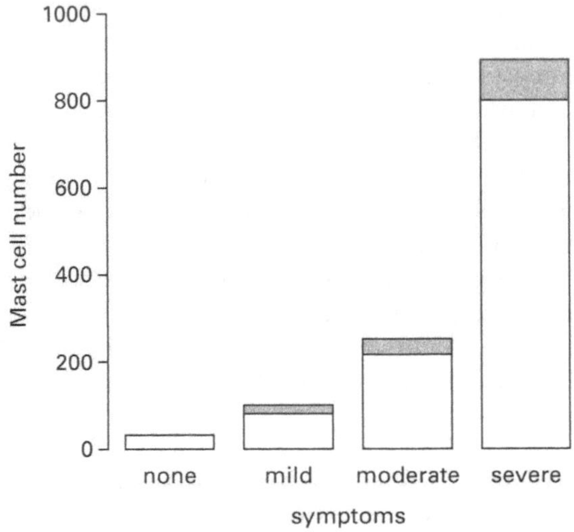

Figure 8. Relationship between nasal symptom score and abundance and type of mast cells in nasal scrapings in allergic rhinitis. □ = Formalin-sensitive mast cell; ■ = formalin-resistant mast cell. Reprinted with permission from [44].

afterwards. The maximum numbers appear about 10 h after challenge. The appearance of eosinophils does not seem to be closely related to hyper-responsiveness or to leakiness of the epithelium indicated by the presence of albumin in nasal washings [3]. The output of eosinophils into nasal secretions can be prevented by pretreatment with corticosteroids.

Eosinophils release various mediators, mainly from preformed granules. These mediators include major basic protein, PAF, leukotrienes and prostaglandins [46]. Presumably these mediators play a major part in the pathology of allergic inflammation. Recently the importance of cytokines released from eosinophils has been emphasised [47].

Lymphocytes have been studied far less in the nose than in the bronchial tree. The equivalent of BALT has been described for the nose, and termed nasal-associated lymphoid tissue (NALT) [48]. This has been studied mainly in monkeys and rats and is presumed to have the same properties as BALT. Thus NALT contains T-cell and B-cell lymphocytes, as well as macrophages and dendritic cells, and is situated very close to the epithelium [48]. The cells express IgG or IgM, other immunoglobulins being rare. Dendritic cells links the NALT to mast and other migratory cells.

3.3. Perennial Allergic Rhinitis

Many of the cellular patterns of this conditions are similar to those found in seasonal allergic rhinitis [38]. There is an increased number of mast cells in the mucosa, although there seem to be fewer in the epithelium compared with the seasonal variety. There may be increased eosinophilia and neutrophilia, with the associated mediators released from these cells. Mucosal lymphocytes, especially T cells, are also abundant.

Nasal hyperresponsiveness to allergens or mediators such as histamine is pronounced in perennial allergic rhinitis [17]; but in general both the epidemiology and the pathophysiological responses are similar to those seen in the seasonal variety, although of course, as the allergen is not seasonal, the condition and symptoms are present throughout the year.

3.4. Nonallergic Noninfectious Rhinitis

This is sometimes referred to as vasomotor rhinitis, but the whole question of nomenclature of different forms of rhinitis is contentious [9–11]. Certainly more than the nasal vasculature is involved in the condition, since there may well be a considerable increase in secretions especially when there is coincident infection [38].

Nonallergic rhinitis is usually classified by exclusion of allergic and other factors, and its pathophysiology has been less studied then that of allergic rhinitis. Hyperresponsiveness is characteristic, with many triggers including common irritants, such as cigarette smoke, cold air, food and spices. Patients can usually be placed in one of two categories, those with nasal blockage and those with increased secretions. However, no difference in pathophysiology has been determined for the two categories. There is no clear picture of the histopathology, except for the presence of mucosal oedema and some cellular infiltrations.

4. Conclusion

The pathophysiology of rhinitis is now an enormously broad topic especially when cellular, inflammatory and immunological aspects are included, and a comprehensive treatment would require consulting many thousands of references. In general all forms of rhinitis are based on abnormal changes in target tissues such as the vascular bed of the mucosa, glandular secretions and epithelial function. The role of sensory nerves, both in causing local neurogenic inflammation and in setting up reflexes, including sneezing, is being increasingly emphasised. However, this component of nasal pathophysiology is only part of a far larger picture that includes the actions and interactions of a very large number of inflammatory and immunological mediators. Classification of different forms of rhinitis still depends far more on case history and response to challenges and therapies than on well-defined histopathological features.

References

1. Widdicombe JG, Wells UM. Airway secretions. In: Proctor DF, Andersen IB, editors. The nose: upper airway physiology and the atmospheric environment. Amsterdam: Elsevier Biomedical Press, 1982: 215–244.
2. Baraniuk JN, Kaliner MA. Pharmacological control of nasal secretions. In: Chung FK, Barnes PJ, editors. Pharmacology of the respiratory tract. New York: Marcel Dekker, 1993: 551–581.
3. Persson CGA. Airway mucosal exudation of plasma. In: Takishima T, Shimura S, editors. Airway secretion. New York: Marcel Dekker, 1994: 451–67.
4. Persson CGA, Greiff L, Andersson M, Erjefält I, Svensson C, Alkner U, et al. Mucosal exudation of plasma in asthma and rhinitis. In: Busse WW, Holgate ST, editors. Asthma and rhinitis. Boston: Blackwell Scientific Publications, 1995: 733–741.
5. Widdicombe JG. Microvascular anatomy of the airways. In: Busse WW, Holgate ST, editors. Asthma and rhinitis. Boston: Blackwell Scientific Publications, 1995: 722–732.
6. Widdicombe JG. Why are the airways so vascular? Thorax 1993; 48: 290–295.
7. Wells U, Widdicombe JG. Lateral nasal gland secretion in the anaesthetized dog. J Physiol 1986; 374: 359–374.
8. Widdicombe JG, Wells UM. Airway secretions. In: Proctor DF, Andersen IB, editors. The nose: upper airway physiology and the atmospheric environment. Amsterdam: Elsevier Biomedical Press, 1982: 215–244.
9. Mygind N, Anggard A, Druce HM. Definition, classification and terminology. In: Mygind N, Weeke B, editors. Allergic and vasomotor rhinitis: clinical aspects. Copenhagen: Munksgaard, 1985: 15–20.
10. Mackay IS. Introduction. In: Mackay I, editor. Rhinitis. London: Royal Society of Medicine Services, 1989: 1–10.
11. Van Cauwenberge PB, Ingels KJAO. Rhinitis: the spectrum of the disease. In: Busse WW, Holgate ST, editors. Asthma and rhinitis. Boston: Blackwell Scientific Publications, 1995: 6–12.
12. Widdicombe J. Nasal and pharyngeal reflexes: protective and respiratory functions. In: Mathew OP, Sant'Ambrogio G, editors. Respiratory function of the upper airway. New York: Marcel Dekker, 1988: 233–258.
13. Widdicome JG, Sant'Ambrogio G, Mathew OP. Nervous receptors of the upper airway. In: Mathew OP, Sant'Ambrogio G, editors. Respiratory function of the upper airway. New York: Dekker, 1988: 193–231.
14. Lacroix JS, Lundberg JM. Neural reflex pathways in rhinitis. In: Busse WW, Holgate ST, editors. Asthma and rhinitis. Boston: Blackwell Scientific Publications, 1995: 686–690.
15. McDonald DM. The concept of neurogenic inflammation in the respiratory tract. In: Kaliner MA, Barnes PJ, Kunkel GHH, Baraniuk JN, editors. Neuropeptides in respiratory medicine. New York: Marcel Dekker, 1994: 321–349.
16. Barnes PJ. Airway neuropeptides. In: Busse WW, Holgate ST, editors. Asthma and rhinitis. Boston: Blackwell Scientific Publications, 1995: 667–685.
17. Andersson M, Mygind N. Nasal hyperresponsiveness. In: Busse WW, Holgate ST, editors. Asthma and rhinitis. Boston: Blackwell Scientific Publications, 1995: 1057–1066.
18. Schellenberg RR. Mechanisms of airway hyperresponsiveness. In: Page CP, Gardiner PJ, editors. Airway hyperresponsiveness: is it really important for asthma? Oxford: Blackwell Scientific Publications, 1993: 33–54.
19. Cauna N, Hinderer KH. Fine structure of blood vessels of the human nasal respiratory mucosa. Ann Otol Rhinol Laryngol 1969; 78: 865–879.
20. Hill P, Goulding D, Webber SE, Widdicombe JG. Blood sinuses in the submucosa of the large airways of the sheep. J Anat 1989; 162: 235–247.

21. Eccles R, Bende M, Widdicombe JG. Nasal blood vessels. In: Mygind N, Pipkorn U, editors. Allergic and vasomotor rhinitis: pathophysiological aspects. Copenhagen: Munksgaard, 1987: 63–76.
22. Malm L. Response of resistance and capacitance vessels in feline nasal mucosa to vasoactive agents. Acta Otolaryngol 1974; 78: 90–97.
23. Druce HM, Baraniuk JN. Asthma and rhinitis. In: Busse WW, Holgate ST, editors. Neuroregulation of mucosal vasculature. Boston: Blackwell Scientific Publications, 1995: 742–751.
24. Atkinson TP, Kaliner MA. Vascular mechanisms in rhinitis. In: Busse WW, Holgate ST, editors. Asthma and rhinitis. Boston: Blackwell Scientific Publications, 1995: 777–788.
25. Borum P, Drettner B, Mygind N, Malmberg H. Anticholinergic agents. In: Mygind N, Weeke B, editors. Allergic and vasomotor rhinitis: clinical aspects. Copenhagen: Munksgaard, 1985: 151–158.
26. Pretolani M, Vargaftig BB. Platelet-activating factor as a mediator of allergic diseases. In: Busse WW, Holgate ST, editors. Asthma and rhinitis. Boston: Blackwell Scientific Publications, 1995: 884–891.
27. Malm L, Druce HM, Holgate ST. Vasoconstrictors and antihistamines. In: Mygind N, Weeke B, editors. Allergic and vasomotor rhinitis: clinical aspects. Copenhagen: Munksgaard, 1985: 140–150.
28. Estelle F, Simons R. New medications for rhinitis. In: Busse WW, Holgate ST, editors. Asthma and rhinitis. Boston: Blackwell Scientific Publications, 1995: 1325–1336.
29. Shimura S, Takishma T. Airway submucosal gland secretion. In: Takishima T, Shimura S, editors. Airway secretion. New York: Marcel Dekker, 1994: 325–398.
30. Johnson CW, Larivee P, Shelhamer JH. Epithelial cells: regulation of mucus secretion. In: Busse WW, Holgate ST, editors. Asthma and rhinitis. Boston: Blackwell Scientific Publications, 1995: 584–598.
31. Pell J, Phipps RJ, Wells UM, Widdicombe JG. Control of mucoglycoprotein output from the rabbit nose. J Physiol 1984; 353: 339–353.
32. Widdicombe J. The tracheobronchial vasculature: a possible role in asthma. Microcirculation 1996; 3: 1–13.
33. Gerth van Wijk RG, Dieges PH. Comparison of nasal responsiveness to histamine, methacholine in allergic rhinitis patients and controls. Clin Allergy 1987; 17: 563–570.
34. Borum P. Nasal methacholine test: a measurement of nasal reactivity. J Allergy Clin Immunol 1991; 87: 457–467.
35. Druce H, Wright R, Kossof D, Kaliner M. Cholinergic nasal hyperreactivity in atopic subjects. J Allergy Clin Immunol 1985; 76: 445–452.
36. Andersson P, Pipkorn U. The effect of platelet activating factor on nasal hypersensitivity. Eur J Pharmacol 1988; 35: 231–235.
37. Bisgaard H, Gronborg H, Mygind N, Dahl R, Venge P. Allergen-induced increase of eosinophil cationic protein in nasal lavage fluid: effect of the glucocorticoid budesonide. J Allergy Clin Immunol 1990; 85: 891–895.
38. Andersson M, Greiff L, Svensson C, Wollmer P, Persson CGA. Allergic and nonallergic rhinitis. In: Busse WW, Holgate ST, editors. Asthma and rhinitis. Boston: Blackwell Scientific Publications, 1995: 145–155.
39. Tyrrell D. Common colds and respiratory viruses. In: Busse WW, Holgate ST, editors. Asthma and rhinitis. Boston: Blackwell Scientific Publications, 1995: 1219–1228.
40. Gwaltney Jr JM, Hayden FG. The nose and infection. In: Proctor DF, Andersen IB, editors. The nose. Amsterdam: Elsevier Biomedical Press, 1982; 399–422.
41. Sibbald B, Strachan DP. Epidemiology of rhinitis. In: Busse WW, Holgate ST, editors. Asthma and rhinitis. Boston: Blackwell Scientific Publications, 1995: 32–43.
42. Davies RJ, Devalia JL. Epithelial cell dysfunction in rhinitis. In: Busse WW, Holgate ST, editors. Asthma and rhinitis. Boston: Blackwell Scientific Publications, 1995: 612–624.
43. Busse WW, Holgate ST, editors. Asthma and rhinitis. Boston: Blackwell Scientific Publications, 1995.
44. Sulakvelidze I, Marshall JS, Dolovich J. Mast cells in rhinitis. In: Busse WW, Holgate ST, editors. Asthma and rhinitis. Boston: Blackwell Scientific Publications, 1995: 231–241.

45. Rottem M, Metcalfe DD. Development and maturation of mast cells and basophils. In: Busse WW, Holgate ST, editors. Asthma and rhinitis. Boston: Blackwell Scientific Publications, 1995: 167–181.
46. Feather IH, Wilson SJ. Eosinophils in rhinitis. In: Busse WW, Holgate ST, editors. Asthma and rhinitis. Boston: Blackwell Scientific Publications, 1995: 347–363.
47. Togias AG. The role of environmental allergens in rhinitis. In: Busse WW, Holgate ST, editors. Asthma and rhinitis. Boston: Blackwell Scientific Publications, 1995: 1009–1029.
48. Howarth PH, Varley J. Animal models of rhinitis. In: Busse WW, Holgate ST, editors. Asthma and rhinitis. Boston: Blackwell Scientific Publications, 1995: 978–986.
49. Baraniuk JN, Kaliner MA. Functional activity of upper-airway nerves. In: Busse WW, Holgate ST, editors. Asthma and rhinitis. Boston: Blackwell Scientific Publications, 1995: 652–666.

Rhinitis: Immunopathology
and Pharmacotherapy
ed. by D. Raeburn and M. A. Giembycz

CHAPTER 3
Immunology of the Nose

Glenis K. Scadding

Royal National Throat, Nose and Ear Hospital, London, UK

1. Introduction

Nasal breathing is essential for neonates and for most vertebrates. Mouth breathing in man can sustain life but is both unpleasant and damaging. The nose acts as a gateway for the respiratory tract and filters, warms and humidifies approximately 10,000 l of air each day in the average normal human subject.

Suspended particles in air tend to be deposited behind constrictions and where there are changes in the direction of flow. The nasal cavity, with its slitlike orifice, large surface area, turbinates and bend into the nasopharynx, provides an excellent filter as demonstrated by Proetz [1]. The majority of particles greater than 10 µm are filtered out, whereas 1 µm particles pass through to the lower airways [2] (Figure 1). Gases can also be retained; sulphur dioxide for example, is more than 99% retained in the nose, not reaching the lungs even at concentrations of 25 ppm [3]. The *British Medical Journal* of 1895 characterized the nose as "one of the dirtiest organs of the body" (see [1]) and suggested regular washing. In fact the

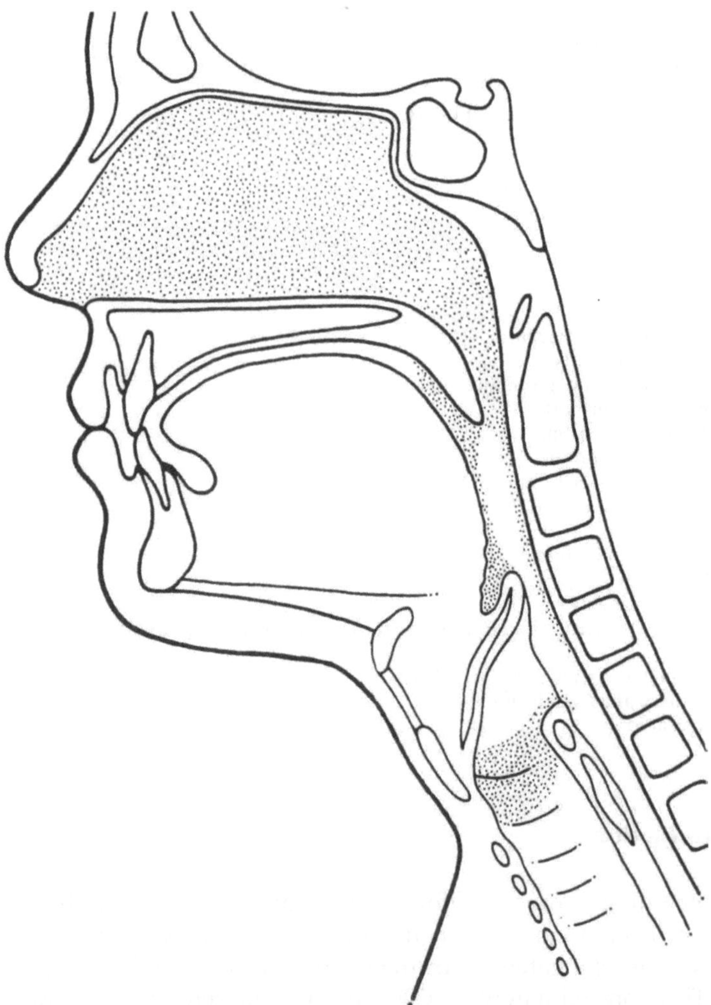

Figure 1. Sites of deposition of airborne powder on a model of the upper respiratory tract, based on a photograph by Proetz (1953) [1]. Most of the particles are deposited in the nose, but a small proportion land on the pharynx and larynx due to turbulence and impingement.

Table 1. The ability of the nose to warm and humidify inspired air

	Temp. (°C)	Relative Humidity (%)
Room air	23	43
Subglottic space following nasal breathing	32	98
Subglottic space following oral breathing	30	90
Subglottic space following 10 min of nasal breathing of cold air (–4° to 0 °C)	31	98

(reproduced with permission from [4]).

nose (in common with the pharynx, larynx, tracheobronchial tree, sinuses and eustachian tube) possesses a remarkable self-cleansing mechanism: the mucociliary system.

Magendie (see [4]) first suggested that the function of the nose was to warm and humidify the inspired air. Ingelstadt [4] demonstrated that this occurred by sampling in the subglottic space (Table 1). This function depends upon a number of factors including nasal secretions from goblet cells and seromucous glands, a larger surface area increased by turbinates and by microvilli, by a profuse and adaptable nasal blood supply including arteriovenous anastomoses and by condensation of expired air in the anterior part of the nose.

In addition, the nose also serves as a major defence mechanism against respiratory tract pathogens. Together with factors such as lysozyme, lactoferrin, interferon and complement, and cells such as neutrophils and mast cells found in nasal secretions, the mucociliary escalator provides the innate intrinsic defence. Superadded are the components of acquired immunity, immunoglobulins and lymphocytes, which have gradually evolved since organisms became more complex and emerged from water to dwell on land and which possess both specificity and memory.

2. Non-specific Immunity

2.1. Mechanical Factors

The nasal epithelium provides a physical barrier function. The nasal vestibule is lined by skin-bearing hairs which provide a barrier to relatively large objects. The remainder of the nasal and paranasal sinus mucosa, with the exception of the specialized olfactory region, is lined with a pseudostratified respiratory epithelium of approximately 120 cm^2. This consists of four types of cells: ciliated and non-ciliated epithelial cells, goblet cells which are unicellular mucous glands and basal cells from which the former cell types develop [5] (Figure 2).

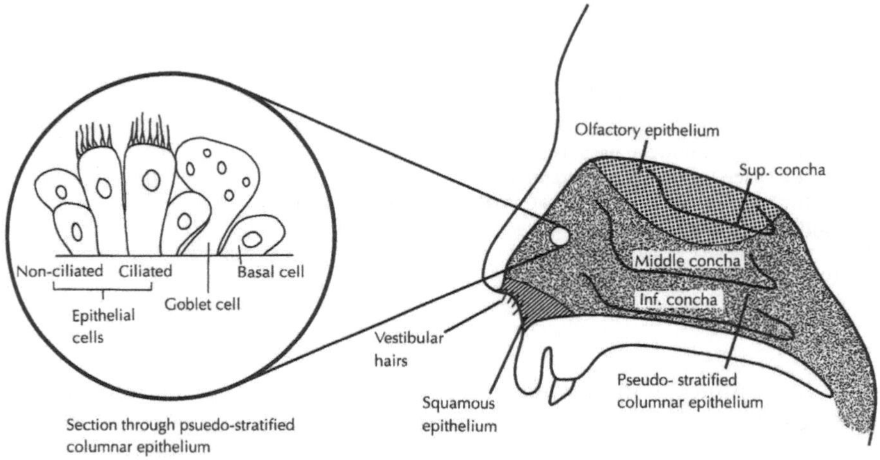

Figure 2. Lateral view of the nasal cavity showing the distribution of the pseudostratified columnar epithelium. The inset shows the epithelial cells in more detail. (Reproduced by kind permission of Kluwer Academic Publishers, Lancaster, England, from Immunology of ENT Disorders, ed. G.K. Scadding, 1994).

The major defence mechanism is mucociliary clearance, which reduces colonization by micro-organisms and enhances their expulsion. In the nasal fluid are secretions of goblet cells, seromucous glands and lacrimal glands as well as condensed vapour from humidified expired air, fluids transported across the epithelial cells and any micro-organisms or deposited particles. In 1934 Lucas and Douglas [6] developed a two-layer concept of respiratory mucus in which the cilia are surrounded by a periciliary fluid layer (sol) and are covered by a thicker mucus layer (gel) which interacts with the tips of the cilia. The cilia beat at 12–15 Hz with a rapid, stiff-armed, forward stroke during which clawlike projections from their tips propel the viscid gel layer towards the nasopharynx. They subsequently bend and return more slowly to their original position (Figure 3). The motion of the adjacent cilia on an individual cell (on which there will be 50–100 cilia) are coordinated, as is the motion among cilia on adjacent cells, in a metachronistic fashion, similar to the "Mexico wave" seen at ball games.

Each cilium is 5–6 μm in length and 0.33 μm in diameter. Electron microscopy shows an organized structure of a ring of nine paired outer microtubules surrounding two central microtubules, the whole enclosed in a surface membrane (Figure 4). The outer tubules are linked by nexin with central spokes linking outer and inner tubules. Each pair of outer tubules has an inner and outer dynein arm. During ciliary movement these arms link and break in a process which derives energy from the dynein-induced breakdown of adenosine triphosphate (ATP) and which is magnesium-dependent. The dynein arms are absent in Kartagener's syndrome of

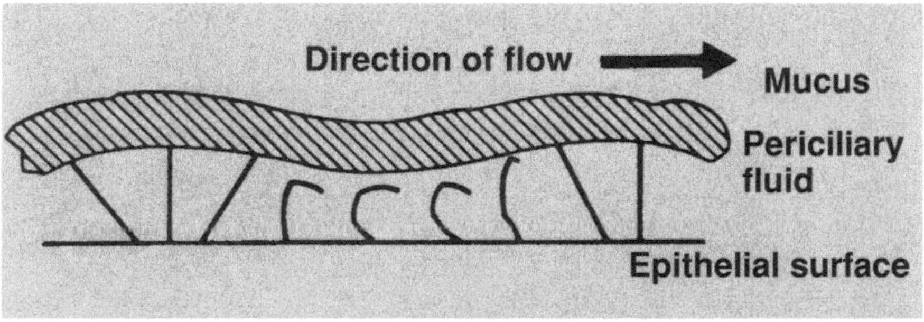

Figure 3. Ciliary action. Ciliary beating occurs with a rapid, stiff-armed, forward stroke in which the gel layer of mucus is moved forward by microscopic hooks present at the tips of the cilia. The recovery phase, during which the cilia bend down into the sol phase of the mucus, is much slower. It is possible to measure ciliary beat frequency by the interruption of a beam of light. (Reproduced by kind permission of Kluwer Academic Publishers, Lancaster, England, from Immunology of ENT Disorders, ed. G.K. Scadding, 1994).

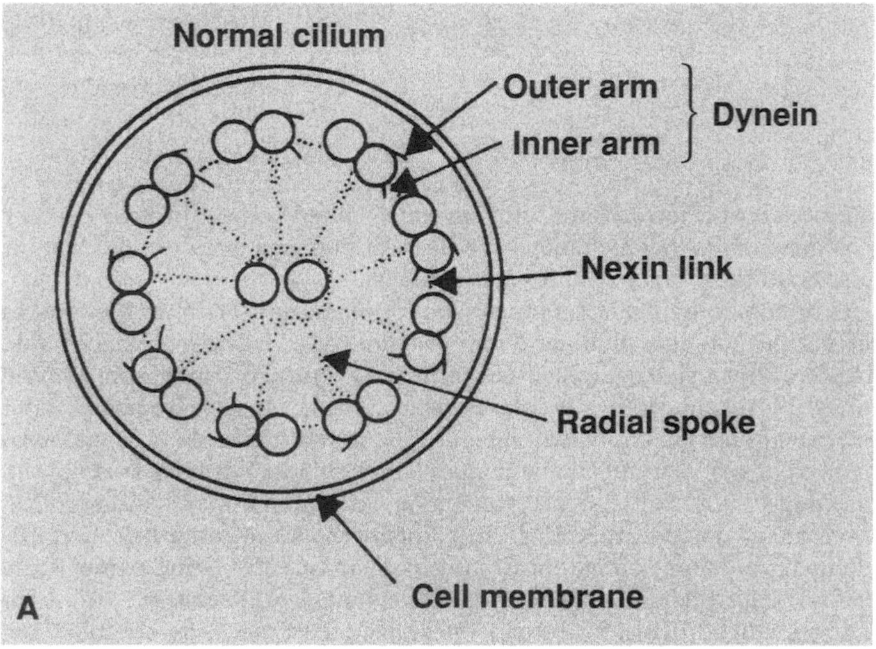

Figures 4 A and B. A: Schematic drawing of a cross-section through a cilium. B: Transverse section of a cilium demonstrating the two central microtubules linked by spokes to nine paired outer microtubules. The inner and outer dynein arms present on the outer microtubules are absent in various forms of primary ciliary dyskinesia. (Reproduced by kind permission of Kluwer Academic Publishers, Lancaster, England, from Immunology of ENT Disorders, ed. G.K. Scadding, 1994).

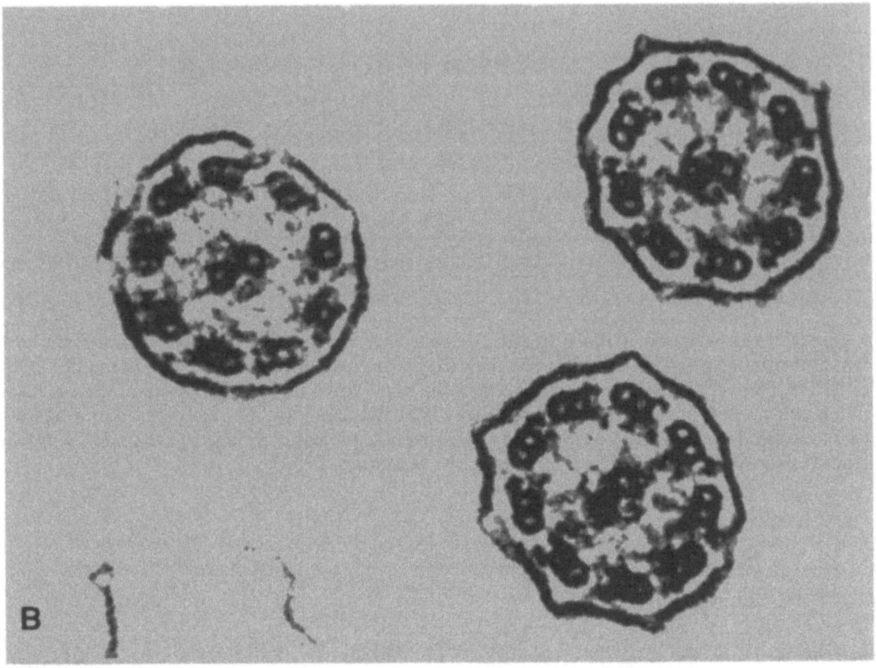

Figure 4B.

sinusitis, bronchiectasis and situs inversus. Other forms of primary ciliary dyskinesia exist in which either the inner or the outer arms are missing, or abnormalities of microtubules are involved.

In normal individuals the time taken for mucus to flow from the front to the back of the nose at about 6 mm per min varies between 5 and 20 min. This is easily tested using the saccharin test (Figure 5). The nasal mucus is joined by mucus from the sinuses which drains through ostia and, after passing around the eustachian tube orifice, is swallowed. *In vitro* measurement of ciliary activity can be undertaken by photometric methods [7, 8]. Secondary causes of ciliary dysfunction, which are far more common than are primary defects, include drying, upper respiratory tract infection, the allergic response, apposition of mucosal surfaces, extremes of pH and certain topical applications such as adrenaline and cocaine [9, 10]. After therapy with corticosteroids for 1 week, the rate of saccharin clearance has been shown to be reduced [11]; however, the effect of 1 year's therapy with fluticasone propionate in allergic rhinitis patients was an improvement in mucociliary clearance (Table 2). Benzalkonium chloride, a preservative common to most nasal sprays, has not been shown to affect mucociliary clearance adversely in normal subjects [12, 13].

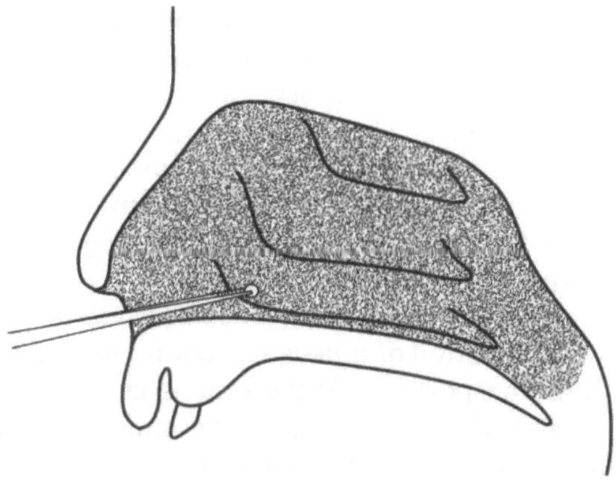

Figure 5. The saccharin clearance test used to measure nasomucociliary clearance. A quarter of a tablet of saccharin is placed about 1 cm back on the medial surface of the inferior turbinate after the subject has blown his or her nose. The length of time taken for the patient to experience a sweet taste is then noted. Patients should be unaware of the taste sensation expected and should not eat, drink, sneeze or blow their nose during the test. The normal time is under 20 min. (Reproduced by kind permission of Kluwer Academic Publishers, Lancaster, England, from Immunology of ENT Disorders, ed. G.K. Scadding, 1994).

Table 2. Saccharin clearance time in 35 patients before and 1 year after regular therapy with fluticasone propionate aqueous nasal spray 400 µg daily. At the end of 1 year saccharin clearance time has improved, showing that long-term use of intranasal steroid is not harmful to the nasal mucosa.

Saccharin clearance times (min)	
Pre-intranasal corticosteroids	After 1 year of treatment
19.6 ± 10.2	14.6 ± 8.3 *

* $p < 0.05$ vs pre-treatment.

Secondary defects in mucociliary clearance are common in patients with chronic or recurrent nasal infection. These are probably caused by toxins produced by certain bacteria such as *Pseudomonas* and *Haemophilus influenzae* [14]. We [15] have recently demonstrated that prolonged low-dose antibiosis over 3 months can return ciliary beat frequency to normal.

2.2. *Mucus*

The thickness of the mucus layer may influence its propagation, i.e. surface particles move faster at a critical mucus thickness. Transport is at its fastest when the mucus has high elasticity and low viscosity [16]. Primary abnormalities of mucus do occur. Cystic fibrosis is a genetically acquired autosomal recessive disease occurring in approximately 1 in 2000 of the

Caucasian population. There is an excessive production of viscid mucus in the respiratory tract together with asociated pancreatic dysfunction. Chronic sepsis of the upper respiratory tract is frequently associated, as in primary ciliary dyskinesia. The major responsible gene has now been identified, and trials of genetic therapy, both inhaled and systemic, are underway. In Young's syndrome [17] there is abnormally viscid mucus with frequent respiratory tract infections. In addition, the patient is usually infertile. The underlying pathogenesis is unknown.

Secondary abnormalities of mucus also occur. *Pseudomonas aeruginosa* has been linked with alteration of mucus secretion, making it more viscous, less elastic and less transportable. If the mucus layer becomes too thick, uncoupling may occur; the cilia transport the underlying sol, but the gel layer, with adherent bacteria, remains stationary. Increasing the sodium content of the mucus also increases its spinability and improves mucociliary transport (P. Cole, personal communication). This may be one reason why nasal douching with saline solutions is helpful in chronic rhinosinusitis.

2.3. Lysozyme, Lactoferrins and Interferons

Lysozymes, enzymes which can split bacterial cell wall mucopeptides, are particularly toxic to gram-positive bacteria lacking capsules. They can also kill damaged gram-negative organisms. As well as being produced by macrophages, lysozymes are found in serous gland secretions, including those of the nose, and are present in tears.

Lactoferrins present in saliva, nasal secretions and in milk, are produced by glandular epithelium. Like transferrin they are capable of binding iron and thus inhibit the growth of certain bacteria, particularly *Staphylococci* and *Pseudomonas* species.

Interferons (IFN) are important in defence against viruses as well as forming part of the cytokine network. Three varieties, IFNα, IFNβ and IFNγ, are produced by different cell types (leucocytes, fibroblasts and T cells respectively). Their mechanisms of action include the induction of intracellular proteins that block viral replication, induction of major histocompatibility (MHC) proteins in the infected cell (rendering it susceptible to T-cell cytotoxicity) and enhancement of macrophage plus natural killer (NK) cell function.

2.4. Complement

The complement system involves over 30 glycoproteins and forms a major defence system which can be activated either directly by the surface of certain bacteria and fungi (alternative pathway) [18] or following the bind-

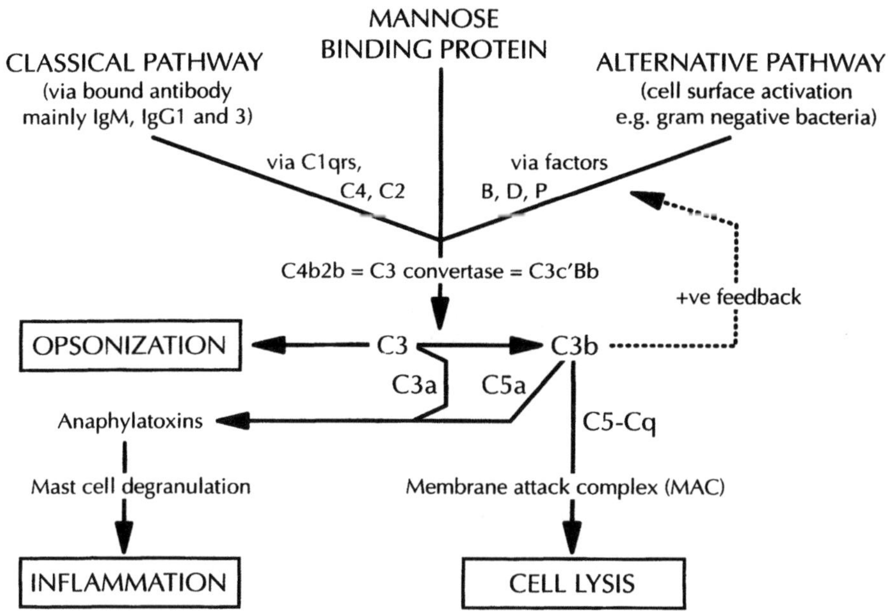

Figure 6. The pathways of complement activation.

ing of antibody to cell surfaces (classical pathway) [19]. Recently a third pathway involving mannose binding protein has been described (Figure 6). The consequences of complement activation include not only cell lysis [20] but opsonization the (process of attachment of bacteria to neutrophil) and cellular activation (Figure 7). Complement has an important role in the clearance and destruction of both gram-negative and gram-positive bacteria, parasites and viruses. Most gram-negative bacteria can activate complement directly by the alternative and by the classical pathway and are usually destroyed by lysis. Gram-positive bacteria activate only the classical pathway following antibody binding and are thus opsonized for phagocytosis. The major phagocytic adherence receptors are FcR (which recognizes the Fc portion of antibody), CR1 and CR3, whose ligands are breakdown products of the third complement component C3b and inactivated C3b. Target organisms which are highly antibody coated will be phagocytosed; those with only low levels of antibody may not effectively bind and stimulate phagocytes. The antibody, however, can activate complement with the subsequent deposition of C3 and C4 fragments; this amplifies the opsonization signal and enhances the efficiency of binding and uptake by phagocytes.

Complement activation also triggers and amplifies inflammation via three anaphylatoxins which stimulate the chemotaxis of leukocytes plus the degranulation of mast cells and basophils. The anaphylatoxins induce vaso-

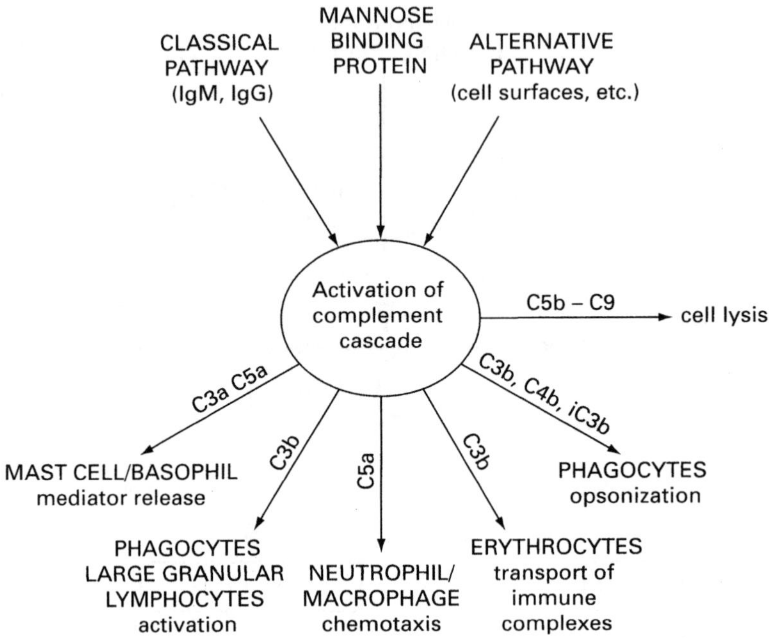

Figure 7. Complement activation and its consequences.

dilatation, increased vascular permeability and smooth muscle contraction via the release of mediators from mast cells and basophils. One anaphylatoxin, C5a, induces the potent pre-inflammatory cytokine interleukin (IL)-1 and causes a number of adherence receptors, including CR1 and CR3, to be displayed on the surface of phagocytes, thus enhancing adherence in phagocytosis. Ligation of complement receptors on neutrophils and monocytes may also stimulate the release of granule contents and free-radical production by the respiratory burst.

Genetic deficiencies of complement occur and have provided evidence of the function of various components. Individuals with a homozygous deficiency in any of the early classical pathway components such as C1q, r or s (breakdown products of C 1, the first component of complement), D4, C2 and C43 show a high incidence of immune complex disease consistent with the importance of the classical pathway in preventing the formation and deposition of large immune complexes. Deficiency of the central component C3 or of its inactivator C3bi is very rare and is associated with recurrent severe pyogenic infection. Low levels of later components from C5 onwards; i.e. loss of the lytic pathway, are associated with neisserial disease.

2.5. Cells

The cellular components of the first line of host defence are macrophages, monocytes, neutrophils, eosinophils, basophils, platelets, neutrophils and endothelial cells. These either produce or interact with soluble factors including complement and acute phase proteins, cytokines and arachadonic acid metabolites. Their interactions are regulated by cell surface receptors and adhesion proteins. When a tissue site is invaded by microbes, an acute inflammatory focus is created with a rapid increase in vascular permeability, changes in blood flow and the local accumulation and activation of white blood cells, largely neutrophils and monocytes (Figure 8).

2.5.1. Polymorphonuclear granulocytes: These cells are produced in the bone marrow at a rate of approximately 80 million per min under the control of cytokines such as IL-3, granulocyte macrophage colony-stimulating factor (GM-CSF) and granulocyte colony-stimulating factor (G-CSF) [21] and are short-lived. Released as mature cells, granulocytes make up approximately two-thirds of the total intravascular white cell pool. The mature cells have a multilobed nucleus with numerous proteolytic and hydrolytic enzyme-containing granules. Granulocytes are classified as neutrophils, eosinophils and basophils according to their staining reactions. Their effects are non-specific, although the involvement of antibody may confer specificity: interaction with antibody and complement is important in their protective role.

2.5.1.1. Neutrophils. These 12- to 16-µm diameter cells make up over 90% of the circulating granulocytes and have an important role in phagocytosis. At sites of inflammation neutrophils become adherent to the local vascular endothelium via a leucocyte function – associated molecule (LFA)-1 (CD11–18) which adheres to the intercellular adhesive molecule (ICAM)-1 or ICAM-2 on the endothelial cell. Expression of ICAM molecules has been shown to be increased in inflammation. The neutrophils then migrate between epithelial cells and down a chemotactic gradient to the site of inflammation. Chemotactic factors include C5a derived from complement, the leukotriene LT B4 produced following mast cell degranulation, and the bacterial peptide F Met Leu Phe (fMLP). These all have defined receptors on the leucocyte surface. In addition, local cytokines such as Il-8 from macrophages or tumour necrosis factor (TNF) from monocytes produced at the site of inflammation may cause non-specific neutrophil accumulation [22].

At the site of inflammation the major function of neutrophils is to phagocytose and destroy bacteria. Phagocytosis can be difficult when organisms have a sugar-containing capsule, as do many upper respiratory tract pathogens such as pneumococcus. Opsonization is enhanced if the bacteria

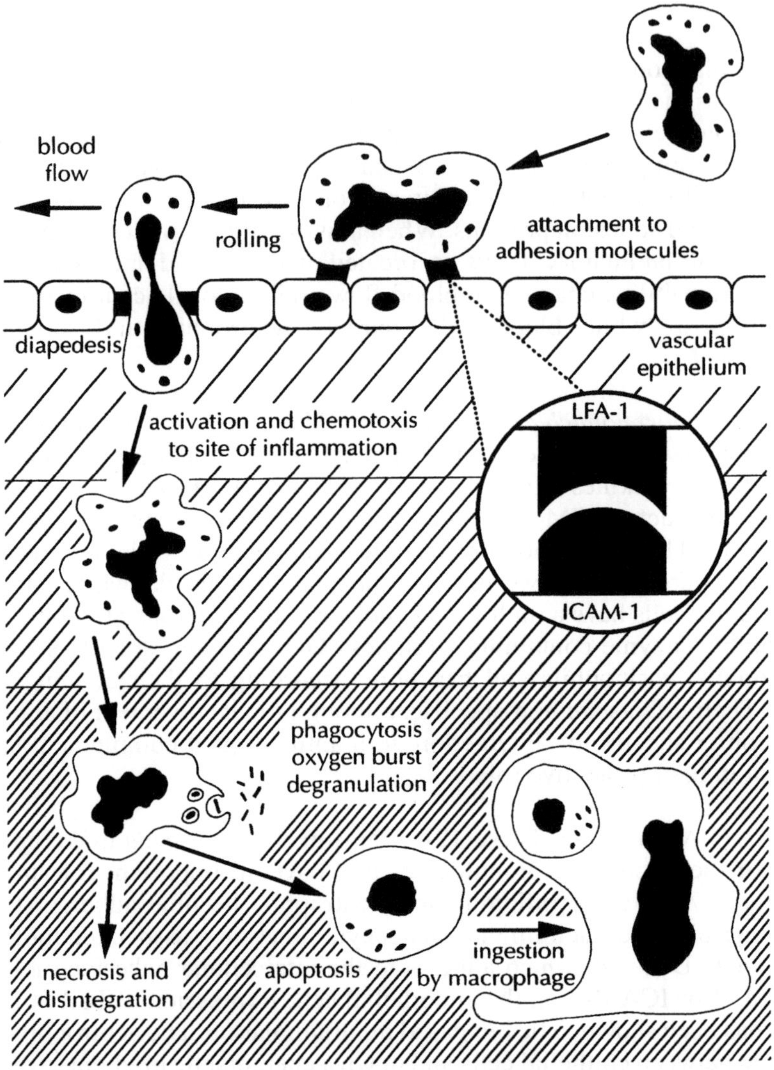

Figure 8. Circulating neutrophils are attracted to the vascular endothelium because of the expression of adhesion molecules in response to cytokines from a local inflammatory site. They diapedese through the endothelium and follow the chemotactic gradient, denoted by shading, becoming activated in the meanwhile. At the site of inflammation they may engulf bacteria and destroy them by oxygen-dependent or independent mechanisms. The subsequent fate of the neutrophil may be apoptosis and ingestion by macrophages or necrosis and disintegration at the reaction site. Fine control of this reaction is essential, underactivity leading to bacterial infection, overactivity to inflammation and destruction by neutrophils which forms part of many disorders, including emphysema and, possibly, Wegener's granulomatosis.

are coated by antibody, since the neutrophil can then become attached via its Fc receptors [23]. Complement coating of bacteria also improves phagocytosis since the neutrophil bears complement receptors. Expression of Fc and complement receptors together with MHC class 1 receptors on the neutrophil surface is increased in the presence of bacterial lipopolysaccharide (LPS), TNF or platelet-activating factor (PAF). These agents cause little secretion by themselves but prime the neutrophils so that subsequent exposure to C5a, immune complexes or fMLP result in a marked increase in secretion.

After internalization of the bacterium the phagosome fuses with lysosomes, and killing mechanisms are usually activated. There involve both oxygen-independent (enzyme-killing mechanisms) and reactive oxygen intermediates (ROI) [24, 25]. The relative importance of these two systems depends on the type of organism involved.

2.5.1.1.1. Oxygen-independent mechanisms. Initially the pH in the phagolysosome rises, and at this stage cationic peptides are released from the azurophil granules; these can damage bacterial permeability. At around 15 min the pH falls, and this in itself can damage organisms. In addition, lysozyme becomes active and is capable of killing gram-positive organisms with readily accessible peptidoglycan. Lactoferrin binds iron and makes it unavailable to bacteria; β-cathepsin has a broad spectrum of antimicrobial activities.

2.5.1.1.2. Oxygen-dependent mechanisms. The neutrophil plasma membrane bears an NADPH oxidase system which generates superoxide ($\cdot O_2^-$). This is converted into toxic oxygen derivatives such as singlet oxygen ($^1O_2$), O-hydroxyl radicals ($OH^\cdot$) and hydrogen peroxide (H_2O_2). Oxygen radicals can cause damage to protein and DNA and can catalyse lipid peroxidation. In addition, if lysosomal fusion occurs, the presence of halides plus peroxidase may produce additional toxic molecules such as hypohalite. These powerful substances can cause damage if released into the environment as can occur if the neutrophil is incapable of phygocytosing and containing the organism (frustrated phagocytosis) [26]. Matrix proteins can be degraded by neutrophil or eosinophil enzymes into chemotactic fragments which can amplify the inflammation. Both neutrophils and eosinophils are implicated in the pathogenesis of certain allergic and autoimmune disorders.

Ageing neutrophils undergo apoptosis (programmed cell death). In this process endonucleases become activated, causing recognition of the cell by macrophages which then ingest and destroy it without releasing toxic substances. Apoptosis is inhibited by some inflammatory mediators such as LPS, prolonging local tissue neutrophil survival. Neutrophils are a frequent component of the nasal smear found in the normal nose, but increase their number during infections and also in the allergic response, although in the latter eosinophils are the most characteristic cells [27]. Eosinophils and basophils will be considered in more detail in the chapter on allergic rhinitis.

2.5.2. Mononuclear phagocytes: Bone marrow stem cells can also develop into cells of the monocyte-macrophage series. These cells are widely distributed throughout the body and are recruited to sites of inflammation. Monocytes (10–18 µm diameter cells with a bilobed nucleus) enter the bloodstream during foetal and adult life in an immature form and differentiate into resident macrophages when they enter the tissues after approximately 10 h in the blood. They can become associated with epithelia, e.g. Langerhans cells in the skin, and can survive for several weeks or months. A local inflammatory stimulus will recruit additional monocytes to the site from the blood, and these cells may have different properties from the resident macrophages (Figure 9).

This mononuclear phagocyte system has two major functions: (1) antigen presentation to specific lymphocytes, and (2) removal of particulate antigens [27]. In addition, they have proinflammatory activity via the secretion of bioactive substances [28]. Antigen presentation is in the form of peptides into which the antigen has been degraded internally by the monocyte. These peptides are presented in association with the major histocompatibility system (Figure 10).

Particulate antigens are removed by phagocytosis; the tissue macrophages form a reticulo-endothelial system, a network which is found in many organs. Phagocytosis may occur following attachment via mannosyl fucosyl receptors on monocytes which bind to the sugars on non-encapsulated organisms or via fibronectin receptors. Opsonization occurs in the same way as for neutrophils by antibody and complement.

Phagocytosis usually involves pseudopodia moving around each side of the organism and fusing distally. Coiling phagocytosis is a variant which occurs with particular intracellular parasites. Complement receptors play a major role in phagocytosis which is much diminished in the absence of serum. Monocytes and activated macrophages can secrete complement components, keeping up the levels at sites of inflammation where continual consumption would otherwise diminish them.

Microbicidal mechanisms after phagocytosis are similar to those of the neutrophil. However, some pathogens, such as *Leishmania* and *mycobacteria* can resist intracellular killing and are disseminated via the mobility of the phagocytes. Recently certain pre-existing (innate) defence mechanisms have been described that are important in resisting such organisms. The N-ramp gene (natural resistance-associated membrane protein) encodes a molecule which appears to form a membrane channel through which nitric oxide (NO) can pass across the membrane of lysosomes. Gene deletion leads to susceptibility to BCG (Bacille

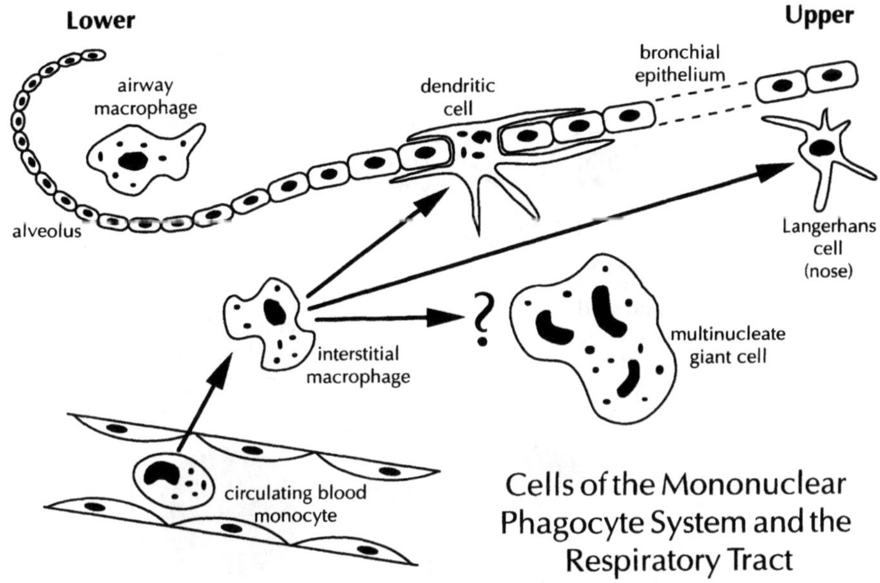

Figure 9. Circulating blood monocytes become macrophages when they migrate into the tissues. Subsequently, some may become specialized antigen-presenting cells such as intra-epithelial dendritic cells in the lung and Langerhans-type cells in the nasal mucosa. Fused macrophages probably form the multinucleate giant cells which are seen in diseases such as sarcoidosis and tuberculosis. In the lower airways macrophages exist within the lumen of the alveoli.

Calmette-Guérin), *Salmonella* and *Leishmania* in mice, humans and cattle [29].

Nathan [30] has produced a mouse deficient in the iNOS (inducible nitric oxide synthase) gene, which renders it susceptible to *leishmanial* infections.

3. Acquired Immunity

Unlike innate immunity acquired immunity is specific, involving immunological memory, which confers improved resistance on subsequent infection with the same organism. The ability to identify and remember antigenic structures resides within the lymphocytes.

3.1. Lymphocytes

Lymphocytes are produced from bone marrow stem cells and are of two types, B cells, which develop in the bone marrow or foetal liver and dif-

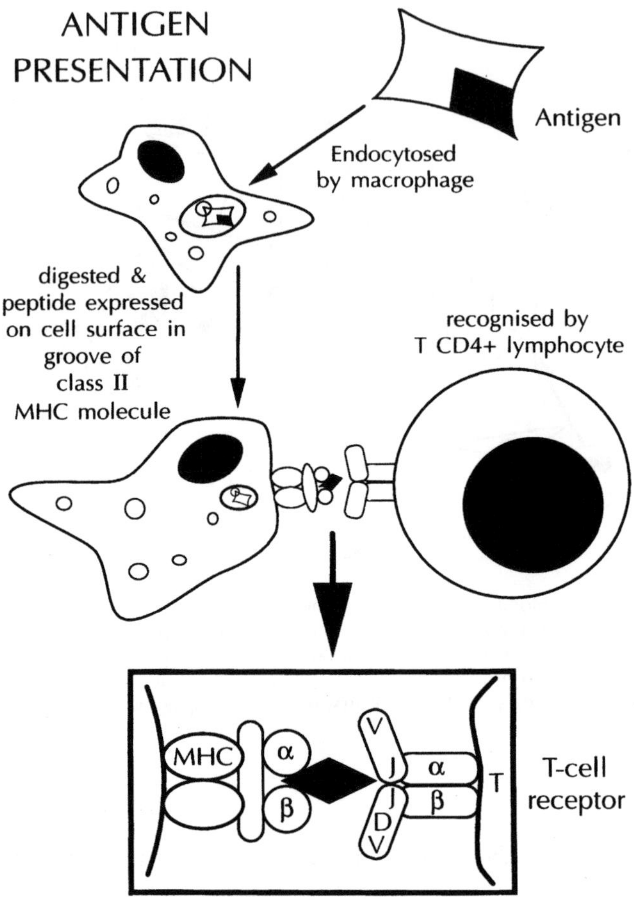

Figure 10. Cells of the mononuclear phagocyte system are ubiquitous and are frequently located near portals of entry of the body. Here they can take up foreign matter, digest it and present peptides in association with class 2 MHC antigens on their surface to CD4-positive T lymphocytes. These in turn become activated and can interact with B lymphocytes, resulting in antibody formations, they also produce various cytokines.

ferentiate into antibody-forming cells and T cells, which differentiate in the thymus and have several functions, including help for B-cell antibody production, cytotoxicity, stimulation of other immune cells and immune regulation. The bone marrow and thymus are known as primary lymphoid organs; other tissues to which lymphocytes migrate in large numbers are the spleen, lymph nodes and the mucosal associated lymphoid tissue (MALT); collectively these are known as the secondary lymphoid organs. In the adult, lymphocytes make up about 20% of the circulating blood cells, and the total lymphocyte load is about 10^{12} cells. These cells may survive for several years as memory cells and can communicate with each other and with other immune cells by cognate (cell-cell contact) or non-cognate (soluble factors) methods. During development in the primary lymphoid organs the lymphocytes develop their repertoire of specific antigen receptors and become self-tolerant. T and B cells can recognize antigen, each cell carrying one type of receptor and being able to recognize one particular epitope, the receptors on different cells having different specificities. The wide range of receptors is generated before antigen contact by somatic mutation and recombination from a relatively small number of germ-line genes [29].

3.1.1. B Lymphocytes: B-lymphocyte antigen recognition is via surface immunoglobulin, which is a cell surface form of the same antibody which the cell is capable of secreting. B cells recognize antigens in their native conformation in solution, on cells or membranes. In contrast, the T-cell receptor is encoded by different genes and recognizes processed or degraded antigen which is physically associated with molecules encoded by MHC [31] (Figure 10). MHC molecule are extremely polymorphic, presumably in order to be able to present many different antigens. Different MHC haplotypes vary in their ability to bind and present different peptides and thus control immune responses at the level of T-cell antigen recognition. Thus an individual's MHC status will determine his ability to respond to certain pathogens and his susceptibility to autoimmune diseases.

3.1.2. T Lymphocytes: T lymphocytes form the majority of lymphocytes in the blood and are also widely distributed throughout the body in lymphoid organs and at mucosal surfaces. They can be divided broadly into functional subsets based on surface markers (Figure 11). The first major division depends on the two polypeptide chains that form the antigen receptor; most T cells use $\alpha\beta$ chains, where a minority use $\gamma\delta$ chains. Those bearing $\alpha\beta$ chains can be further divided into CD4 or CD8 positive cells (rarely cells express both or neither). CD4-positive T lymphocytes are proinflammatory, helping B cells to produce antibody and also producing a variety of cytokines. Characteristically, CD4-positive T cells recognize peptides in conjunction with MHC class II molecules. A division into T-helper (TH)1 and TH2 subsets with different functional properties has recently been proposed [32].

CD8-positive T cells usually recognize antigenic peptides in conjunction with class I MHC molecules and are cytotoxic. They kill by cell contact, innocent bystander cells being spared, and probably elaborate perforins which form a hole in the cell membrane. CD8-positive cells recognize changes in surface markings of cells which have become transformed by viruses or have undergone neoplastic change. They also recognize heterologous transplanted cells.

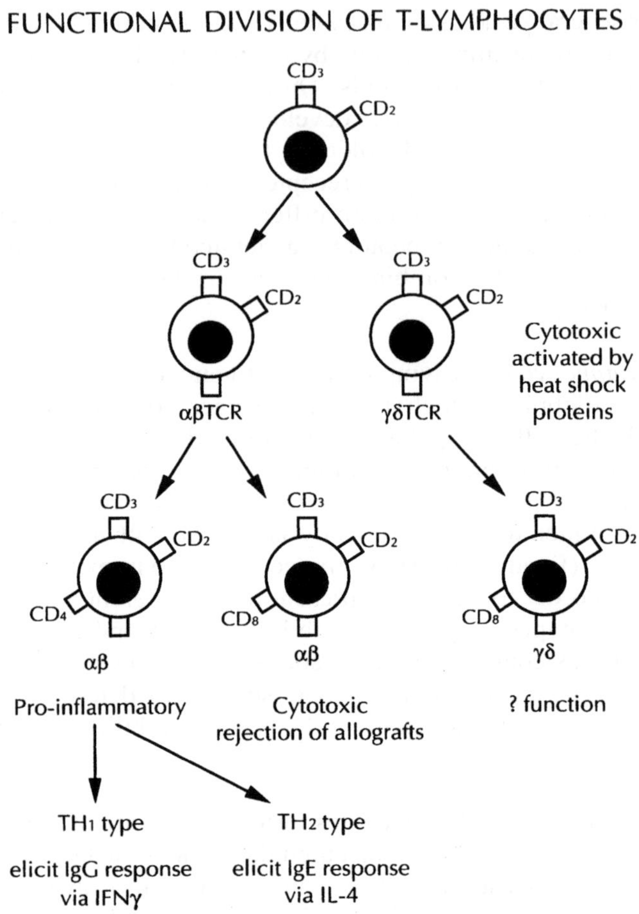

Figure 11. All T lymphocytes express CD2 and CD3 surface markers. The majority of T cells possess an $\alpha\beta$ T-cell receptor, and this subgroup is further divided into CD4-positive cells, which are proinflammatory, and CD8-positive cells, which are cytotoxic. The former usually recognize antigen in association with MHC class II, the latter with class 1. Recently, a further division of CD4-positive cells into TH1 and TH2 types has been noted in mice and humans. TH1 T cells produce any IgG response from B cells via cytokines which include interferon γ; TH2-type lymphocytes elicit IgE responses from B cells via cytokines including IL-4.

A subgroup of T cells possess a $\gamma\delta$ T-cell receptors; these are cytotoxic cells but do not need MHC class 1 recognition. They are activated by heat shock proteins. A subgroup of these cells is CD8-positive; their function is unknown. Recently murine $\gamma\delta$ T-cell clones were found to recognize empty class II molecules from the side rather than the top. Gamma delta recognition was more similar to that of immunoglobulin than $\alpha\beta$, i.e. low frequency/broad recognition. The receptor saw multivalent molecules, cells, tissues and large pathogens which could be recognized without the requirement for antigen processing.

The function of T $\gamma\delta$ cells is largely unknown [33]. They are found predominantly in mucosal surfaces, especially the gut, and are cytotoxic, but this cytotoxicity is not class I restricted. They are activated by heat shock proteins, highly conserved proteins produced during infection and inflammation.

3.1.3. T cell antigen receptor: The peptide chains which make up the antigen receptor are formed from a number of genes on chromosomes 7 and 14 [34]. As in B cells, each complete chain is encoded by three or four gene segments which are brought together by enzymatic splicing of the DNA as the T lymphocyte develops; once a productive rearrangement occurs, the gene is expressed and further development ceases. There are three hypervariable regions, two in contact with the MHC and one in contact with antigenic peptide [35].

The antigen receptor is largely extracellular, and once contacted, intracellular signalling is largely via the associated CD3 molecule. CD4 or -8 probably creates further contact with the MHC molecule and acts as an associative ligand.

After the random acquisition of antigen specificity in the thymus, any T lymphocytes with self-reactivity are eliminated by apoptosis. Those with reactivity against foreign antigens in association with cell MHC are positively selected. Later expansion of these clones probably occurs in the periphery.

Initial contact with antigen will result in stimulation of only the very few lymphocytes which are capable of interacting. These cells respond by proliferation and further differentiation, forming a clone of cells with the capacity to recognize that antigen. Some of these will remain as memory cells, which on second encounter with the antigen will form a larger clone of specific cells which may be further differentiated. This secondary response is faster and more effective than the primary response and forms the basis for immunization.

3.1.3.1. Structure of antibody. Antibody molecules, or immunoglobulins, are glycoproteins present in plasma and tissue fluids of all mammals. Their basic structure is one of four polypeptide chains, two identical heavy (H) and two identical light (L) chains linked by disulphide bonds (Figure 12). Cleavage with the enzyme papain at the hinge region produces three fragments: two identical Fab fragments and one Fc fragment. The Fab fragments bind antigen but cannot precipitate it because they are univalent. The Fc fragment mediates effector functions such as binding to cells and complement fixation [36].

Immunoglobulins are members of the immunoglobulin superfamily [37], which contains all antibodies, together with many cell receptors (e.g. MHC classes I and II, CD3, -4 and -8), and adhesion molecules such as LFA-3 and CD2, together with some central nervous system CNS molecules such

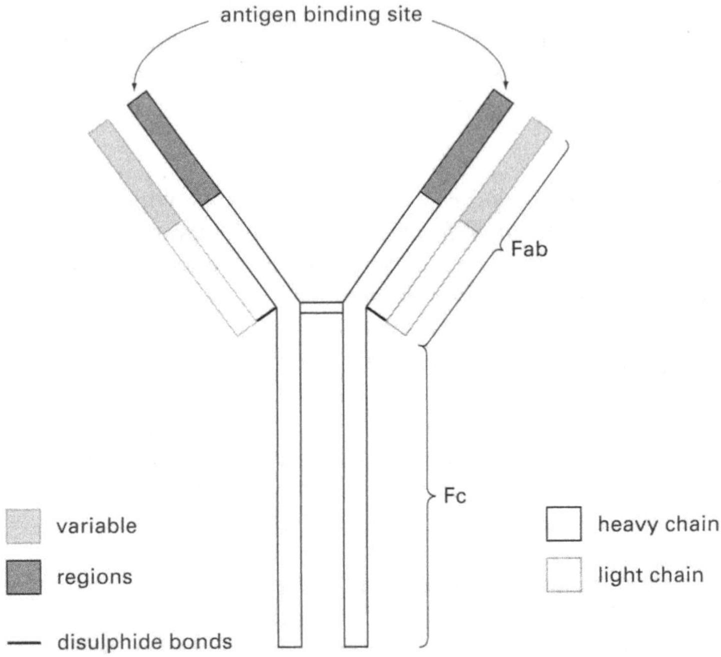

Figure 12. The basic structure of immunoglobulin. Each antibody consists of two light and two heavy chains. The light chains comprise a variable and a constant domain ($V_L + C_L$); the heavy chain comprises one variable region and three or four constant regions ($V_H - C_{H\,1,2,3\text{ and }4}$). The variable regions contain a hypervariable portion which forms the antibody combining site. The tail or Fc portion of the molecule is responsible for many of its functional properties, such as binding to neutrophils or to complement.

as MAG (myelin-associated glycoprotein) and NCAM (neural adhesion molecule). All of these contain one or more domains, compact units of about 100 amino acids formed into antiparallel β-pleated sheets, stabilized by disulphide bonds.

Antibody light chains, which have a molecular weight of approximately 22 kDa, consist of variable (V_L) and constant (C_L) domains, each of approximately 110 amino acid residues. Heavy chains, with a molecular weight of 50–77 kDa, consist of one VH and a number of CH domains which vary with antibody class. There are five different classes of antibodies, IgG, M, A, D and E.

IgG is the major immunoglobulin in normal human serum. It is present in both intra- and extravascular pools and makes up about 75% of the total immunoglobulin content. There are three heavy chain domains which by variation in amino acid composition divide into four classes, γ 1, 2, 3 and 4. These form approximately 66, 23, 7 and 4% of the total IgG respectively. Since the immune response to a particular organism may lie largely within one subclass, a subclass deficiency can lead to a failure of immunoprotection. Carbohydrate-coated antibodies such as *Haemophilus influenzae* and *Streptococcus pneumoniae* elicit mainly IgG2 antibodies. Approximately 5% of patients with chronic lower respiratory tract infections are IgG2-deficient. IgG1 and -3 are effective at complement fixation; IgG2 is moderately effective, and IgG4 does not fix complement.

IgM, which is important in the primary response, is pentameric, the individual units being joined by J chains. IgM forms approximately 10% of the immunoglobulin pool and is largely intravascular. It is extremely effective at fixing complement.

IgA forms approximately 20% of human serum immunoglobulin found in the serum as a monomer. It is also present in secretions largely as a dimer, again joined by a J chain and protected by secretory piece. It does not activate complement.

IgD is present on the membrane of many circulating B cells but forms less than 1% of circulating immunoglobulin. Its role appears to be largely in B-cell differentiation. IgD is found increased in the human tonsil, especially following repeated infections, possibly because certain bacteria possess Fc receptors for IgD.

IgE is present in the serum only in nanogram amounts, but is found extensively cell-bound, especially to high-affinity receptors on the surfaces of mast cells and basophils. Its function is probably in protection against multicellular organisms, but its major interest is as the sensitizing antibody for allergic reactions.

The major functions of antibody are neutralization, opsonization for phagocytosis and preparation of the cell surface for killing either by cellular cytotoxicity (antibody-dependent cellular toxicity) or by complement-mediated lysis (Table 3).

4. Mucosal Immunity

Brandtzaeg [38] has identified three main components of mucosal immune defence: immune exclusion, immune regulation and immune elimination. Immune exclusion is mediated largely by secretory IgA, which was first identified in the 1960s, although in 1938 Walsh and Cannon [39] first noted that intranasal immunization resulted in local antibody formation.

Nasal secretions contain mostly secretory IgA and IgM, which are actively transported across the epithelium; there are also significant amounts of IgG due to passive leakage. IgA also participates in immune exclusion in the upper respiratory tract, whereas in the gut it is rapidly degraded.

Table 3. Functions of antibody

Each immunoglobulin molecule is bifunctional, with the $F(ab)_2$ portion of the molecule concerned with binding to antigen and the Fc region with binding to host tissues, including phagocytes and lymphoid cells, and to the first component of complement. The ability of each immunoglobulin molecule to undertake these functions is determined by its Fc structure. Complement activation is most effective with IgM, IgG1 and IgG3. IgG2 is less effective, whilst IgG4, IgA, IgD and IgE do not bind complement. IgG of all subclasses crosses the placenta, providing the newborn with passive immunity.
Via Fab-antigen interaction
Neutralization, e.g. toxins (IgG)
Prevention of attachment (IgA, IgG)
Recognition/antigen presentation by B cells
Via Fc binding
Attachment to neutrophils → phagocytosis (IgG)
Complement activation (classical path) (IgM, G)
Binding to T and B lymphocytes (immune regulation: IgA, M, G, E)
K-cell cytotoxicity (IgG)
Degranulation of mast cells/basophils (IgE)
Attachment of epithelial cell and transfer into secretions (IgA)
Placental transfer (IgG)

4.1. Secretory Immunoglobulins

IgA is the main immunoglobulin secreted by mucosal-associated lymphocytes. It acts as "mucosal antiseptic paint", combining with pathogens or toxins and either preventing attachment and absorption or rendering them harmless. Human IgA occurs in polymeric and monomeric forms and in two subclasses, A1 and A2 which show differential distribution between the mucosal and systemic immune systems. Secretory IgA is a dimer held together by a J chain which is also formed by the plasma cell. In the nasal mucosa, IgA-producing cells show 98% J-chain expression; most nasal IgM and IgD immunocytes are also J chain-positive, together with 46–79% of IgG cells. This J-chain positivity is decreased in rhinitis, where there is an increased production of monomeric IgA [38].

The nasal mucosa contains 90–95% IgA1 immunocytes, in contrast to the gut where IgA2 immunocytes predominate. This is surprising, since many bacterial species, including *Haemophilus influenzae* and *Streptococcus pneumoniae* elaborate IgA1 proteases which cleave one of the Pro-Thr or Pro-Ser bonds of the hinge region to yield Fab and Fc fragments. These proteases appear to be virulence factors, since non-pathogenic strains do not make them. The Fab antibody fragments may coat the organism, rendering it invulnerable to other defence mechanisms. IgA2 is also a more efficient inhibitor of carbohydrate (mannose)-dependent bacterial adherence.

4.2. *Epithelial Transport*

Dimeric IgA and pentameric IgM use a common transport mechanism in which, after J-chain incorporation, a binding site is induced in the quaternary structure allowing IgA and IgM to combine non-covalently with the poly-Ig receptor on the abluminal surface of the plasma membrane. They are endocytosed and transported across the epithelial cell to the luminal surface, where the vesicle fuses with the plasma membrane, releasing the antibody combined with a secretory component derived from cleavage of the poly-Ig receptor. This probably protects the immunoglobulin from enzymic digestion. This process takes place mainly in the serous-type nasal acinar and duct cells (Figure 13).

Polymeric immunoglobulins, even if of low affinity for antigen, posses high avidity due to the presence of many antigen binding sites per molecule. Polymeric IgA and IgM are more effective in virus neutralization than in monomeric IgA and are also bound more effectively by phagocytes, T cells and hepatocyte receptors.

4.3. *Quantitative Aspects*

In nasal secretions total IgA is usually between 0.5 and 2.2 g. Since monomeric IgA can arrive from serum by passive diffusion, it is probably important to estimate the amount of secretory IgA. This represents about 75% of the total IgA content in nasopharyngeal secretions from children with secretory otitis media [38]. It has been shown to be depressed in children with severe protein-calorie malnutrition, returning to normal 4 weeks after treatment [40].

Only traces of IgM are found in normal nasal secretions, but levels are elevated in a proportion of patients with selective IgA deficiency. This is the commonest humoral immune deficiency, affecting between 1 in 500 and 1 in 700 of the population. This can be transient in children due to late maturation, normal levels of IgA not being reached until about 7 years of age. Roughly half of selective IgA-deficient individuals suffer an increase in respiratory tract infections; the remainder appear unaffected.

It is possible that substitution of secretory IgM is protective, whereas the substitution of IgD is not. An alternative explanation is that more affected individuals have a concomitant IgG subclass deficiency. IgA deficiency is also associated with atopy and, in some patients, with autoimmunity.

4.4. *Immune Regulation*

Antigen presented to the nasal mucosa is probably taken up by antigen-presenting cells, which can be macrophages, dendritic cells or possible

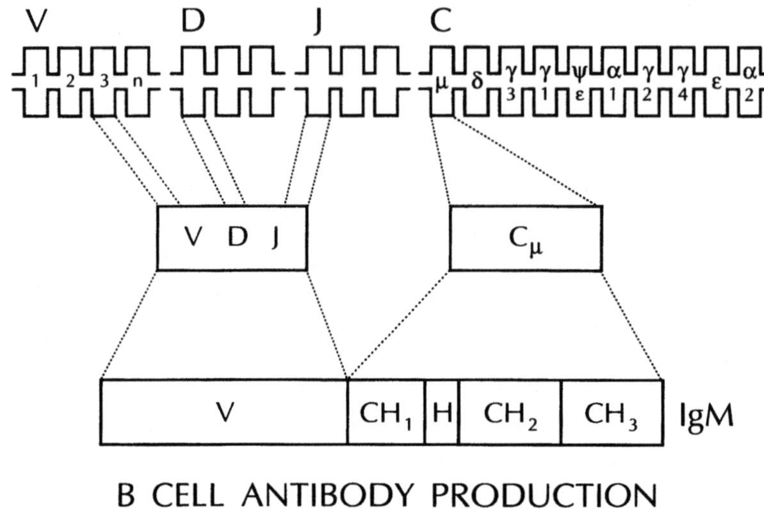

Figure 13. DNA recombination takes place during B-cell development and maturation in two stages. First there is the combination of one of many germ line V genes with one of a few J genes (light chain) or with one of several D and then a heavy J gene (heavy chain). This occurs during the transition from lymphoid stem cell to B lymphocyte. In the light chain the VJ region then combines with a constant region gene which can be κ or λ. In the heavy chain the constant C region genes are several kilobases downstream from the V domains, and a VDJ segment may link with any one of the C genes. The order of these genes is shown in the figure; initially a B cell uses the C gene to produce IgM, but can later switch to a different isotype, e.g. IgG, thus changing antibody class whilst retaining antigen specificity. Sequential switching is thought to occur in the upper respiratory tract, although recent direct switching from IgM to IgE has been reported.

epithelial cells which have become human leukocyte antigens (HLA) class 2-positive [41]. It is likely that they are then transported to mucosa-associated lymphoid tissue. As there are no lymphoepithelial structures typical of MALT in the nose, it is likely that the tonsils and adenoids fulfil this function for the upper respiratory tract. At this site antigenic peptides derived from antigen breakdown within the antigen presenting cell (APC) are presented on the cell surface together with MHC antigens to T lymphocytes. Only those lymphocytes which bear a receptor which will fit the peptide and MHC are capable of responding; second signals (ligation of CD 40 and CD28) are necessary, together with proinflammatory cytokines such as IL-1, in order for the T lymphocyte to respond. In the absence of these factors T-cell anergy occurs.

Once stimulated, T cells release a variety of cytokines, which then affect T and B cells. The pattern of cytokine release affects the class of antibody which is subsequently produced by the B cells. Recently, TH1 and TH2 T cell subsets have been described; TH1 subsets release predominantly IL-2 and interferon γ and result in IgG class antibody production. TH2 T cells secrete predominantly IL-4, -5 and -10 and result in B-cell IgE production.

Cognate interaction takes place between the activated T helper cell and local B cells in the MALT. B cells recognize antigen, internalize and digest it, then present it to T cells in the form of MHC-associated peptide (Figure 13). Only B cells bearing the relevant antigen receptor will be stimulated to proliferate. Some of these then migrate to secretory tissue, i.e. the nasal mucosa, where "second signals" (ligation of CD40 further antigen contact, cytokines) induce local proliferation of immunocytes: IgA-producing cells being present in the glandular areas and IgG-producing cells in the stroma beneath the surface epithelium. The former are mainly responsible for local secretory immunity, the latter for immune elimination, which is increased in rhinitis. Occasional IgE-producing cells are found in the nasal mucosa of allergic individuals. There is a proportion of IgD-producing cells associated with the glandular areas, and these are increased in most subjects with selective IgA deficiency. In the remainder IgM immunocytes are increased, and these individuals do not have recurrent infections of the upper respiratory tract. This is thought to be because IgM can function as a secretory antibody, whereas IgD does not fix complement and may itself block other protective antibodies such as IgG and -M.

The class of antibody produced is dependent upon the constant heavy chain (CH) gene used by the B cell [42] (Figure 13). Initially the μ gene is used to produce IgM, but subsequently the B cells can switch to produce an isotype further down the gene (the order is shown in Figure 14). It was assumed that sequential switching took place in the tonsils, nasal mucosa, lacrimal glands and bronchial-associated lymphoid tissue, whereas in the gut, a direct switch occurred from μ to ε. In fact a direct switch from μ to ε in the upper respiratory tract has recently been reported. The immunoglobulin isotype produced probably depends upon local T-cell cytokines and other environmental factors [43, 44].

4.5. Common Mucosal Immune System

Mucosal associated lymphoid tissue is found in association with the upper and lower respiratory tract (bronchial associated lymphoid tissue, BALT) and also with the gut (gastrointestinal associated lymphoid tissue, GALT) and urinary tract. Animal studies demonstrate that the antigen-driven expansion of B-cell clones taking place in these tissues induces a very high proportion of IgA-immunocyte precursors. This is distinct from immune responses in the systemic immune system (peripheral lymph nodes and spleen), where IgG production predominates.

Initial B-cell stimulation takes place in the MALT, and subsequently migration occurs via lymph and blood to secretory sites all over the body.

It appears that there is a tendency for the B lymphocyte to home back to its tissue of origin, possibly guided by endothelial surface determinants. Differences between upper respiratory tract and gut mucosa, such as the subclass distribution of IgA immunocytes, and the occurrence, or lack of, IgG immunocytes, suggests that the gut receives most of its B cells from GALT and the respiratory tract from BALT and tonsils [45, 46]. Salivary and mammary glands probably receive precursor cells from both.

Mucosal immunization or infection results largely in a local antibody response, mainly polyclonal or IgA. A systemic response does not usually occur unless the antigen is live. Conversely, parenteral immunization induces a circulatory IgA response but is an inefficient route of immunization for the mucosa. In recent years the experimental presentation of specific immunogenic peptides via the nasal or oral route has been shown to exert an immunoregulatory effect upon certain autoimmune disorders both in animal models and more recently in humans. Oral cholera toxin β subunit (a mucosa-binding molecule), together with myelin basic protein (MBP), prevents experimental autoimmune encephalomyelitis in Lewis rats, and oral cholera toxin β together with insulin prevents diabetes in non-obese diabetic (NOD) mice [47]. In humans feeding keyhole limpet haemocyanin (KLH) causes a specific reduction in T-cell responses following subcutaneous antigen. Current human trials of oral tolerance include MBP for multiple sclerosis and collagen II for rheumatoid arthritis [48]. The mechanism(s) of this is as yet unknown but may involve a switch from a TH1 to a TH2 type of response.

4.6. Antigen-Presenting Cells

Langerhans cells in the human nasal mucosa have recently been shown to be HLA-DR positive, to possess high-affinity IgE receptors and to be exquisitely steroid-sensitive [49]. Murine class 2 positive dendritic cells possess antigen-presenting ability. Dendritic cells resident in the airway epithelium effectively uptake and process antigen but cannot present (25% of dendritic cells in pathogen-free rats are MHC class 2 low or negative). After stimulation by GM-CSF or TNF, they drain to the regional lymph nodes where they become paracortical interdigitating dendritic cells and are effective antigen presenters but are poor at antigen uptake and processing [50]. Thus dendritic cells perform a sentinel function at epithelial surfaces. They are rapidly upregulated during acute inflammation, with kinetics similar to those of the neutrophil response [50].

4.7. T Cells

T lymphocytes are found scattered in the human nasal mucosa, both CD4- and CD8-positive, with a ratio of about 3:1 in the subepithelium. Between the glands the ratio is 0.8 : 1, CD4 to CD8. In the epithelium itself there are very few T cells, mainly CD4-positive [38]. This is in marked contrast to the intestinal epithelium, where CD8-positive T lymphocytes are found. The proportions of T lymphocytes are altered in certain conditions such as allergic rhinitis. The nature of the class 2-positive cell encountered and the local T-cell cytokine production may well be determining factors in the type of antibody produced.

4.8. Immune Elimination

If foreign material penetrates the mucosal barrier, it is dealt with by the specific immune system, involving both antibodies and lymphocytes. These will assist non-specific mechanisms such as phagocytosis and complement activation to break down and destroy any antigenic material. If elimination cannot be achieved, possibly due to recurrent presentation of foreign material, then the resulting inflammation may become pathological due to an excess of complement-activating immune complexes and enzyme-releasing phagocytes. This situation may lead to enhanced mucosal permeability to a variety of inhalant and infectious agents. Chronic, non-allergic rhinitis is probably largely mediated by such mechanisms.

4.9. IgE

IgE diffuses passively into nasal secretions. In atopic individuals there is also evidence for mucosal synthesis of IgE by local immunocytes. This antibody is known predominantly for its role in allergic rhinitis, but its function is probably in immune elimination where vasodilatation, plasma leakage, histamine release and subsequent sneezing are designed to eliminate foreign material. The recruitment of eosinophils with their capacity to phagocytose IgE-coated material or to kill IgE-coated metazoan parasites such as schistosome larvae has a protective function under the right circumstances.

4.10. Olfactory mucosa

This specialized region in the vault of the nose contains, besides olfactory receptors and supporting tissues, all the immunological defence mechanisms found in the remainder of the nasal mucosal [51]. Despite this the olfactory mucosa has been suggested as a route of entry of neurotropic arbovirus into the CNS [52] and as the route of invasion or aetiological factors responsible for diseases such as Parkinson's and Alzheimer's [53].

5. Immune Deficiency and Ear, Nose and Throat (ENT) Disorders

Recurrent upper respiratory tract infections are a common mode of presentation in immune-deficient individuals. Figure 14 shows the major immune abnormalities which may be found in such patients. The categories are not exclusive, since antibody-mediated deficiency can lead to secondary ciliary and mucosal problems via repeated infection.

True γ-globulin deficiency, with a serum IgG of less than 3 g/l, is very rare, occurring in approximately 1 in 50,000 individuals. However, it is probably underdiagnosed, and many patients initially present with recurrent sinusitis. It has become increasingly clear that decreased serum levels of single or multiple IgG subclasses may be associated with susceptibility to infections on or via mucosal membranes [54]. In a few patients immunoglobulin gene deletions have been described [55], but the majority of IgG subclass-deficient individuals are probably suffering from regulatory defects. IgG subclass deficiency is difficult to define since reference materials vary between laboratories and the clinically relevant cut-off levels for various subclasses are not well known. The diagnosis should be based on more than one determination of serum levels since variation can occur e.g. due to infection or surgery. A further confounding factor is that sometimes even a total lack of a subclass can be found in healthy individuals [56]. IgG2 subclass deficiency is the predominant form among children, with a sex distribution of 3 boys to 1 girl; after puberty IgG3 deficiency is more common and affects 1 male to 3 females [57].

Nielson et al. [58] found that chronic lung disease was common in patient groups with selective serum IgG1 deficiency or with combined IgG1 plus IgG3 deficiencies, whereas patients with other subclass abnormalities had mainly upper airway and other mild infections. Serum IgG2 or -G3 deficiency was usually expressed at the cellular level in rectal mucosa; conversely, the nasal proportion of IgG3 cells was unaffected by the deficiency of this subclass in serum and rectal mucosa [57]. It is possible that local antigenic stimulation overrides a B-cell maturation defect.

We have found IgG3 deficiency to be the commonest abnormality in a group of patients with chronic or recurrent rhinosinusitis [59]. On test immunization with tetanus and with pneumococcal polysaccharide approximately 50% of our patients with chronic or recurrent purulent upper respiratory tract infections show a poor response to carbohydrate antigen. In a pilot study of intravenous γ-globulin replacement therapy, clinical improvement was noticed in about 50% of patients with an abnormal subclass level or test immunization response. Interestingly, the response rate was not different in patients in whom no immune abnormality could be detected.

In a double-blind cross-over study of immunoglobulin prophylaxis over 2 years in 43 IgG subclass-deficient adult patients, a significant decrease in the number of days of infection was seen in the whole group and among

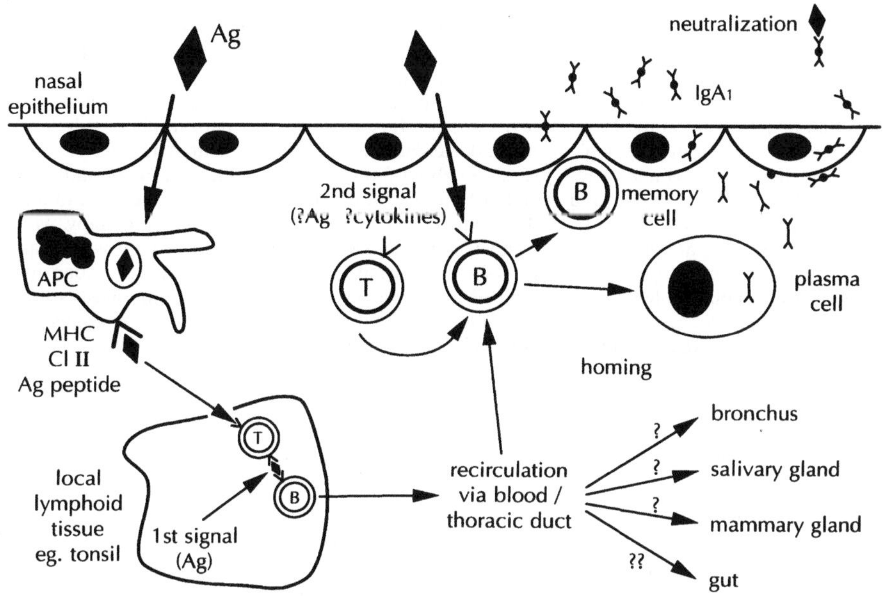

Figure 14. Antigen contact at mucosal surfaces results in uptake via antigen-presenting cells which then migrate to local lymphoid tissues and present antigenic peptides to T cells. Here B cells are also sensitized by antigen. They leave via the blood or thoracic duct and circulate before homing to mucosal sites. There is evidence for preferential homing of respiratory tract cells to the respiratory tract, but some may go to salivary and mammary glands and possibly to the gut. B cells in the mucosa receive their second signal, involving CD40 ligation, possibly either further antigen contact or cytokine which stimulates them to become antibody-secreting plasma cells. In the mucosal system IgA is the predominant antibody produced, and this is passed through the epithelial cell gaining secretory piece on the way. It is secreted into the lumen where it is able to neutralize further antigen or prevent antigenic attachment and ingress.

the IgG1 deficient patients. The 22 asthmatics also had fewer days with bronchial constriction; acute bronchitis was significantly less frequent in the IgG3-deficient patients [57].

The most severely affected patients have IgA deficiency in association with an IgG subclass abnormality; these tend to have recurrent respiratory infections, and lung function impairment is noticeable in about 50%. In a small study, Petruson et al. [60], studies 18 IgA-deficient patients and 22 with common variable immune deficiency (IgG or G subclass together with IgM or IgA). The results are shown in Table 4. It is noticeable that the common variable immunodeficient patients are more likely to have chronic rhinosinusitis and to be carrying pathogenic bacteria in their nasopharynx.

Investigation of the IgA system requires assessment of both secretory and serum IgA because of their dissociation. Patients with serum IgA

Table 4. Immunodeficiency and ENT disorders. The major immune defects leading to ENT disorders are shown. Abnormalities of cilia and mucus are very likely to result in chronic nose and sinus infections. Approximately half the patients with primary ciliary dyskinesia show situs inversus (Kartagener's syndrome). Affected individuals are frequently sterile, as are those with Young's syndrome, in which a mucus abnormality is postulated. There are two types of well-defined acquired immune deficiencies: selective IgA deficiency occurs in about 0.3% of a population, and common variable immune deficiency (CVID), in which there is a deficiency of IgG together with IgM and/or IgA, occurs in about 0.002% of a population. In any individual with recurrent ENT infections, a sample of clotted blood should be sent for serum immunoglobulin determination, since affected individuals can benefit from replacement therapy, which can now take place at home. Early diagnosis and treatment confer a better prognosis, probably because chronic infections leads to secondary irreversible changes in the mucosa. Abnormalities of IgG subclasses have been described in chronic rhinosinusitis; the commonest is probably IgG3. This contrasts with IgG2 deficiency, which is present in 5% of individuals with chronic lower respiratory tract infections. The significance of subclass abnormalities remains to be defined.

Innate immune system		
Ciliary dysfunction		– 1° (± situs inversus) – 2° to infection, pollution, allergy
Mucus abnormalities		– cystic fibrosis ?Young's syndrome
Complement deficiencies		– C_3 or C_3 inactivation → severe infections C_5–C_9 → neisserial infections
Neutrophil abnormalities		– ?lazy leukocyte syndrome
Acquired immune system		
Humoral (antibody-mediated)		
	may occur together	→ IgA IgG ± IgA ± IgM deficiencies (CVID) → IgG subclass
		Dysfunctional hypergammaglobulinaemia (AIDS)
Cellular	– minor T/B abnormalities occur in CVID – marked abnormalities (1° or 2°) associated with severe infections, e.g. mycobacteria, fungi, viruses	

deficiency (<0.05 g/l) usually have undetectable IgA in nasal secretions [58, 59] but can have normal secretory IgA [61–62]; the reverse situation has also been described [63, 64].

Hypogammaglobulinaemic and IgG subclass-deficient patients frequently show minor abnormalities of B- and T-lymphocyte numbers or function. Severe cell-mediated immune defects are usually associated with major infections, notably with fungi, mycobacteria and viruses as well as an increase in neoplastic disease.

5.1. HIV

The human immunodeficiency virus (HIV) is an acquired cause of immune deficiency which may present to the ENT specialist. The infections observed are with organisms normally controlled by the T cell and macrophage arm of the immune system, i.e. predominantly intracellular organisms, in particular viruses (herpes simplex, varicella zoster, cytomegalovirus and polyomavirus) fungi (*Candida, Cryptococcus, Histoplasma*) and protozoa (*Pneumocystis carinii, Toxoplasma* and *Cryptosporidium*). *Salmonella* and *mycobacteria*, which are facultative intracellular bacteria, can also cause disease. Bacterial infections which are usually controlled by antibody, complement and phagocytes are not problematical in adults unless a new antigen is encountered when the lack of CD4-positive T cells may prevent a proper antibody response. In children infected with HIV *in utero*, disseminated bacterial infection is a common cause of mortality since the antibody repertoire has not been developed and the children are unable to mount an immune response to the bacteria [65].

The majority of opportunist infections in HIV-positive patients are due to reactivation of previously acquired infection rather than *de novo* disease. Superadded to the viral-induced immune deficiency is the effect of bone marrow suppressive drugs used in treatment which can induce neutropenia.

Common ENT presentations are candidiasis in the mouth and pharynx or hairy oral leukoplakia. Kaposi's sarcoma can be found anywhere in the mouth, tongue and throat. Oral ulceration is common and may be associated with drug-induced neutropenia.

Table 5. Immunodeficiency and sinuses [55]. The prevalence of ENT infections was determined in a group of individuals with IgA deficiency and in a group with CVID, and these data were compared with those from normal controls. Recurrent rhinosinusitis was defined as more than one acute purulent rhinosinusitis per year. Chronic rhinosinusitis required radiologic signs of infections showing no improvement over a period of 6 months or more. Chronic rhinosinusitis was present in 50% of the patients with CVID, three quarters of whom were carrying pathogenic bacteria in their nasopharynx.

Immune Status	Recurrent rhinosinusitis	Chronic rhinosinusitis	Nasopharyngeal bacteria*	Histology
IgA deficiency ($n = 18$)	10	0	12	↑ goblet cells
Common variable immunodeficiency ($n = 22$)	7	11	16	↑ submucous glands
Normal ($n = 20$)	0	0	4	normal

* *Haemophilus influenzae* was the most common isolate, followed by *Staph. aureus* and *Strep. pneumoniae.*

In the nose, allergic rhinosinusitis is a common problem, possibly due to poor regulation of IgE synthesis [66]. The treatment is standard, but long-term high-dose topical corticosteroids should be avoided because of the dangers of additional immunosuppression. Interferon γ has reportedly been helpful. Infective sinusitis is seen with the same spectrum of bacteria that cause sinusitis in the immunocompetent host (*Haemophilus influenzae, Streptococcus pneumonii, Staphylococcus aureus*), but with a much higher incidence. This may be due to the dysfunctional hypergammaglobulinaemia which is polyclonal, but which may hide an IgG subclass deficiency [67].

The diagnosis of infection in HIV-infected individuals is difficult because the lack of an inflammatory response makes histological diagnosis difficult and the failure of antibody production means that serology cannot be relied upon. Direct identification of organisms is necessary, and it should be recognized that multiple infections are frequent [68].

5.2. Granulomatous Disease in the Nose

Two conditions which are associated with a disordered immunity are Wegener's granulomatosis and sarcoidosis. In the former, antinuclear cytoplasmic antibodies (ANCA) have been described [69]. These are not specific for Wegener's but can also occur in microscopic polyarteritis and certain other forms of vasculitis [70]. About 60% of patients with Wegener's disease localized to the respiratory tract are seropositive for ANCA. The antigenic target is a 29-kDa serine proteinase in neutrophil primary granules [71]. Histologically, the staining pattern is cytoplasmic, and the antibody is known as C-ANCA.

The pathogenicity of ANCA is unproven, but there is some evidence for their having a role in disease causation. A fourfold rise in ANCA titre predicted clinical relapse [72], and ANCA are more readily detected in patients with active disease [69]. However, ANCA can be positive without overt disease. Incubation of C-ANCA with normal neutrophils primed with TNF leads to neutrophil degranulation and a respiratory burst [13]. There is also some evidence that ANCA can stimulate primed neutrophils to cause endothelial cell injury [74].

Sarcoidosis is a cause of florid nasal symptoms, particularly mucopurulent catarrh, and may present to the ENT surgeon. The current concept of the pathogenesis of this disease is that persistent antigen of some form stimulates an antigen-presenting cell, probably a macrophage. This results in an IL-1/IL-2-driven T-lymphocyte proliferation. Monocytes are attracted to the site by a monocyte chemotactic factor (IL-8) and are held at the site of the reaction by macrophage migration inhibition factor. Monocyte activation by IFN-γ occurs, and this stimulates calcitriol production, which in turn causes macrophage fusion to epithelioid cells and granulomata.

There is a bias in the T-cell receptor variable region gene expression, with many patients showing an increase in the number of cells expressing Vβ8 [75]. Analysis of the c-DNA clones produced from mRNA extracted from such cells reveals homology in gene sequence in the hypervariable regions, suggesting preferential T-cell selection or replication. In a different sub-group of patients there were expanded numbers of T cells expressing the β receptor. Studies of the β chain constant region showed a preferential bias of $C\beta1$ over $C\beta2$ (>3 standard deviations above the mean) in the lung T lymphocytes of sarcoid patients compared with their blood cells, normal blood and normal lung [76].

These studies suggest not only that sarcoidosis results from antigen triggering, but that the antigen (or epitope) may be different in different groups of patients. The possibility that an atypical mycobacterium could be the initiating organism has recently been reviewed, since many nasal granulomata are the result of specific infections with inability of the immune system to completely remove the invading organism, which has usually taken up residence in cells of the monocyte/macrophage series.

6. Summary and Conclusions

The upper respiratory tract mucosa is protected against infections by inborn, non-specific and by acquired, specific defence mechanisms which interact in a complex manner. The epithelial lining, covered by mucus, is the first non-specific barrier. In the mucus are various antimicrobial substances including lysozyme, lactoferrin and interferon. Granulocytes are also located here, and their phagocytic function is improved if bacteria are coated with antibodies and/or complement.

Continual movement of mucus towards the pharynx is effected by beating cilia, which move in low viscosity periciliary fluid. Bacteria are trapped in the mucus layer and are prevented from attaching to epithelial cells and causing infection.

Specific defence mechanisms arise from T and B lymphocytes and involve mucosal IgA, which is produced by B lymphocytes belonging to the mucosal-associated lymphoid tissue. IgG is found in secretions when plasma leakage, which is increased in infection, occurs.

Recurrent or chronic infections of the nose and sinuses occur when these defence mechanisms fail. Primary abnormalities of mucociliary clearance cause severe and permanent impairment; secondary abnormalities may arise as a consequence of chronic infection with subsequent mucosal damage. Probably the most common cause of dysfunction is a viral upper respiratory tract infection, followed often by a secondary bacterial infection, frequently with bacteria which were previously being carried harmlessly in the nasopharynx [77].

IgG subclass deficiencies, or frank hypogammaglobulinaemia, may be found in patients with chronic rhinosinusitis. Since these are treatable conditions, especially if diagnosed early, it is important to check the immune status of such patients.

References

1. Proetz AW. Applied physiology of the nose. St. Lous: Annals Publishing Co., 1953.
2. Muir DCF. Clinical aspects of inhaled particles. London: Heinemann, 1972.
3. Andersen I, Lundqvist GR, Jensen PL, Proctor DF. Human response to controlled levels of sulfur dioxide. Arch Environ Hlth 1974; 28: 31.
4. Ingelstedt S. Studies on the conditioning of air in the respiratory tract. Acta Otolaryngol, suppl 131, 1956.
5. Jeffery PK, Reid L. New observations of rat airway epithelium: a quantitative and electron microscopic study. J Anat 1975; 120: 295–320.
6. Lucas AM, Douglas LC. Principles underlying ciliary activity in the respiratory tract. Arch Otolaryngol 1934; 20: 518–541.
7. Rutland J, Cole PJ. Non-invasive sampling of nasal cilia for measurement of beat frequency and study of architecture. Lancet 1980; 2: 564–565.
8. Greenstone M, Logan-Sinclair R, Cole PJ. An automated method of recording nasal ciliary beat frequency. IRCS Med Sci 1984; 12: 715–716.
9. Wilson R, Cole PJ. The effect of bacterial products on ciliary function. Am Rev Respir Dis 1988; 138: 549–553.
10. Holmstrom M, Lund VJ, Scadding GK. Nasal ciliary beat frequency following nasal allergen challenge. Am J Rhinol 1992; 6: 101–105.
11. Holmberg K, Pipkorn U. Mucociliary transport in the human nose: effect of topical glucocorticoid treatment. Rhinology 1985; 23: 181–185.
12. Braat JPM, Ainge G, Bowles JAK, Richards DH., Van Riessen D, Visser WJ et al. The lack of effect of benzalkonium chloride on the cilia of the nasal mucosa in patients with perennial allergic rhinitis: a combined functional, light and transmission electron microscopy study. Clin Exp Allergy 1995; 25: 957–965.
13. McMahon C, Ryan R, Darby YC, Scadding GK. The effect of benzalkonium chloride-containing nasal sprays upon normal human nasal mucociliary clearance *in vivo*. Clin Otolaryngol 1996: in press.
14. Cole P, Wilson R. Host-microbial relationships in respiratory disease. Chest 1989; 95 (suppl): 217 s–221 s.
15. Scadding GK, Lund VJ, Darby YC. The effect of long-term antibiotic therapy upon ciliary beat frequency in chronic rhinosinusitis. J Laryngol Otol 1995; 109: 24–26.
16. Wanner A. Clinical aspects of mucociliary transport. Am Rev Respir Dis 1977; 116: 73–125.
17. Young D. Surgical treatment of male infertility. J Reprod Fertil 1970: 23: 541–542.
18. Fearon DT. Activation of the alternative complement pathway Crit Rev Immunol 1979; 1: 1.
19. Porter RR, Reid KBM. Activation of the complement system by antigen-antibody complexes: the classical pathway. Adv Protein Chem 1979; 33: 1.
20. Muller-Eberhard HJ. The membrane network complex of complement. Ann Rev Immunol 1986; 4: 503.
21. Haslett C, Savill JS, Meagher L. The neutrophil. Curr Opin Immunol 1989; 2: 10–18.
22. Hugli TE. Chemotaxis. Curr Opin Immunol 1989; 2: 19–27.
23. Unkeless JC, Wright SD. Phagocytic cells: Fc γ and complement receptors. In: Galein JI, Goldstein IM, Snyderman R, editors. Inflammation: basic principles and clinical correlates, chap 21. New York: Raven Press, 1988.

24. Henson PM, Henson JE, Fittschen C, Kimani G, Bratton DL, Riches DHW. Phagocytic cells: degranulation and secretion. In: Galein JI, Goldstein IM, Snyderman R, editors. Inflammation: basic principles and clinical correlates; chap 22. New York: Raven Press, 1988.
25. Klebanoff SJ. Phagocytic cells: products of oxygen metabolism. In: Galein JI, Goldstein IM, Snyderman R, editors, Inflammation: basic principles and clinical correlates, chap 23. New York: Raven Press, 1988.
26. Weiss SJ. Tissue destruction by neutrophils. N Engl J Med 1989 1989; 320: 365–376.
27. Johnson RB. Monocytes and macrophages: current concepts. New Engl J Med 1988; 318: 747–753.
28. Nathan CF. Secretory products of macrophages. J Clin Invest 1987; 79: 319–326.
29. Skamene E, Templeton J, Adams L. Data presented at IXth International Congress of Immunology; 1995 August; San Francisco. Immunologists 1995; 3: 198
30. Nathan CF. Secretory products of macrophages. J Clin Invest 1987: 79: 198.
31. Marrack P, Kappler J. The antigen-specific major histocompatibility complex-restricted receptor on T cells. Adv Immunol 1986; 38: 1–30.
32. Mosmann TR, Coffman RL, Th1 and Th2 cells: different patterns of lymphokine secretion lead to different functional properties. Annu Rev Immunol 1989; 7: 145–73.
33. Janeway CA, Jones B, Hayday A. Specificity and function of cells bearing $\gamma\delta$ receptors. Immunol Today 1988; 9: 73–76.
34. Kronenberg M, Sul G, Hood KE, Shastri N. The molecular genetics of T cell antigen recognition. Ann Rev Immunol 1986; 4: 529–591.
35. Allison JP, Lanier LL. The structure, function and serology of the T cell antigen receptor complex. Ann Rev Immunol 1987: 5: 503–540.
36. Burton DR. The conformation of antibodies. In: Metzger H, editor. Fc receptors and the action of antibodies. Washington DC: American Society for Microbiology, 1990: 31–56.
37. Williams AF. A year in the life of the immunoglobulin superfamily. Immunol Today 1987; 8: 298–303
38. Brandtzaeg P. The immune system of the nose and nasopharynx. In: Mygind N, Pipkorn U, editors. Allergic and vasomotor rhinitis: pathophysiological aspects; chap 6. Copenhagen: Mungsgaard, 1987: pp 91–120.
39. Walsh TE, Cannon PR. Immunization of the respiratory tract: a comparative study of the antibody content of the respiratory and other tissues following active, passive and regional immunization. J Immunol 1938; 25: 31–46.
40. Reddy V, Raghuramulu N, Bhaskaram C. Secretory IgA in protein calorie malnutrition. Aut Dis Child 1976; 51: 871–874.
41. Steinman RM. The dendritic cell system and its role in immunogenicity. Ann Rev Immunol 1991; 9: 271–274.
42. Alt FW, Blackwell TK, Definho RA, Reth MG, Yancopoulos, GD et al. Regulation of genome rearrangement events during lymphocyte differentiation. Immunol Rev 1987; 89: 5–30.
43. Mayer L, Posnett DN, Kunkel HG. Human malignant cells capable of inducing an immunoglobulin class switch. J Exp Med 1985; 161: 134–144.
44. Cebra JJ, Fuhrman JA, Horsfall DJ, Shahin RD. Natural and deliberate priming of IgA response to bacterial antigens by the mucosal route. In: Robbins JB, Hill JC, Sundoff JL, editors. Seminars in infectious disease, vol 4, bacterial vaccines. New York: Thieme, 1982: 6–12.
45. Chin Y-H, Rasmossen R, Cakiroglu AG, Woodruff JJ. Lymphocyte recognition of lymph node high endothelium. VI. Evidence of distinct structures mediating binding to high endothelial cells of lymph nodes and Peyer's patches. J Immunol 1984; 133: 2961–2965.
46. Van der Brugge-Gamelkoorn GJ, Kraal G. The specificity of the high endothelial venule in bronchus-associated lymphoid tissue (BALT). J Immunol 1985; 134: 3746–3750.
47. Sun JB, Holgrem J, Czerkinsey C. Cholera toxin in B subunit: an efficient transmucosal carrier delivery system for induction of peripheral immunological tolerance. Proc Natl Acad Sci USA 1994; 91: 10795–10799.
48. Elson C. Oral tolerance. Data presented at 8th International Congress of Mucosal Imunology, August 1995, reported in Immunology News 1995; 2(6): 219.

49. Godthelp T, Holm AF, Blom H, Klein JAN, Rijntjes E and Fokkens WJ. The effect of fluticasone propionate aqueous nasal spray on nasal mucosal inflammation in perennial allergic rhinitis. Allergy 1995; 50(23): 21–24.
50. Holt PG, Haining S, Nelson DJ, Sedgwick JD. Origin and steady state turnover of Class II MHC-bearing dendritic cells in the epithelium of the conducting airways. J Immunol 1994; 153: 256–261.
51. Mellert TK, Getchell M, Sparks L, Getchell TV. Characterization of the immune barrier in human olfactory mucosa. Otolaryngol Head Neck Surg 1992; 106: 181–188.
52. Monath TP, Cropp CB, Harrison AK. Mode of entry of a neurotropic arborus into the central nervous system: reinvestigation of an old controversy. Lab Invest 1983; 48: 399–410.
53. Shipley MT. Transport of molecules from nose to brain: transneuronal anterograde and retrograde labeling in the rat olfactory system by wheat-germ agglutinin-horse radish peroxidase applied to the nasal epithelium. Brain Res Bull 1985; 15: 129–142.
54. Terry WD. Variations in the subclasses of IgG. In: Bersome D, editor. Imunology deficiency diseases in man, vol 4, New York: Liss, 357.
55. Carbonara AO, Demarchi M. Ig isotype deficiency caused by gene deletions. In: Hanson LA, Soderstrom T, Oxelius V-A, editors. Immunoglobulin subclass deficiencies. Monographs in Allergy, vol 20, Basel: Karger, 1986: 13.
56. Madassery JV, Kwon OH, Lee SY, Nahm MH. IgG2 subclass deficiency: IgG subclass assays and IgG2 concentrations among 8015 blood donors. Clin Chem 1988: 347–1047.
57. Hanson LA, Soderstrom R, Nilssen DE, Theman K,Bjorkander J, Sodenstrom T et al. IgG subclass deficiency without IgA deficiency. Clin Immunol Immunopathol 1991; 61: 570–577.
58. Nilssen DE, Soderstrom R, Brandtzaeg P, Kett K, Helgeland L, Karlsson G. Isotype distribution of mucosal IgG-producing cells in patients with various IgG subclass deficiencies. Clin Exp Immunol 1991; 82: 17–24.
59. Scadding GK, Lund VJ, Darby YC, Navas Romero J, Seymour N, Turner MW. IgG subclass levels in chronic rhinosinusitis. Rhinology 1994; 32: 15–19.
60. Petruson B, Karlsson G, Hanson HA. Immunodeficiency and sinusitis. ORL Tokyo, 1988; volume suppl 7: 70–73.
61. Stanley PJ, Cole PJ. The concentrations of IgA and free secretory piece in the nasal secretions of patients with recurrent respiratory infections. Clin Exp Immunol 1985; 59: 197–202.
62. Amman AJ, Hong R. Selective IgA deficiency: presentation of 30 cases and review of the literature. Medicine 1971; 50: 223–236.
63. Srober W, Krakauer R, Klaeveman HL, Reynolds HY, Nelson DL. Secretory component deficiency: a disorder of the IgA immune system. N Engl J Med 1976; 294: 251.
64. Stockley RA, Burnett D, Afford SC. The immunological measurement of "free" secretory piece and its relationship to local IgA production. Clin Exp Immunol 1981; 45: 124.
65. Parkin JM. The ENT presentation of HIV infection and the acquired immunodeficiency syndrome. In: Scadding G, editor. Immunology of ENT disorders. Lancaster: Kluwer, 1994.
66. Parkin JM; Eales L-J, Galazka AR, Pinching AJ. Atopic manifestations of AIDS: response to interferon gamma. Br Med J 1987; 194: 1185.
67. Parkin JM, Helbert M, Hughes C, Pinching AJ. Association of IgG subclass deficiency and pyogenic infections in patients with AIDS. AIDS 1989; 3: 37.
68. Herdman G, Forster J, Stafford ND, Pinching AJ. The recognition and management of the otolaryngological manifestations of AIDS. Clin Otolaryngol 1989; 14: 323–332.
69. Van der Woude FJ, Rasmussen N, Lobatto S, Wik A, Permin H, Van-Es LA et al. Autoantibodies against neutrophils and monocytes: tool for diagnosis and marker of disease activity in Wegener's granulomatosis. Lancet 1985; i: 425–429.
70. Savage CO, Winearls CG, Jones S, Marshall PD, Lockwood CM. Prospective study of radioimmunoassay for antibodies against neutrophil cytoplasm in diagnosis of system vasculitis. Lancet 1987; i: 1389–1393.
71. Niles JL, McClusky RT, Ahmad MF, Arnaout MA. Wegener's granulomatosis autoantigen is a novel neutrophil serine protease. Blood 1989; 74: 1888–1893.
72. Cohen-Tervaert JW. Association between active Wegener's granulomatosis and anticytoplasmic antibodies. Arch Intern Med 1989; 149: 2461–2465.
73. Falk RJ. ANCA-associated renal disease. Kidney Int 1990; 38: 998–1010.

74. Savage CO, Pottinger BE, Gaskin G, Pusey CD, Pearson JD. Autoantibodies developed to mycloperoxidase and proteinase 3 in systemic vasculitis stimulate neutrophil cytotoxicity towards cultured epithelial cells. Am J Pathol 1992; 141: 335–342.
75. Moller DR, Konishi K, Kirby M, Balbi B, Crystal RG. Bias toward use of a specific T cell receptor B chain variable region in a subgroup of individuals with sarcoidosis. J Clin Invest 1988; 82: 1183–1191.
76. Tamura N, Moller DR, Balbi B, Crystal RG. Preferential use of the T cell antigen receptor B chain content region CB1 element by lung T-lymphocytes of patients with pulmonary sarcoidosis. Am Rev Respir Dis 1991; 143; 635–639.
77. Openshaw PJM. When we sneeze, does the immune system catch a cold? Br Med J 1991; 303: 935–936.

Rhinitis: Immunopathology
and Pharmacotherapy
ed. by D. Raeburn and M. A. Giembycz

CHAPTER 4
Inflammation in Rhinitis

Morgan Andersson*[1], Christer Svensson[1], Lennart Greiff[1], Jonas Erjefält[2], and Carl G. A. Persson[3]

[1]Department of Otorhinolaryngology, [2]Department of Physiology and Neuroscience, [3]Department of Clinical Pharmacology, University Hospital, Lund, Sweden.

1. Introduction

Rhinitis and asthma are common diseases which are increasing both in terms of occurrence and severity. The pathophysiology and pharmacology of these diseases suggest that inflammatory processes have a primary pathogenic importance.

The inflammatory process in allergic rhinitis may involve several phases and functions which, in some respects, may be better investigated under laboratory conditions than during natural disease. Thus it has been demonstrated that when the nose of the allergic patient is challenged with allergens, an immediate nasal response occurs. This "early allergic reaction" is characterized by nasal symptoms such as itching, sneezing, increased nasal obstruction and watery discharge. Histamine, probably released from mast cells, is considered the most important mediator for this early event [1]. The early allergic reaction gradually abates, and other symptoms may follow later. In contrast to the dual allergic response of the lower airways the "nasal late phase" does not exert any clear biphasic event; rather it is a continuous process characterized by symptoms of milder degree for a longer time period. When the allergic nasal mucosa is re-exposed to pollens as well as certain non-specific stimuli, an increased responsiveness to allergens "priming" [2] and non-specific stimuli occurs [3]. In natural allergic rhinitis, symptomatology and pathophysiology may con-

* Author for correspondence.

stitute a mixture of early and late responses with added chronic features of inflammation. Hence, inflammatory processes and associated clinical symptoms are far more complicated events than those which can be achieved in the laboratory.

How do we describe the signs and characteristics of inflammation? The classical signs of inflammation (rubor, tumor, calor, dolor and function laesa) are unfortunately not very relevant for rhinitis and other inflammatory airway diseases. Rubor (redness), tumor (swelling) and calor (warmth) are not specific signs and may in part reflect increased blood pooling. Furthermore, these functions are components of the normal physiological changes in the vascular tonus, "the nasal cycle", and are dependent on neural control. Dolor (pain) is not a typical feature of nasal inflammation. On the contrary, it is very seldom that patients complain of nasal pain, except of course in the case of trauma or local infections in the nose. Instead of functio laesa (loss of function), the final classical sign, we often discover mucosal hyperfunction such as hyperresponsiveness seen in rhinitis. Consequently we may have to look for other signs more applicable to inflammation in rhinitis. This chapter discusses potentially appropriate indices of the inflammatory process in rhinitis. The emphasis is on mucosal end-organ functions *in vivo*, reflecting the focus of the airway research group in Lund.

2. Plasma Exudation in Rhinitis

Studies of human airways have shown that it is difficult to find a correlation between inflammatory cells and clinical signs of the allergic disease, even though the presence of inflammatory cells in the airways has been accepted as a definition of an ongoing allergic processes (reviewed by [4]). This may not always be a complete description. Cells can be present in the airways without exerting any deleterious effect on the host or they may fulfill low-grade defence and repair functions. We think it is important to find factors which can determine whether the airway mucosa itself is affected by an inflammatory process. Increased secretion, increased pooling of blood and changes in the mucociliary transport are examples of activities in allergic rhinitis which are of a non-specific character. These are effects that can be evoked equally by non-inflammatory irritants, and they may represent normal ongoing activities. The exudation of bulk plasma, in contrast, is a specific tissue response to different inflammatory insults [5, 6]. It is not an increase of the normal exchange in the capillary bed of fluid and solved solutes. Thus exudative indices can quantitatively reflect the intensity and time course of allergic and other inflammatory processes both in natural rhinitis (allergic rhinitis, common cold), and in experimental challenge – generated rhinitis [5, 6]. This is shown in Figure 1. In contrast to the number of inflammatory cells, exudative indices may correlate well to patients' clinical symptoms [5–7].

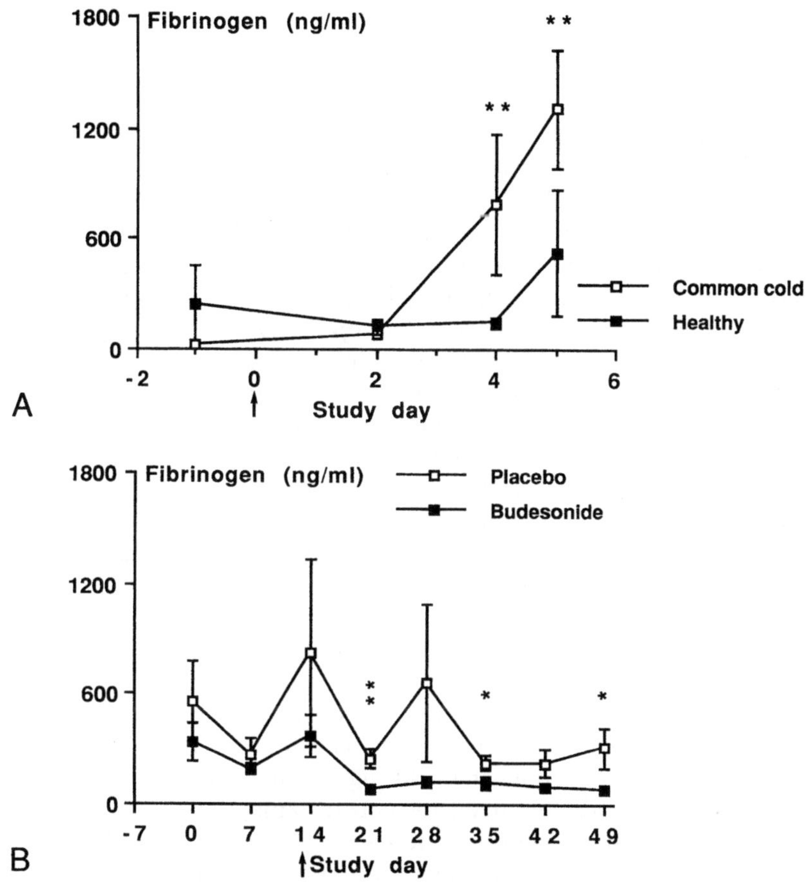

Figure 1. Exudation of plasma occurs both in allergic and infectious rhinitis. A: Nasal lavage of fibrinogen in healthy control subjects and corona virus-induced common cold. Only subjects with common colds exhibited an increase in nasal lavage levels of fibrinogen compared with healthy subjects, (*, $p<0.05$; **, $p<0.01$). Arrow indicates virus inoculation. B: Fibrinogen levels in nasal lavages of allergic subjects ($n = 22$) during a birch pollen season. Half of the patients received a topical glucocorticoid (budesonide, 400 µg daily) and the rest placebo. Budesonide significantly decreased the levels of fibrinogen compared with placebo on study days 21, 35 and 49. No difference was seen in the run-in period. Arrow indicates treatment start (day 14). Data taken from [7] and [36].

The profuse airway mucosal microcirculation has several important functions in health and disease. One of its major roles lies in the process of extravasation of bulk plasma. This response is produced by allergic reactions, infectious processes, occupational disease factors, inflammatory factors and epithelial shedding. In contrast, simple neurogenic irritants are without exudative effects [8, 9]. The extravasated plasma harbours adhesive and leukocyte-activating proteins (such as fibrinogen and fibronectin), proteases, immunoglobulins; cytokines and cytokine-modulating proteins;

and an endless variety of biologically active peptides. This dynamic molecular milieu may explain in part why any translation of *in vitro* cell data to *in vivo* function may be fraught with disaster.

Epithelial restitution, after shedding, suggests a paramount role of plasma exudation also in mucosal repair. Shedding-like removal of the epithelial lining promptly induces extravasation and luminal entry of bulk plasma. A plasma-derived gel thus covers the denuded but intact basement membrane until a new flat epithelium has been established. The gel is rich in fibronectin-fibrin and other repair-promoting plasma-derived agents, potentially explaining why re-epithelialisation *in vivo* occurs both promptly and at exceedingly high speeds. The epithelial restitution process involves several physiological responses (plasma extravasation, secretory effects), cellular responses (migration and activation of neutrophils and eosinophils, and proliferation of fibroblasts and smooth muscle cells) and extracellular matrix effects (thickening of reticular basement membrane and regional lymph nodes). Hence, shedding-restitution processes, as they evolve under *in vivo* conditions, evoke several disease-like effects (reviewed by [10]). Protecting the epithelial lining from damage and shedding appears an increasingly important goal of the treatment of rhinitis and asthma.

Patients' symptoms in asthma and rhinitis display a marked diurnal variation with increased symptomatology during the morning hours. The exudative inflammatory processes may follow the same diurnal rhythm. In infectious rhinitis significantly more plasma exudate is found in the airway lumen during morning hours than during the rest of the day [11]. This observation underscores the need for anti-inflammatory treatments to be effective during night and morning hours.

When guinea-pig and rat airways are exposed to local irritating substances such as capsaicin, an exudative inflammation occurs. Hence, based on animal data, "neurogenic airway inflammation" has become an established concept widely believed to be significant in rhinitis. This concept of the presence of neurogenic inflammation in human airways may, however, have been prematurely accepted. Nasal provocation with irritating agents like nicotine and capsaicin simply causes pain and nasal secretion. No exudative inflammation is produced [8, 9] nor is there any exaggertion of inflammation in ongoing allergic rhinitis [9]. Thus, we propose that neurogenic inflammation is not relevant to human nasal airways. It must be stressed that traditional paradigms based on animal data cannot be directly interpreted as relevant for human airways. We recommend early studies in the accessible human nose [12] to assess novel ideas about airway inflammation. Relevance of mechanisms observed in animal models or in cells *ex vivo* to the human airway could be promptly corroborated or refuted in the human nose, thus avoiding premature conclusions about their importance for disease and future treatment.

3. Cells and Cytokines in Allergic Rhinitis

The kinetics of inflammatory cell traffic and its relation to airway mucosal changes in reactivities have been widely investigated in allergic rhinitis [13–19]. After allergen exposure there is a fairly rapid increase in the number of eosinophils on the mucosal surface. There is also a time-related relationship between the influx of cells and the increase in nasal responsiveness to secretory stimuli. Hence, when the allergic mucosa is challenged with methacholine (a secretory stimulus in the upper airways), an increased volume of nasal secretions is produced compared with the response in non-allergic, non-inflamed nasal mucosa. It seems, however, that these two events appear at the same time, since no individual relationship between these two events could be seen. Hence there were patients with a rapid increase in the number of eosinophils and a much later occurring secretory hyperresponsiveness and *vice versa* [17].

Anti-inflammatory treatment with topical glucocorticoids raises further questions about the role of the eosinophil as inducer of hyperresponsiveness. Short pretreatment with topical glucocorticoids totally abolished allergen challenge-induced increase in nasal responsiveness ("priming") but had no effect on the signs of eosinophil activation. Hence, in nasal washings the levels of eosinophil cationic protein were still augmented at the later ongoing inflammatory period [16]. Similarly, we have shown that two different antihistamines (terfenadine and cetirizine) reduced secretory hyperresponsiveness to methacholine but did not affect the increased number of eosinophils [18]. The phenomenon of hyperreactivity surely involves more than just recruitment and activation of eosinophils.

Studies of cell products have made an important contribution to the understanding of the pathophysiology of allergic airway diseases. In contrast to the exudation of plasma, these data demonstrate the potential of the allergic mucosa for allergic response rather than the actual intensity of an ongoing allergic inflammation.

Allergic and infectious rhinitis conditions share features such as plasma exudation and exudative hyperresponsiveness. Recently we demonstrated an increase of granulocyte macrophage colony stimulating factor (GM-CSF) but not other cytokines such as interleukin (IL)-1, IL-6 and tumour necrosis factor α (TNFα) in nasal lavage fluid levels from patients with allergic rhinitis [19]. On the contrary, patients with infectious (common cold) rhinitis had increased levels of interferon (IFN) γ. These observations indicate that different inflammatory stimuli like allergens and viruses cause different cytokine response in inflamed nasal mucosa, as shown in Figure 2. It could be speculated whether other forms of rhinitis (such as vasomotor rhinitis) differ in their cytokine profile.

Bone marrow-derived circulating myeloid progenitor cells are affected in patients with allergic inflammation (reviewed by [20]). The number of progenitors and their sensitivity for GM-CSF stimulation *ex vivo* changes

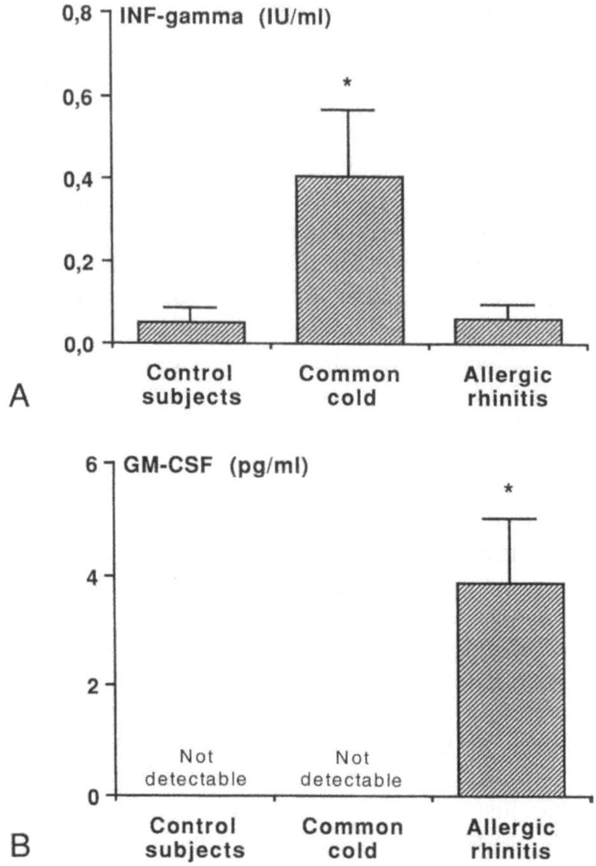

Figure 2. Differences in nasal cytokine profile in allergic rhinitis and corona virus-induced common cold. A: Significantly increased nasal lavage levels of IFN-γ were found at the height of the infection compared with allergic and healthy control subjects. B: In allergic subjects, however, significantly increased levels of GM-CSF following a nasal allergen challenge were demonstrated. * $p<0.05$. Data taken from [19].

during the pollen season in allergic rhinitis [21]. At the height of the pollen season the number of circulating progenitors and the levels of GM-CSF in nasal lavage samples increased and decreased towards the end. Furthermore, sensitivity to *ex vivo* stimulation of the blood progenitors by GM-CSF was reduced at the height of the season compared with increased sensitivity to GM-CSF prior to and at the end of the season. These results suggest a role for GM-CSF as one of the regulator molecules involved in mobilisation and activation of eosinophilic progenitors in allergic rhinitis, although the true nature and significance of myeloid precursors are still unknown.

4. The Barrier Function of the Airway Mucosa in Health and Disease

It has generally been claimed that the airway mucosa develop an abnormal increased absorption permeability for inhaled material during active allergic disease. Hyperreactivity and other features of the allergic airway mucosa could thus be explained by simple changes in perviousness. This hypothesis has been widely disseminated, although the underlying *in vivo* observations which support the increased absorption theory are few and contradictory. With new and specific methods we have demonstrated that the airway mucosa is in fact functionally tighter in patients with allergic rhinitis at the end of the pollen season compared with its healthy condition outside the season [22] (Figure 3). Furthermore, the absorption barrier seems unaffected in corona virus-induced rhinitis as well as in wild, not specified clinical common cold [23, 24]. Even the exposure of the nasal mucosa to cigarette smoke failed to reveal increased absorption across the airway mucosa [25]. These human *in vivo* data seriously question the hypothesis of increased absorption permeability in the pathogenesis and progress of airway inflammatory diseases.

One possible explanation for an improved absorption barrier in active nasal inflammation could be our observation that plasma-derived extracellular matrix proteins such as fibrinogen are laid down in the lamina propria, in the basement membrane, in the epithelium and on the epithelial surface [26]. These extracellular proteins may exert important functions both in the repair phase of the epithelium and as a barrier to inhaled material in active rhinitis inflammation. Indeed, the dramatically high speed of epithelial restitution (after shedding) *in vivo* and the establishment of flat, tight and large repair cells together with some metaplasia might also explain why an inflamed mucosa with epithelial shedding may develop into an abnormally tight mucosa.

5. Hyperfunctions in Nasal Mucosal End Organs

Hyperreactivity to unspecified local provocations may be considered a cardinal sign of asthma and rhinitis [27]. In contrast to studies in the lower airways, the nose offers excellent opportunities for specific functional measurement of different aspects of hyperreactivity. Investigations can also be performed without any interactions with smooth muscle contractions. By using different kinds of challenge agents, specific nasal mucosal end-organ hyperreactivities (microcirculation, glands and nerves) can be monitored [12]. Thus when the allergic mucosa is challenged with methacholine, an augmented secretory response occurs. Furthermore, this methacholine-induced hypersecretion is significantly reduced by topical glucocorticoid treatment [28]. Microvascular exudative responsiveness can be investigated by topical application of histamine to the nose. At the end

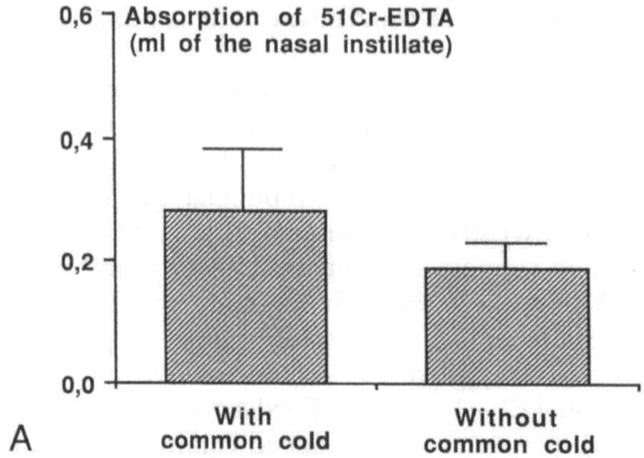

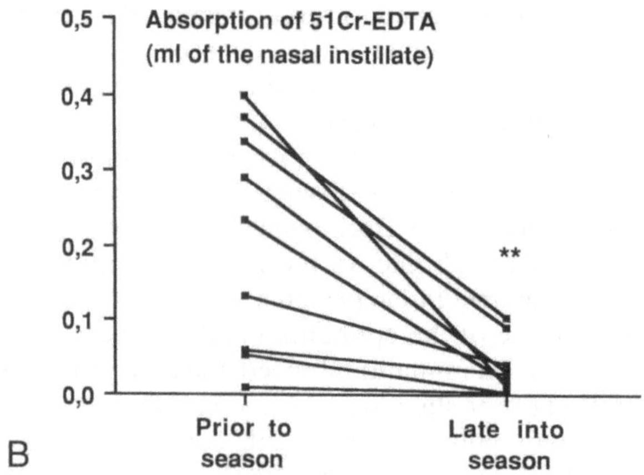

Figure 3. A: Absorption of 51-Cr EDTA across the nasal mucosa in healthy subjects and in corona virus-induced common cold. No differences in the absorption rate was found. B: Nasal absorption of 51-Cr EDTA in allergic subjects prior to and at the end of a pollen season. As seen, there is significantly reduced absorption of the tracer at the end of the pollen season. ** $p<0.01$. Data taken from [22] and [23].

of the pollen season, when patients have been exposed to pollens for several weeks, there is an increased exudative responsiveness to histamine as compared with reactions outside the pollen season, when patients are asymptomatic [29]. We have demonstrated similar features of increased exudative responsiveness in corona virus-induced common cold [23] (Figure 4). At the height of the infection there was an increased exudative hyperresponsiveness as compared with asymptomatic non-infectious conditions.

Sensory C-fibers of the nasal mucosa may be stimulated by capsaicin, the pungent agent of hot pepper. Topical provocation with capsaicin induces

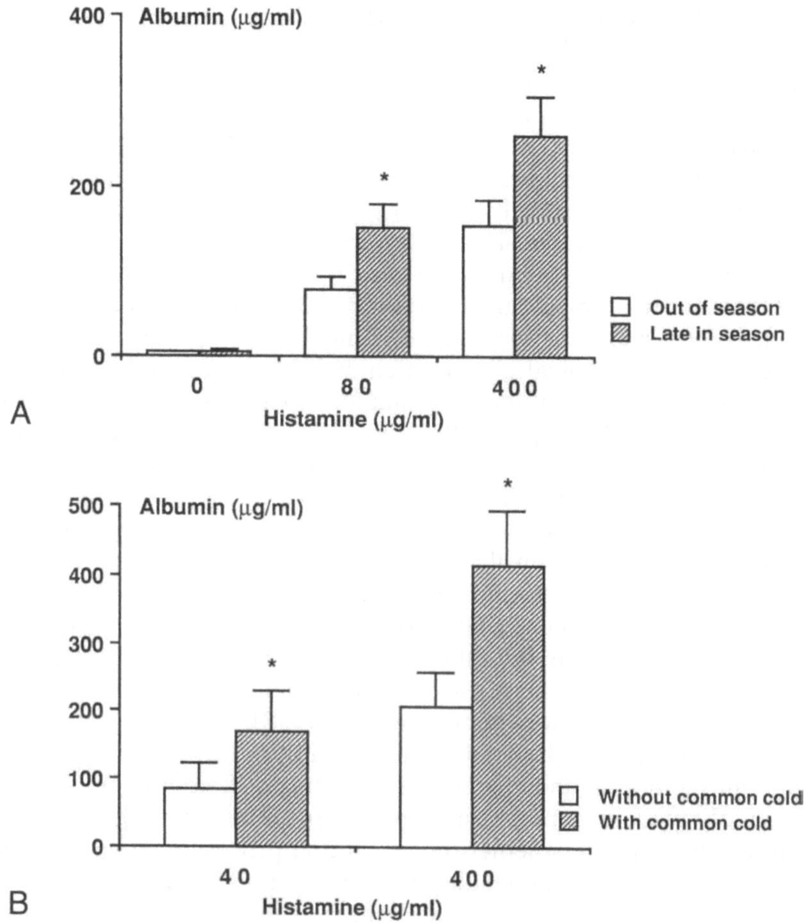

Figure 4. Exudative hyperresponsiveness after instillation of increasing doses of histamine in infectious and allergic rhinitis. A: Significantly more albumin is exuded to the nasal mucosal surface in the presence of histamine in corona virus-induced common cold compared with healthy controls. B: Late into the pollen season significantly more albumin is exuded in the presence of histamine compared with outside the pollen season. * $p<0.05$.

pain in the nose. At the end of the pollen season a hyperreactivity of the sensory nerves to nasal topical capsaicin provocation occurred compared with outside the pollen season [9]. A sensory neurogenic hyperreactivity also occurs similar to microvascular exudative and glandular secretory hyperreactivity and may be considered as a characteristic sign in allergic rhinitis. It must, however, be emphasised that the neurogenic responses in human airways include no tendency whatsoever to an inflammatory exudative response [9].

6. Anti-Inflammatory Treatment in Rhinitis

Anti-inflammatory treatment with glucocorticosteroids is currently the most efficacious management of allergic and non-allergic rhinitis [1] see also accompanying chapters. When topical glucocorticoid treatment is initiated and continued for a prolonged period before a nasal allergen provocation, both the early allergic nasal symptoms and concomitant release of mediators into the nasal mucosa surface are reduced [30]. Later-occurring symptoms and ongoing mediator release are reduced after shorter pretreatment times with topical glucocorticoids [31]. Allergen-induced hyperresponsiveness and accompanying inflammatory cell influx seem also to be highly sensitive to topical glucocorticoids [32]. In natural allergic rhinitis topical glucocorticoids reduce the number of nasal epithelial mast cells [33] and eosinophils [28] as well as the signs of eosinophil activation [34] and the number of antigen-presenting cells [35]. Reduction in the number of T lymphocytes has also been observed [35].

Topical glucocorticoids inhibit the exudation of plasma and the formation of potent peptides on the nasal mucosal surface in natural ongoing allergic rhinitis [36]. In contrast to animal studies [37], however, the anti-exudative effect of topical glucocorticoids seems not to be a direct acute effect on the vasculature but rather reflects the inhibition of inflammatory processes that involve the release of mediators, cytokines and proteases, which in turn affect airway microcirculation [38].

Continuous epithelial shedding and restitution processes may also be important factors in, and characteristic features of, active rhinitis and are particularly evident in polyps and in sinusitis and asthma [39]. Thus it is important to examine whether the restitution process may be affected by glucocorticoids. Although results are still lacking from nasal studies, topical glucocorticoids did not have any negative effect on the repair process in the guinea-pig trachea, where topical budesonide did not interfere with the high speed and efficient restitution of the airway epithelium after shedding and denudation [40].

Topical glucocorticoids exert their clinical effects primarily locally, not systemically. When the same dose of glucocorticosteroids were given orally and intranasally, only the intranasal treatment were clinically effective [41, 42]. In contrast to topical antihistamines, topical glucocorticoids reduce both baseline symptoms and allergen challenge-induced acute inflammation (exudation) in seasonal allergic rhinitis [43].

7. Summary and Conclusion

The term "rhinitis" refers to several different disease classifications of the nose; whether all these nasal disorders actually also reflect inflammatory processes is not known. We particularly lack information about potential inflammatory components in non-allergic "vasomotor" rhinitis. In natural allergic rhinitis the function of the nasal mucosa is characteristically altered. There are signs of increased levels of inflammatory cells and cell activation, increased exudation of plasma proteins and hyperreactivity of the nasal mucosal end organs (glands, microcirculation, and sensory nerves) but reduced absorption. Anti-inflammatory treatment with topical glucocorticoids abolishes or reduces these signs in the inflamed nasal mucosa.

References

1. Mygind N, Dahl R, Pedersen S, Thestrup-Pedersen K. Essential Allergy. Oxford: Blackwell Science, 1996.
2. Connel JT. Quantitative intranasal pollen challenges: the priming effect in allergic rhinitis. J Allergy 1969; 43: 34–44.
3. Andersson M, Andersson P, Pipkorn U. Allergen-induced specific and non-specific nasal reactions: reciprocal relationship and inhibition by topical glucocorticosteroids. Acta Otolaryngol 1989; 107: 270–277.
4. Persson CGA, Alkner U, Andersson M, Erjefält I, Erjefält J, Greiff L, et al. What is airway inflammation? In: Bousquet J, editor. Airway inflammation: the trigger of asthma and rhinitis. Research Clin Forum 1992; 14: 33–47.
5. Greiff L, Erjefält I, Svensson C, Wollmer P, Alkner U, Andersson M, et al. Plasma exudation and solute absorption across the airway mucosa. Clin Physiol 1993; 13: 19–233.1.
6. Persson CGA, Greiff L, Andersson M, Erjefält I, Svensson C, Alkner U, et al. Mucosal exudation of plasma in asthma and rhinitis. In: Busse WW, Holgate ST, editors. Asthma and rhinitis, Blackwell, Boston: 1995: 733–741.
7. Åkerlund A, Greiff L, Andersson M, Bende M, Alkner U, Persson CGA. Mucosal exudation of fibrinogen in coronavirus induced common cold. Acta Otolaryngol 1993; 113: 642–648.
8. Greiff L, Erjefält I, Wollmer P, Andersson M, Pipkorn U, Alkner U, et al. Effects of nicotine on the human nasal mucosa. Thorax 1993; 48: 651–655.
9. Greiff L, Svensson C, Andersson M, Persson CGA. Effects of topical capsaicin in seasonal allergic rhinitis. Thorax 1995; 50: 225–229.
10. Persson CGA, Erjefält JS. Airway epithelial restitution following shedding and denudation. In: Crystal JG, West JB, Barnes PJ, editors. The lung. Raven Press: New York. 1997: 2611–2627.
11. Greiff L, Åkerlund A, Andersson M, Svensson C, Alkner U, Persson CGA. Day-night differences in mucosal exudation of bulk plasma in coronavirus-induced common cold. Acta Otolaryngol 1995; 96: 85–90.
12. Persson CGA, Svensson C, Greiff L, Andersson M, Wollmer P, Alkner U, et al. The use of the nose of study the inflammatory response in the respiratory tract. Thorax 1992; 47: 993–1000.
13. Godthelp T, Holm AF, Fokkens WJ, Doorenbal P, Mulder PGH, Hoefsmith ECM, et al. Dynamics of nasal eosinophils in response to a nonnatural allergen challenge in patients with allergic rhinitis and control sunjects: a biopsy and brush study. J Allergy Clin Immunol 1996; 97: 800–811.
14. Lim MC, Taylor RM, Naclerio RM. The histology of allergic rhinitis and its comparison to cellular changes in nasal lavage. Am J Respir Crit Care Med 1995; 151: 136–44.
15. Bentley AM, Jacobson MR, Cumberworth V, Barkans JR, Moqbel R, Schwartz LB, et al. Immunohistology of the nasal mucosa in seasonal allergic rhinitis: increases in activated eosinophils and epithelial mast cells. J Allergy Clin Immunol 1992; 89: 877–883.
16. Andersson M, Andersson P, Venge P, Pipkorn U. Eosinophils and eosinophil cationic protein (ECP) in nasal lavages in allergen-induced hyper-responsiveness: effects of topical glucocorticosteroid treatment. Allergy 1989; 44: 342–348.

17. Klementsson H, Andersson M, Baumgarten C, Venge P, Pipkorn U. Changes in non-specific nasal reactivity and eosinophil influx and activation after allergen challenge. Clin Exp Allergy 1990; 20: 539–47.
18. Klementsson H, Andersson M, Pipkorn U. Allergen-induced increase in non-specific nasal reactivity is blocked by antihistamines without a clearcut relationship to eosinophil influx. J Allergy Clin Immunol. 1990; 86: 466–72.
19. Linden M, Greiff L, Andersson M, Svensson C, Åkerlund A, Bende M, et al. Nasal cytokines in common cold and allergic rhinitis. Clin Exp 1995; 25: 166–72.
20. Denburg JA, Dolovich J, Harnish D. Basophil mast cell and eosinophil growth and differentiation factors in human allergic disease. Clin Exp Allergy 1989; 19: 249–54.
21. Linden M, Svensson C, Andersson M, Greiff L, Andersson E, Denburg JA, et al. GM-CSF may regulate circulating eosinophil progenitors in seasonal allergic rhinitis. Am Rev Respir Dis Abstract 1995; 151: A240.
22. Greiff L, Wollmer P, Svensson C, Andersson M, Persson CGA. Effect of seasonal allergic rhinitis on airway mucosal absorption of chromium-51 labelled EDTA. Thorax 1993; 48: 648–650.
23. Greiff L, Andersson M, Åkerlund A, Wollmer P, Svensson C, Alkner U, et al. Microvascular exudative hyperresponsiveness in human coronavirus-induced common cold. Thorax 1994; 49: 121–127.
24. Lunell E, Molander L, Andersson M. Relative biovailability of nicotine from a nasal spray in patients experiencing rhinitis: interactions with a nasal decongestant. Eur J Clin Pharmacol 1995; 48: 71–75.
25. Greiff L, Wollmer P, Andersson M, Persson CGA. Human nasal absorption of Cr_{51}-EDTA in smokers and control subjects. Clin Exp Allergy 1994; 24: 1036–40.
26. Greiff L, Erjefält J, Andersson M, Svensson C, Persson CGA. Nasal polyps: microvascular exudation of plasma and epithelial shedding-restitution processes as causative events in inflammatory airway diseases. In: Mygind N, Lindholt T, editors. Nasal polyposis. Copehagen, Denmark: Munksgaard. In press.
27. Andersson M, Mygind N. Nasal hyperresponsiveness. In: Rhinitis and asthma: similarities and differences. Busse W, Holgate S, editors. Oxford: Blackwell Scientific Publishers 1995; 1057–67.
28. Klementsson H, Svensson C, Andersson M, Venge P, Pipkorn U. Eosinophils, secretory responsiveness and glucocorticoid-induced effects on the allergic nasal mucosa during a weak pollen season. Clin Exp Allergy 1991; 21: 705–10.
29. Svensson C, Andersson M, Greiff L, Alkner U. Persson CGA. Exudative hyperresponsiveness to histamine in seasonal allergic rhinitis. Clin Exp Allergy 1995; 25: 942–50.
30. Pipkorn U, Proud D, Lichtenstein LM, Kagey-Sobotka A, Norman PS, Naclerio RM. Inhibition of mediator release in allergic rhinitis by pretreatment with topical glucocorticosteroids on human nasal mediator release after antigen challenge. N Engl J Med 1987; 316: 1506–10.
31. Pipkorn U, Proud D, Lichtenstein LM, Schleimer RP, Peters SP, Adkinson NF, et al. Effect of short-term systemic glucocorticoid treatment on human nasal mediator release after antigen challenge. J Clin Invest 1987; 80: 957–61.
32. Andersson M, Andersson P, Pipkorn U. Topical glucocorticosteroids and allergen-induced increase in nasal reactivity: relationship between treatment time and inhibitory effect. J Allergy Clin Immunol 1989; 82: 1019–26.
33. Gomez E, Clague J, Gatland D, Davies R. Effect of topical glucocorticosteroids on seasonally induced increase in nasal mast cells. Br Med J 1988; 246: 1572–1573.
34. Svensson C, Andersson M, Alkner U, Venge P, Persson CGA, Pipkorn U. Albumin bradykinins and eosinophil cationic protein on the nasal mucosal surface in patients with hay fever during natural allergen exposure. J Allergy Clin Immunol 1990; 85: 828–33.
35. Holm AF, Fokkens WJ, Godthelp T, Mulder PG, Vroom TM, Rijntjes E. Effect of 3 months' nasal steroid therapy on nasal T cells and Langerhans cells in patients suffering from allergic rhinitis. Allergy 1995; 50: 204–09.
36. Svensson C, Klementsson H, Andersson M, Pipkorn U, Alkner U, Persson CGA. Glucocorticoid-induced attenuation of mucosal exudation of bradykinins and fibrinogen in seasonal allergic rhinitis. Allergy 1994; 49: 177–83.

37. Erjefält I, Persson CGA. Anti-asthma drugs attenuate inflammatory leakage of plasma into airway lumen. Acta Physiol Scand 1986; 128: 653–54.
38. Greiff L, Andersson M, Svensson C, Alkner U, Persson CGA. Glucocorticoids may not inhibit plasma exudation by direct vascular antipermeabilty effects in human airways. Eur Respir J 1994; 7: 1120–24.
39. Erjefält J. Airway epithelial shedding: morphological and functional aspects *in vivo* thesis: Lund University, 1996.
40. Erjefält J, Erjefält I, Sundler F, Persson CGA. Effects of topical budesonide on epithelial restitution *in vivo* in guinea-pig trachea. Thorax 1995; 50: 785–92.
41. Kwaselow A, Maclean J, Busse W. A comparison of intranasal and oral flunisolide in the theraphy of allergic rhinitis. J Allergy Clin Immunol 1985; 40: 363–67.
42. Lindqvist N, Bende M, Andersson M, Löth S, Pipkorn U. The clinical effect of budesonide treatment in hay fever is dependent on topical nasal administration. Clin Allergy 1989; 19: 71–76.
43. Andersson M, Svensson C, Greiff L, Blychert L, Alkner U, Persson CGA. Effects of topical levocabastine and budesonide on nasal responses during a Swedish birch pollen season. Eur Respir J 1995: 8(suppl 19) : A136.

Rhinitis: Immunopathology
and Pharmacotherapy
ed. by D. Raeburn and M.A. Giembycz

CHAPTER 5
Allergic Rhinitis

Moisés A. Calderón and Robert J. Davies *

Department of Respiratory Medicine and Allergy, St. Bartholomew's Hospital, London, UK

* Author for correspondence.

1. Introduction

Rhinitis is a very common disease, but surprisingly little is known about its epidemiology, probably due to the fact that diagnosis relies on recognition of a symptom complex of varying severity. Surveys of normal subjects not considered to suffer from rhinitis have shown that nevertheless 40% had experienced nasal symptoms the previous day. There may be a continuum in the frequency and severity of nasal symptoms from subjects with no detectable illness to those with severe disease. Changing patient behaviour, diagnostic fashion and research methods may explain much of the variation in the prevalence of rhinitis between populations and over time.

Allergic rhinitis is characterised by infiltration of the nasal mucosa with inflammatory cells including mast cells, eosinophils, basophils, T lymphocytes, and upregulation of the vascular endothelial expression of leucocyte adhesion molecules. Clinical features of rhinitis may occur in relation to exposure allergens, most frequently pollens (seasonal allergic rhinitis); house dust mite and household pets (perennial rhinitis).

Because allergic rhinitis is so common and the symptoms are variable, it is essential that treatment be fast acting, well tolerated and above all safe. In addition, it is unlikely that sufferers will take treatment on a regular basis unless symptoms are particularly severe. Therefore, treatment for this condition must be effective when taken irregularly. At the present time there is no single treatment which encompasses all these criteria. Although claims have been made that many treatments for allergic rhinitis have additional therapeutic activities, for example histamine receptor antagonists (antihistamines) with antiallergic activity, such mechanisms are often only demonstrable *in vitro*.

2. Allergen Avoidance

Avoidance of exposure to allergens is the first prophylactic measure advised in the management of allergic diseases, including allergic rhinitis. Allergens in the home, working place or school not only cause worsening of symptoms immediately after acute exposure but can also prolong the clinical symptoms of allergic rhinitis.

Vigorous allergen control measures can make a real difference in symptoms and significantly reduce the need for pharmacological treatment. The beneficial results of this approach may take several weeks or months to be observed. Due to practical and economic reasons it may be difficult completely to eradicate offending allergens from the patient's environment, but avoidance measures are helpful. Control measures for indoor allergens should be applied even if their efficacy is not complete. Allergen control/avoidance measures should be undertaken in homes of sensitive individuals with allergic rhinitis. It is worth noting that it is more difficult

Table 1. Allergen avoidance

House dust mite control measures
Use allergen-impermeable mattress, duvet and pillow covers.
Vaccum the mattress, pillows, around the base of the bed and bedroom floor weekly.
Remove feather pillows, woollen blankets and eiderdowns; replace with synthetic ones. Remove carpeting if possible.
Wipe all surfaces weekly with a damp cloth.
Use a vacuum cleaner with disposable paper bags and a filter.
Wear a mask whilst cleaning.
Chemical agents (acaricides) to reduce house dust mites may be helpful.
Affected children should be out of the room when cleaning is being done and should no return for 2 hours.
Toys should be vacuumed, tumble-dried or put in the deep-freeze overnight to reduce mites. Children should not sleep with furry toys in their beds.
Pollen avoidance measures
Monitor pollen forecasts.
Stay inside when pollen count is high or avoid high pollen areas.
Consider using glasses outside.
Control of pet allergens
Remove pets (if possible); do not replace animal.
No pets in the bedroom at any time. Wash pet regularly.
Allergic families should avoid having furred or feathered pets; since allergic sensitivity to them may develop in time, even if not immediately apparent.

to reduce exposure to pollens and outdoor allergens than it is to control exposure to indoor allergens [1].

Control of symptoms of allergic rhinitis have been reported in different clinical trials after reducing house dust mite (HDM) allergen exposure. These measure include the use of vinyl or cork flooring, the use of mattress covers [2] and high-efficiency particulate air filters [3]. More recently, a single treatment with Acarosan, an acaricidal cleaning formulation, has been claimed to improve symptoms in allergic rhinitis [4, 5]. Recommendations regarding allergen avoidance for the control of perennial and seasonal allergic rhinitis are outlined in Table 1.

3. Antihistamines

Histamine is released form mast cells and basophils in response to allergen. While a number of other mediators are released simultaneously, histamine had been most consistently linked with allergic symptoms such as itching, sneezing and pain through stimulation of the afferent nerve endings of the trigeminal nerve situated in the nasal epithelium. Histamine also acts on the subepithelial blood vessels, causing vasodilatation, hyperaemia and oedema through plasma exudation. This action contributes to the symptoms of nasal blockage and rhinorrhoea. Contrary to previous experimental work *in vivo*, we have reported that histamine does not directly influence epithelial permeability *in vitro* [6]. Exudation of plasma into the nasal cavity results from extravasated fluid from postcapillary venules exerting a lateral pressure load an epithelial cells causing temporary and reversible separation of the tight junctions [7].

Antihistamines are widely used in allergic disease. There are two types of antihistamine drugs, H_1- and H_2-receptor antagonists (blockers). Both types act by a reversible and competitive blocking of histamine binding at the respective receptor sites. Most antihistamines used to treat allergies are histamine (H_1)-receptor antagonists and can be categorized as either first- or second-generation H_1 antagonists. The most important difference between the two groups relates to the presence or absence of unwanted sedative effects. Since their discovery, more than 50 competitive H_1-receptor antagonists have been used as antiallergic and anti-inflammatory agents. These have been shown to be very effective drugs in the management of allergic rhinitis.

3.1. First-Generation H_1 Antagonists

First-generation H_1 antagonists have a rapid onset of action, reaching their peak plasma concentrations in 1–2 h. They are effective over a 4- to 6-h period after oral or parenteral administration. Chemically the first-generation H_1 antagonists can be classed into several groups including ethanolamines, ethylenediamines, alkylamines, piperidines and phenothiazines. These agents are lipophilic and thus cross the blood-brain barrier, attaching to H_1 receptors on brain cells [8]. They can also cross the placenta. All first-generation H_1 antagonists are metabolized by the hepatic cytochrome P-450 system.

3.1.1. Side effects: The major disadvantage of these drugs is the sedative effects that they produce. These are caused by their interactions with the central nervous system. The sedative or hypnotic effects result from central inhibitory activity. These effects may be transient and sometimes unrecognized. Potential psychomotor changes may influence activities that require attentive and motor skills [8, 9]. The first-generation H_1 antagonists also have other unwanted side effects such as a blockade of muscarinic cholinoceptors, α-adrenoceptors and 5-hydroxytryptaminergic receptors as well as local anaesthetic effects. This limits the dose of these compounds which may be administrated safely to humans. The anticholinergic effects include palpitations, tachycardia, constipation, urinary retention (in the presence of prostatic hypertrophy), vertigo and clouded vision [10].

3.1.2. Drug interactions: Antihistamines may intensify or prolong the effects of drugs such as monoamine oxidase (MAO) inhibitors, tricyclic antidepressants, barbiturates, tranquilizers and narcotics, all of which are used in the treatment of mental disorders. They can also increase the effects of anti-Parkinson drugs and alcohol. Additionally, these antihistamines can also cause inhibition of the action of anticoagulants and may reduce the effectiveness of oral contraceptives, progesterone, reserpine and thiazide diuretics [11].

3.2. Second-Generation H_1 Antagonists

These antihistamines are well absorbed when taken orally and have a rapid onset of action after dosing reaching peak plasma concentrations after 1.5–4 h. Astemizole (peaking 4–8 h after dosing) is slower in onset. All are well distributed in the body and most are metabolized in the liver and excreted by the renal or gastrointestinal route (Table 2). These agents are

Table 2. Pharmacokinetics of second-generation H_1 antagonists

	Peak plasma conc. (h)	Plasma half-life (h)	Liver metabolism	Excretion
Acrivastine	1.5	1.5	–	urine
Astemizole	4–8	19 days	+	urine/faeces
Azelastine	4–5	25–35	++ [*]	urine/faeces
Cetirizine	<1	11	–	urine
Ebastine	3	10–14	?	?
Levocabastine		[Topical application]	+	
Loratidine	<2	12–18	++[*]	urine/faeces
Terfenadine	2	16–24	++ [*]	urine/faeces

[*] Active metabolite.

lipophobic and hence are, less likely to cross the blood-brain barrier. They also have limited affinity for brain H_1 receptors. In view of these properties they cause little sedation and few if any psychomotor changes. They have little or no anticholinergic activity and are safe for patients who have glaucoma or prostatic hypertrophy. They have few known adverse drug interactions [12]. The rate of metabolism of these drugs varies, but most tend to be long acting. The pharmacological properties of the second generation of H_1 antagonists are shown in Table 3.

Table 3. Pharmacological properties of second-generation H_1 antagonists

	Histamine (H_1) antagonism	α-adrenoceptor effects	5-HT	anti-PAF	anti-SRS-A	Calcium blocking	Muscarinic cholinoceptor effects
Astemizole	+	±					–
Azelastine	+	–	+	+	+	+	
Cetirizine	+						
Classical H_1 antihistamine	+	±	+			±	+
Loratidine	+	+	+	+			
Terfenadine	+	–	+	+	+	+	

5-HT: 5-hydroxytryptamine receptors; PAF: platelet activating factor; SRS-A: slow-reacting substance of anaphylaxis.

3.2.1. Mode of action:

3.2.1.1. In vitro studies. Studies *in vitro* have shown that high concentrations of H_1 antagonists are able to block mediator release from basophils and human mast cells. For instance, at concentrations ranging from 1 to 50 μM, loratadine blocks the release of histamine from basophils [13]. Similarly astemizole inhibits histamine release from human basophils and mast cells [14], and terfenadine inhibits the release of eoicosanoids from mast cells and macrophages [15]. The mechanisms involved are not completely understood, though Berthon et al. [16] demonstrated that loratadine impairs the increase in intracellular free Ca^{2+} following cell activation, by decreasing the influx of extracellular Ca^{2+} and inhibiting the release of Ca^{2+} from intracellular stores. Loratadine has also been shown to inhibit release of leukotriene (LT) C_4 and histamine from cloned murine mast cells [17]. Azelastine interferes with the synthesis and release of LTC_4 and LTD_4 from neutrophils [18], and blocks Ca^{2+} influx into target tissues. Cetirizine has been shown to inhibit platelet activating factor (PAF)-induced migration of eosinophils, *in vitro* and *in vivo* [19]. Terfenadine and cetirizine have also been shown to be capable of reducing the expression of intercellular adhesion molecule-1 (ICAM-1) on epithelial cell lines *in vitro* [20]. These actions are thought to be separate from the H_1 receptor-blocking activity of the antihistamines.

3.2.1.2. In vivo studies. A number of studies have been performed *in vivo* to assess the clinical effectiveness of antihistamines in inhibiting the allergen-induced inflammatory process in the nasal mucosa and the conjunctiva. In a double-blind, crossover study, Bousquet et al. demonstrated the clinical efficacy of terfenadine (60 mg b.i.d.) and loratidine (10 mg o.d.) during nasal allergen challenge. A significant reduction in the release of prostaglandin (PG) D2 in nasal secretions in the loratidine-treated group was noted [21]. Faraj and Jackson [14] have demonstrated that astemizole (at a concentration range of 33–156 μmol) inhibited allergen-mediated histamine release from blood basophils obtained from patients with allergic rhinitis. In addition, Ciprandi et al. [22, 23] demonstrated that loratidine exerted a significant protective effect both on early and late phase allergen-induced reactions in the conjunctiva, reducing cellular infiltration. The higher concentrations of antihistamines achievable by topical administration should enhance any antiallergic or anti-inflammatory activity possessed by these drugs.

Pazdrak et al. (1993) showed that treatment with levocabastine (0.5 mg/ml solution) caused a significant reduction in nasal symptoms and inflammatory cell influx of eosinophils and neutrophils after allergen challenge when compared with placebo administration. In addition to its H_1-receptor antagonist effect, levocabastine has an inhibitory effect on inflammatory cell influx and hyperresponsiveness to histamine [24]. Van Wauwe, using histamine as well al allergen provocation, showed a marked decrease in vascular permeability after the use of topical levocabastine compared with placebo [25]. In addition to H_1 blockade, cetirizine has been shown to block the influx of eosinophils to the site of an allergic reaction. It also blocks the increased sensitivity to methacholine that occurs 24 h after antigen provocation of the nasal mucosa and decreases levels of albumin and N-α-tosyl-arginine-methyl-esterase (TAME) activity, which are indicators of vascular permeability [26].

3.2.2. Characteristics of second-generation antihistamines: Comparison of second-generation antihistamines is complicated, as not all of these drugs have been studied in the same way, and comparisons between them have varied in methodology. A concise outline of the findings on some commonly used antihistamines is listed in Table 4.

3.2.2.1. Astemizole. Astemizole was one of the first antihistamines introduced as a once-a-day dose for the treatment of allergic rhinitis. Its onset of action is slow, 4–8 h, and therefore it is not an appropriate agent for acute

Table 4. Second-Generation H_1 antagonists

Class	Example	Trade name	Daily dose (adults)
Alkylamines	Acrivastine	Semprex	8 mg t.i.d.
Piperazine	Cetirizine	Zirtek	10 mg o.d.
Piperine	Astemizole	Hismanal	10 mg o.d.
	Loratadine	Clarityn	10 mg o.d.
	Terfenadine	Triludan	60 mg b.i.d.
Miscellaneous	Azelastine	Rhinolast	topical b.i.d.
	Ebastine	–	–
	Levocabastine	–	topical b.i.d.

symptom relief. Astemizole is an specially long-acting antihistamine, with a plasma half-life of approximately 19 days; consequently, skin tests for allergic reactions will not be reliable for up to 6 weeks after its discontinuation. It also appears to stimulate appetite, and weight gain may occur [8, 27].

Astemizole is an effective and generally safe drug for the relief of nasal and ocular symptoms in adults and children with seasonal allergic rhinitis [27–30]. However, overdose with this antihistamine may produce cardiac arrhythmias associated with QT wave prolongation and production of ventricular tachycardia referred to as "torsade de pointes".

3.2.2.2. Loratadine. This is a selective peripheral anti-H_1 receptor which is safe and well tolerated. Loratadine can be administrated on a once-daily basis. Improvement in allergy symptoms may be noticed within the first 4 h of treatment. Loratadine can be used as a prophylactic therapy in seasonal allergic rhinitis, and it provides symptom-free days throughout the pollen season [31, 32]. Due to a lower incidence of sedative and anticholinergic side effects it has also been claimed that loratadine may possess an advantage in the treatment of perennial allergic rhinitis [31, 33, 34].

In a randomized double-blind, parallel group study, 167 adult patients with seasonal allergic rhinitis were treated once daily for 2 months during the pollen season with either loratadine (10 mg o. d.) or astemizole (10 mg o. d.). The physicians' and patients' evaluations of response to treatment were generally higher for loratadine than astemizole [27].

Carlsen et al. evaluated the efficacy of loratadine (10 mg o. d.) and terfenadine (60 md b. i. d.) in 76 patients with perennial allergic rhinitis in a double blind, selected cross-over study. They found a positive correlation between total immunoglobulin (Ig) E levels and reduction in overall symptoms for patients treated with loratadine, whereas a negative correlation was found for patients treated with terfenadine [35].

More recently, in a double-blind, placebo-controlled, multicenter study, 874 patients with moderate to severe symptoms of seasonal allergic rhinitis were treated with a combination of 10 mg of loratadine in an outer coating and 240 mg of pseudoephedrine sulphate in an extended-release core once daily, or placebo, or either of its components alone. The authors found that the combination therapy was consistently superior to placebo or either of the components alone in controlling nasal and non-nasal symptoms in seasonal allergic rhinitis [36].

Loratadine is rapidly and well absorbed, metabolized in the liver, and excreted rapidly in the urine and faeces. A few side effects are reported, such as headache, fatigue, somnolence, dizziness, appetite increases, diarrhoea and dry mouth. No tachyphylaxis has been reported [27, 31, 34].

3.2.2.3. Terfenadine. This is an effective antihistamine broadly used in adults and children. The advised maximum dose for adults in 120 mg a day (given as 60 mg b.i.d. or 120 mg in the morning). In children aged 6–12 years, the dose suggested is 30 mg b.i.d. Terfenadine is also available as a combination with a decongestant (Seldane-D®), as a twice-daily dose. Terfenadine is rapidly absorbed from the gastrointestinal tract and achieves peak plasma concentrations within 2 h. It is extensively metabolized in the liver to from an active metabolite. Terfenadine does not cross the blood-brain barrier. About 97% of the drug is bound to plasma proteins, and it has an elimination half-life of 16–23 h. The drug metabolites are excreted in the urine and faeces.

There is an interaction between terfenadine and ketoconazole, erythromycin and other macrolide antibiotics [37], with the risk of producing QT wave prolongation, and potential ventricular arrhythmias. It is recommended that the maximum dose of 120 mg daily should not be exceeded. Terfenadine is contraindicated in significant liver impairment, pre-existing prolongation of the QT interval, electrolyte imbalance, or in patients taking erythromycin, ketoconazole, itraconazole or drugs with an arrhythmogenic potential [38].

3.2.2.4. Acrivastine. Acrivastine is a short-acting H_1-receptor antagonist with a low sedative potential and antimuscarinic effects. It has a rapid onset of action, estimated by an exponential decay model to be 19 min. In a placebo-controlled, randomized and double-blind 1-day field study, acrivastine (8 mg) was shown significantly to reduce nasal and ocular symptoms by 50% at the median time of 80 min and to improve nasal congestion at 90–120 min (as measured by nasal peak flow) after start of treatment [39]. Peak plasma concentrations are obtained at 1.5 h after single-dose oral administration. The elimination half-life is 1.4–2.1 h.

3.2.2.5. Cetirizine. Cetirizine is a potent non-sedating antihistamine with a half-life of 9 h, allowing once-daily administration. Its onset of action is between 1–2 h and is similar to that of terfenadine and loratidine. It is more potent than astemizole, terfenadine and loratidine. Cetirizine in once-daily dosage of 10 mg has proved to be effective in reducing nasal congestion, nasal itching, rhinorrhoea, lacrimation, ocular itching and particularly postnasal discharge and sneezing [30, 40]. In children (aged 6–12 years) with perennial rhinitis, cetirizine 10 mg once daily significantly reduced nasal and ocular symptoms as compared with the 2.5- and 5-mg daily treatment groups [41].

Sedative effects of cetirizine are minimal, and the drug is well tolerated [42]. This is the only second-generation antihistamine which is not metabolized by the hepatic cytochrome P-450 system [12]. Cetirizine is excreted exclusively by the kidneys; therefore it is essential to confirm that the patient has normal renal function before the drug is prescribed [11].

More recently, Grant et al. [43] conducted a clinical trial in 93 patients with seasonal allergic rhinitis and concomitant mild asthma. In this randomized, double-blind, parallel study, daily cetirizine (10 mg) was compared with placebo treatment for 6 weeks. Cetirizine was found to be safe and effective in relieving both upper and lower respiratory tract symptoms [43]. In a dose-ranging, placebo-controlled study Clement et al. [44] have shown that topical application of a concentration of cetirizine 0.125% nasal spray was clinically and statistically significant by better than topically applied concentrations of 0.06% and 0.25% cetirizine or placebo in reducing symptoms in patients with perennial rhinitis [44].

3.2.2.6. Azelastine. Azelastine inhibits both early and late-phase allergic responses, relieving most of the common symptoms (including rhinorrhoea and nasal obstruction) of both seasonal and perennial allergic rhinitis. Azelastine provides symptomatic relief as early as 2 h postdose, with a maximum effect at 4 h and a duration of action of 12 h [45]. The incidence of adverse effects, which include headache, somnolence, taste perversion and nasal irritation at the site of topical application, caused by treatment with azelastine is low. Azelastine is administered twice daily as an intranasal spray.

Azelastine (nasal spray, 0.28 mg b.i.d.) was compared with the glucocorticoid beclomethasone dipropionate (0.1 mg b.i.d.) in a double-blind, randomized, parallel-group, placebo-controlled study involving 130 patients in the UK [46] where the effect of 6 weeks of treatment on the symptoms of perennial rhinitis was assessed. Efficacy was assessed by patients recording daily the severity of the symptoms of rhinitis on 10-cm visual analogue scales. Analysis of this diary data showed significant reductions in sneezing, blocked nose, running nose and itching nose during azelastine treatment. Patients on beclomethasone dipropionate recorded a consistent reduction in rhinitis symptoms, but these reductions were statistically significant only for sneezing on treatment day 7.

In a randomized, double-blind, placebo-controlled study, Balzano and coworkers [47], showed that after 2 weeks of treatment with azelastine (4 mg b.i.d.) patients with seasonal allergic rhinitis and allergy to *Parietaria* pollen had significantly diminished rhinitis symptoms and a reduced requirement for antihistaminic drugs. Similar results were found by Ratner et al. [48] in their randomized, double-blind, parallel-group study which involved 251 patients, supporting the efficacy and safety of azelastine nasal spray in the treatment of seasonal allergic rhinitis.

Gastpar et al. [49] compared the efficacy of intranasally administered azelastine with oral terfenadine in perennial rhinitic patients. Azelastine showed a trend towards superior relief of rhinorrhoea and nasal obstruction, whereas terfenadine showed a trend towards better control of sneezing and nasal itch. However, in this study no clinically relevant statistically significant differences between the medication treatments were identified.

3.2.2.7. Levocabastine. Levocabastine is a novel topical, long-acting, highly potent, selective antihistamine which is effective and well tolerated in the treatment of allergic rhinitis and allergic conjunctivitis. Onset of action is fast, within 15–30 min of administration [50]. Levocabastine has been shown to be as good or even slightly better than disodium cromoglycate (SCG) [51–54], but less effective than the topical corticosteroids in reducing sneezing, itchy nose, runny nose, itchy eyes, red eyes and lacrimation [50, 55, 56].

In two separate double-blind, parallel-group and randomized studies levocabastine (eye drops and nasal spray) were compared with oral terfenadine (60 mg b.i.d.) in patients with seasonal allergic conjunctivitis. Both studies have shown that levocabastine was significantly better than terfenadine in reducing nasal and ocular symptoms when the pollen count was high [57, 58].

In a multicenter, double-blind, double-dummy, parallel-group trial, 95 patients with seasonal allergic rhinitis, showed that levocabastine eye drops and nasal spray appear to be as effective and well tolerated as oral loratidine [59].

The incidence of adverse effects associated with levocabastine therapy is very low, similar to those presenting after the use of SCG and placebo, for nasal spray as well as eye drops. Nasal and ocular irritation are the most frequent complaints [55, 60]). No tachyphylaxis has been shown during prolonged treatment with levocabastine [50]. Levocabastine has been evaluated in adults, and preliminary data indicate that it can also be effective and safe in children.

3.2.2.8. Ebastine. Ebastine is a new, relatively non-sedating second-generation H_1-receptor antagonist in the piperidine class. Ebastine is absorbed well and has a quick onset of action. Peak plasma concentrations occur approximately 3 h after dosing. This drug has a long duration of action with an average plasma half-life ranging from 10 to 14 h. It is suitable for once-daily administration to adults and children [61, 62]. As yet no adverse effects have been reported.

4. α-Adrenergic Decongestants

4.1. Mode of Action

Decongestants produce their effect by activating postjunctional α-adrenoceptors found on precapillary and postcapillary blood vessels of the nasal mucosa. Activation of these receptors occurs either by direct binding of the sympathomimetic agent to the receptor, or by enhanced release or noradrenaline. This effect produces vasoconstriction, reducing blood flow through the nasal mucosa [63], which results in decreased nasal oedema and rhinorrhoea. Decongestants can be administered orally (systemic nasal decongestants), or topically directly onto the nasal mucosa.

4.2. *Oral Decongestants*

Phenylpropanolamine, pseudoephedrine and phenylephrine are the most commonly used oral decongestants. All are different in their pharmacokinetic and pharmacodynamic properties (Table 5). Both phenylpropanolamine and pseudoephedrine are promptly and completely absorbed, whereas phenylephrine is dependent on intestinal metabolism and is absorbed erratically with an approximate bioavailability of 38%. Peak concentrations are reached between 0.5 and 2 h after administration.

All three drugs are extensively distributed into extravascular sites. Phenylephrine undergoes substantial biotransformation in the intestine and the liver. Phenylpropanolamine and pseudoephedrine are not substantially metabolized, and their elimination is predominantly renal, with urinary excretion being pH dependent. Consequently, these agents should be used with caution in patients with renal impairment. Elimination of phenylpropanolamine and pseudoephedrine may be rapid in children. Interestingly, no direct relationship between nasal decongestant effect and plasma concentration has been established [64].

The decongestant effects of the oral preparations differ from patient to patient some respond rapidly, others poorly or not at all. Phenylpropanolamine and pseudoephedrine are effective decongestants. Phenylephrine is less effective. Slow-release formulations of these drugs allow a longer dosing interval, especially during the night [65].

Since they produce generalized peripheral vasoconstriction (sympathomimetic effect), increase arterial pressure is always of concern. Decongestants must be used carefully at all times and should be avoided in patients with coronary heart disease, hypertension, and in individuals with endocrine or metabolic problems such as hyperthyroidism and diabetes. In addition, the α-adsenoceptor agonist effect can induce contraction of the radial muscle of the iris, producing mydriasis, potentially blocking the exit of aqueous humor from the anterior chamber of the eye. Therefore, indivi-

Table 5. Pharmacokinetics of systemic decongestants

	Peak plasma conc. (h)	Plasma half-life (h)	Hepatic metabolism	Excretion
Phenylephrine	0.5	2.5	+	urine
Phenylpropanolamine	<2	4	+	urine
Pseudoephedrine	<1	6	+	urine

duals with glaucoma should avoid sympathomimetic agents. Stimulation of α_1-adrenoceptors on the trigone and sphincter muscles of the bladder can cause urinary retention, especially in individuals with prostate gland enlargement [63, 66].

4.3. Topical Decongestants

Topical nasal decongestants include the sympathomimetic amines (e.g. phenylephrine) and the imidazoles (e.g. oxymetazoline, xylometazoline and naphazoline). The imidazoline derivatives are mainly α-adrenoceptor agonists, while β-phenylethylamine derivatives are α_1-adrenoceptor agonists (Table 6). The venous erectile tissue is sensitive to both, but resistance vessels are mostly sensitive to α_2-adrenoceptor agonists. This difference in the adrenoceptor activity determines that imidazoline derivatives decrease the mucosal blood flow, whereas the β-phenylethylamine derivatives do not [67].

The imidazoles are more potent and have longer-acting effects. For example, the effect of 0.1 % xylometazoline remains for 8 h, whereas 1 % phenylephrine lasts only 2–3 h. These drugs are beneficial in reducing nasal congestion, consequently permitting other topical preparations to penetrate effectively into the nasal cavity [67, 68].

Overuse of topical decongestants generates a prolonged vasoconstriction, the rebound congestion, in which a reversal effect to vasodilation occurs due to fatigue of the constrictor mechanisms. This is followed by reactive hyperaemia. The mucosa becomes less drug responsive, requiring increasing amounts of the drug to decrease the oedema. This in turn induces the further use of the decongestant, leading to a vicious circle of events.

Topical decongestants are not recommended to be used for more than 7–10 days because of the risk of inducing rhinitis medicamentosa [38], in

Table 6. Topical nasal decongestants

	Adrenoceptor activities	Trade name
β-Phenylethylamine derivates		
Ephedrine HCl	α_1, α_2, β_1, β_2	Ephedrine Nasal Drops
Phenylephrine HCl	α_1	Fenox
Imidazoline derivatives		
Naphazoline HCl	α_2	Privine
Oxymetazoline HCl	α_2	Nezeril
Xylometazoline HCl	α_2	Otrivine Nasal Drops

which nasal obstruction becomes unresponsive to venoconstrictive agents. Damage to the mucosal glands and ephithelial cilia may occur after prolonged use of topical decongestants [11].

To reverse the local rebound effects, the spray or drops must not be used for at least 48–72 h; during this time oral decongestants and topical nasal steroids will be of benefit. Oral decongestants will not produce rebound effects and may be used for extended periods, but their benefits are variable [8]. The imidazole derivatives seem more capable of causing rebound congestion and rhinitis medicamentosa than the sympathomimetic amines, possibly because of their longer duration of effect on mucosal blood flow [67].

MAO inhibitors and tricyclic antidepressants can interact with some nasal decongestants such as phenylpropanolamine reducing their metabolism or preventing their efficacy, producing high levels of the sympathomimetic drug in the blood. Decongestants can interfere with the effect of antihypertensive drugs such as α-methyldopa and β-adrenoceptor antagonists and may also react with indomethacin, general anaesthetics and digoxin. Phenylpropanolamine increases caffeine plasma levels and decreases theophylline clearance.

5. Anticholinergics

Ipratropium bromide and oxitropium bromide inhibit the muscarinic cholinoceptors in the nasal mucosa. Ipratropium bromide is an anticholinergic compound that is chemically related to atropine. Its mechanism of action is by selective blockade of muscarinic receptor sites. These anticholinergic drugs can reduce watery rhinorrhoea, but they have no effect on nasal blockage. They have no influence on sensory nerve endings and consequently no effect on nasal itching or sneezing. Ipratropium bromide absorption is very poor; thus it is unusual to have systemic cholinergic side effects such as dry mouth, urinary retention, tachycardia and disturbances of visual accommodation. Epistaxis, dryness and irritation of the nose are, however, reported as topical side effects.

In a double-blind, placebo-controlled study, Baroody et al. demonstrated that ipratropium bromide administrated as an aqueous nasal spray (42–168 µg per nostril b.i.d. or t.i.d.), significantly decreased methacholine-induced rhinorrhoea in perennial rhinitics [69]. In addition to having a longer duration, the 168-µg-per-nostril dose produced approximately twice the inhibitory effect of the 42-µg dose as measured by reduction of nasal secretions. The higher dose did not cause an increased incidence of side effects [70].

Meltzer et al. [71] conducted a double-blind, multicenter, randomized, placebo-controlled, parallel-group trial in 123 patients with perennial rhinitis naturally exposed to allergen. They studied the effect of ipratropium bromide aqueous nasal spray (21 μg or 42 μg) in the relief of nasal symptoms, quality of life and side effects. They found significantly decreased rhinorrhoea, in both ipratropium bromide treatment groups, with consistently greater improvement in the group treated with the higher dose. Both doses improved quality of life and produced no significant local or systemic adverse effects.

6. Anti-Inflammatory Drugs

6.1. Nedocromil Sodium

6.1.1. Mode of action: Nedocromil sodium is a cromone derivative compound that stabilizes both mucosal and connective tissue mast cells as well as eosinophils, monocytes, epithelial cells and alveolar macrophages [11, 72–74]. Nedocromil also acts as a B-lymphocyte (B-cell) regulatory reagent [75] and it may inhibit interleukin (IL)-4-induced switching of IgE and IgG4 production by affecting the interaction of B cells, T lymphocytes (T cells) and monocytes [76, 77]. Nedocromil sodium has been claimed to inhibit chloride ion channel activity in a mucosal-type must cell line [78].

6.1.2. Use and effects: Nedocromil prevents both the acute and late phases of the allergic response [79–81]. The anti-inflammatory properties of nedocromil seem to be many times greater than those of SCG [80–82) in reducing nasal symptoms in allergic rhinitis [83, 84]. For the control of symptoms in mild to moderate allergic rhinitis, nedocromil should be used regularly throughout the allergic season. Other than its application before an anticipated acute allergen exposure, nedocromil cannot be used on an as-needed basis.

In a double-blind, placebo-controlled trial, Donnelly et al. showed that nedocromil significantly relieved pre-existing seasonal allergic rhinitis symptoms during peak pollen exposures within 2 h of the first dose [79]. They also demonstrated that the beneficial effects of nedocromil can be maintained on a dosing administration of four times a day. Once effective symptom control has been achieved, the maintenance dose may be decreased to a frequency of twice daily. After topical use the small amount absorbed is excreted almost unchanged in the bile and faeces [81].

6.1.3. Adverse effects: Nedocromil is an exceptionally safe drug with a low incidence of reported side effects [85]. Nasal dryness, bitter taste, nausea and headache have been reported, but no systemic symptoms have been reported after topical use.

6.2. *Cromolyn Sodium*

6.2.1. Mode of action: The mode of action of cromolyn sodium is complex and involves the reduction of calcium transport across the cell membranes of a number of cells by inhibiting the calcium-dependent activation process [86]. SCG may also be involved in the inhibition of phosphodiesterases and IgE-dependent mediator secretion by cell types other than mast cells. It may also suppress the effects of PAF. SCG is a highly ionized acid salt, a lipophobic agent that does not readily pass through cell membranes; consequently, it is not metabolized [81]. When it is administered locally, it has the advantage of providing maximal topical effect.

6.2.2. Use and effects: SCG is used for the prevention and treatment of seasonal [87, 88] and perennial [89] allergic rhinitis. Less than 7% of an intranasal dose is absorbed. The majority of an intranasal dose which is swallowed is excreted unchanged in the bile and faeces. SCG is poorly absorbed from the gastrointestinal tract, with a bioavailability of only 1%. Its half-life is about 80 min [81].

The recommended dose of SCG is 10 mg as powder given by nasal insufflation into each nostril up to four times a day. Approximately 2.5 or 5 mg as a 2 or 4% solution is administered as drops or spray into each nostril up to six times a day, until relief evident. Relief normally occurs within 4 to 7 days. In cases of severe seasonal or perennial allergic rhinitis, patients may require 2 or more weeks of treatment for maximum effect. The drug must be distributed broadly over the area involved; thus in patients with nasal congestion to use of a decongestant prior to application of SCG is recommended.

Prophylactic treatment for seasonal allergic rhinitis should begin at least 1 week before exposure to the aggravating allergen and should persist throughout the season on a regular basis [78].

6.2.3. Adverse effects: Intranasal use of SCG may cause transitory irritation, burning and stinging of the nasal mucosa, sneezing and sometimes epistaxis.

7. Corticosteroids

7.1. *Mechanism of Action*

The mechanism of action of corticosteroids, administrated either topically or systemically, involves the passive diffusion of free or unbound glucocorticoid molecules through the cell membrane into the cytoplasm where they attach to the so-called glucocorticoid receptors. These receptors regulate the transcription of several steroid-responsive target genes [90]. This steroid-receptor complex migrates into the cell nucleus, where it attaches firmly to specific nuclear bindings sites on the DNA molecules, leading to mRNA synthesis and protein production [91–93]. The anti-inflammatory effects of steroids may be due to a direct inhibitiory interaction between corticosteroid receptors and other transcription factors, such as activator protein 1 (AP-1) and nuclear factor-kappa B (NF-kB) [90, 94].

In allergic rhinitis, glucocorticoids reduce inflammatory cell infiltration of mast cells, basophils and eosinophils in to nasal mucosa and nasal secretions [95–102]. They also reduce the generation of eosinophil cationic protein (ECP) during natural seasonal exposure to allergen [98, 103) and inhibit prostaglandin and leukotriene generation [104]. Nasal blockage can be diminished by the reduction in capillary permeability and mucus secretion in the nasal mucosa [92]. The effectiveness of corticosteroids exceeds that of antihistamines, decongestants and cromolyn sodium [104].

7.2. Topical Corticosteroids

Since their introduction two decades ago, topical corticosteroids, either alone or as complementary therapy with other drugs, have been well established as an effective treatment for allergic rhinitis. They have significant topical anti-inflammatory potency with low or no systemic effects [11, 105] as compared with oral or parenteral therapy. Topical corticosteroids are therefore widely used in the treatment of allergic rhinitis.

7.2.1. Use and effects: Intranasal corticosteroid therapy can inhibit both early and late inflammatory responses after allergen challenge [104]. Topical corticosteroids are very effective at relieving the symptoms of rhinitis, such as sneezing, itching, rhinorrhoea and nasal blockage [106]. Their effect appears to be due to local activity on the nasal mucosa [107]. After intranasal administration corticosteroids are absorbed via the respiratory tract, but a portion of the dose is swallowed. The systemic absorption of most intranasal corticosteroids is minimal at recommended doses.

It has been shown that beclomethasone dipropionate (beclomethasone) has no effect on histamine-induced secretion, but it seems to have an important effect on the vascular bed, reducing mediator-induced vasodilation in perennial rhinitis [108]. Beclomethasone may downregulate the production of specific IgE after seasonal exposure to allergen [109].

Lozewicz et al. have demonstrated that fluticasone propionate (fluticasone) is a potent topical anti-inflammatory drug that inhibits the activation of eosinophils infiltrating the nasal mucosa during early-phase response to allergen [102]. Nevertheless, it has been shown that fluticasone does not influence mast cell density, tissue histamine concentration, lavage histamine levels or TAME-esterase activity after allergen challenge of the nasal mucosa of allergic rhinitics [110, 111].

It has been shown that budesonide is associated with an inhibition of the allergen-induced increase of eosinophil cationic protein in the nasal mucosa [112]. Triamcinolone acetonide (triamcinolone) reduces specific IgE antibody after seasonal exposure to allergen [109], but less dramatically than beclomethasone. This is probably a result of the lower potency of the dose delivered. Triamcinolone has also been shown to reduce eosinophil counts in nasal smears in allergic rhinitics after natural exposure to allergen [113]. Flunisolide blocks the increase in mediators and the total inflammatory cell influx in nasal secretions obtained from allergic rhinitics during the late-phase reaction after allergen challenge [114].

Achieving the maximum benefit of topical corticosteroids takes several days. This is due to the fact that the likely mode of action of this group of drugs is indirect through the downregulation of proinflammatory mediators and cytokines. The previous administration of a topical decongestant may be necessary if significant nasal blockage is present to allow adequate action of topical corticosteroids.

The risk of adverse effects is low when topical corticosteroids have been used as long-term intranasal treatment in adults [115]. Moreover, while continuing to suppress the nasal symptoms, intranasal corticosteroids do not interfere with skin testing. Corticosteroids are more effective than histamine (H_1) receptor antagonists in treating allergic rhinitis associated with nasal obstruction [107].

7.2.2. Side effects: Inhaled corticosteroids have been prescribed at increasing doses and for longer periods of time. Transient topical symptoms of nasal irritation, burning, dryness, sneezing, epistaxis and sore throat have been reported [91, 93]. There is no evidence of atrophy of the nasal mucosa or nasopharyngeal infection, including candidiasis, after regular and prolonged use (more than 5 years) of beclomethasone or budesonide. If intranasal problems appear due to the use of topical corticosteroids, patients should reduce the dosage, change from a pressurized aerosol to an aqueous spray, or use neutral ointment in the nostril on a regular basis.

The systemic side effects of particular concern after use of high-dose inhaled corticosteroids are adrenocortical suppression, bone resorption, decreased growth in children, skin thinning and cataract formation. Little evidence of significant long-term side effects has been reported with doses up to 1 mg per day of inhaled corticosteroids. In doses above this level effects on adrenocortical function can be seen, but a lack of well-conducted trials makes it impossible to determine whether effects on bone, skin or cataract occur at a result of the use of high-dose inhaled corticosteroids [94, 116]. Hypothalamic-pituitary-adrenal (HPA) suppression has not been shown in adults with the topical use of beclomethasone [117] or triamcinolone [118] at recommended dosages. In children, high-dose inhaled corticosteroids seem to have effects on short-term measures of growth velocity, but no effect on final height [119]. Physicians must be aware of the possible

Table 7. List of topical nasal corticosteroids

Approved name	Trade name	Recommended dose adults
Beclomethasone dipropionate	Beconase AQ nasal spray	400–800 μg/day
Budesonide	Rhinocort nasal aerosol	200–400 μg/day
	Rhinocort Aqua nasal spray	200–400 μg/day
Flunisolide	Syntaris Aqueous nasal spray	200–300 μg/day
Fluticasone propionate	Flixonase Aqueous nasal spray	100–200 μg/day
Triamcinolone acetonide	Nasacort	220–440 μg/day

effects from systemic absorption of topically applied nasal steroids, especially when they have been used for a long term without careful dosage limitation.

7.2.3. Topical Corticosteroid Preparations: Table 7 summarizes the most commonly used preparations of topical corticosteroids in the treatment of allergic rhinitis.

7.2.3.1. Fluticasone. This new, potent topical anti-inflammatory drug inhibits nasal symptoms in patients with perennial [120–122] and seasonal allergic rhinitis [106, 123–126]. In a double-blind, placebo-controlled crossover study, De-Graaf-in't Veld et al. demonstrated that fluticasone that aqueous nasal spray (ANS, 200 μg b.i.d.) significantly inhibited immediate and late allergic response and reduced nasal hyperreactivity in 24 perennial rhinitics [95].

In a randomized, double-blind, double-dummy, placebo-controlled multicent parallel-group study, Darnel et al. compared the efficacy and tolerability of fluticasone ANS (200 μg o.d.) with terfenadine (60 mg b.i.d.) or placebo in 214 rhinitics. They found corticosteroid to be an effective and well-tolerated treatment for seasonal allergic rhinitis and significantly more effective than terfenadine in controlling nasal blockage and rhinorrhoea at all times of the day [127].

Similarly, Charpin and Vervloet reported that fluticasone ANS (200 μg o.d.) was more effective than cetirizine (10 mg o.d.), loratidine (10 mg o.d.), terfenadine (60 mg b.i.d.) and astemizole (10 mg o.d.) in treating seasonal allergic rhinitis in individuals aged 12 years and over [128].

Grossman et al. [129] and Boner et al. [130, 131) evaluated the efficacy and safety of this fluticasone formulation in children as young as 4 years. They found that 100 μg of fluticasone ANS given once daily was as effective, well tolerated and safe as 200 μg given once daily. In two separate double-blind, randomized, placebo-controlled multicenter trials involving 313 patients with seasonal allergic rhinitis [126] and 466 patients with perennial rhinitis [122], the effects fluticasone of ANS given once daily and beclomethasone ANS given twice daily were studied. It was demonstrated that fluticasone ANS (200 µg per day) given once daily was as effective and as safe as beclomethasone ANS (336 µg per day) given twice daily in the treatment of seasonal allergic rhinitis and perennial allergic rhinitis [125].

With fluticasone, the most frequently reported local adverse events are epistaxis, blood in nasal mucous and nasal burning [120]. The systemic activity of fluticasone after topical administration is minimal in adults and in children [129], as any swallowed portion of the dose is poorly absorbed (oral bioavailability < 1 %) [105]. The small amount that is absorbed is metabolized rapidly by hepatic degradation to an inactive metabolite [132, 133].

The fluticasone systemic side effects of were studied in a randomized, double-blind, placebo-controlled study of 24 weeks' duration in 365 patients with perennial rhinitis. Ophtalmic examination of patients treated with fluticasone at 200 µg once daily showed no changes that suggested corticosteroid-induced posterior subcapsular formation. Moreover, the corticosteroid did not appear to affect the HPA axis as determined by morning plasma cortisol concentrations and response to cosyntropin stimulation [12].

Similarly, van As et al. conducted a multicenter, double-blind, parallel-group, dose tolerance study in 97 adult patients with seasonal allergic rhinitis. They demonstrated no evidence of effects on adrenal function in doses up to 1600 µg per day [106]. Fluticasone has less systemic activity than beclomethasone (132).

7.2.3.2. Beclomethasone. Beclomethasone is a potent topical corticosteroid that is effective in reducing sneezing, nasal obstruction and rhinorrhoea during the pollen season. In a randomized, unblinded, parallel-group study, Juniper et al. [134] compared the effects of "regular use" (400 µg daily) and "as needed use" (p. r. n.) of beclomethasone in 60 adults with seasonal allergic rhinitis. They found that control of all nasal symptoms in the regular group tended to be better than in the p. r. n. group, but the majority of differences did not reach conventional statistical significance.

Beclomethasone is available as an aerosol, powder and aqueous nasal solution (0.05%). There is no difference between the three forms in reducing signs and symptoms of allergic rhinitis. The recommended dose to be inhaled per nostril is 42 µg two to four times a day (168–336 µg/day) [93].

In a double-blind, randomized, parallel-group trial, Juniper et al. [135] compared the clinical effect of beclomethasone (400 µg nasal spray), astemizole (10 mg daily) and the combination of both drugs in 90 patients with ragweed pollen-induced rhinoconjunctivitis. They found that sneezing, nasal obstruction and rhinorrhoea were significantly better in subjects taking beclomethasone than in those taking astemizole. Combination of beclomethasone plus astemizole provided no better control of rhinitis than did beclomethasone alone.

Absorption of beclomethasone occurs rapidly from all respiratory tissues, but when delivered intranasally, some of the drugs is swallowed. Swallowed drug is slowly absorbed from the gastrointestinal tract where it is hydrolysed by faecal esterases and biotransformed by oxidation into inactive polar metabolites. Beclomethasone is excreted via the bile, and its plasma elimination time is about 15 h [93, 117].

7.2.3.3. Budesonide. This corticosteroid has very high topical potency in the treatment of seasonal and perennial allergic rhinitis [93, 136]. Budesonide is clinically effective and safe in adults and children [137–139] with allergic rhinitis. Following intranasal administration, peak plasma concentrations are reached within 15–45 min. Budesonide is completely inactivated in the liver. Budesonide has a lower systemic potency than triamcinolone, flunisolide or beclomethasone. The half-life after inhalation is 2–3 h in adults and 1.5 h in children. Plasma elimination time is approximately 2 h. Recommended dosage is 400 µg per day (i.e. two 50-µg inhalations in each nostril b.i.d.) [93, 105, 115, 137].

In a double-blind, parallel-group study Bunnag et al. compared the effects of budesonide nasal spray (400 µg daily) and astemizole (10 mg o.d.) in 69 perennial rhinitis. They found significantly greater improvement in blocked nose, runny nose and eye tearing during the first 2 weeks of budesonide treatment than during the same period on astemizole. After 4 weeks, blocked and runny nose remained significantly less troublesome in the budesonide group [136]. Similarly, Gronborg et al. have reported in their double-blind, crossover trial that budesonide (400 µg daily) was more effective on late response than on early nasal symptom response to allergen challenge [110].

7.2.3.4. Triamcinolone. Triamcinolone is a highly potent, nonpolar, water-insoluble, halogenated topical corticosteroid. It is absorbed very slowly, reaching peak plasma concentrations at 3.5 h after administration. The plasma half-life is 4 h [105). Like other topical corticosteroids, triamcinolone is rapidly metabolized in the liver, but it is less active topically than beclomethasone, flunisolide or budesonide [93]. Triamcinolone is currently recommended for use at once-daily dosages of 220 or 440 µg a day [109, 118, 140].

Welch et al. [141] have conducted a double-blind clinical trial in 93 patients with perennial allergic rhinitis to evaluate the long-term (1 year) safety and efficacy of once-daily therapy with triamcinolone nasal aerosol at three different dosages (100, 200 and 400 µg daily). They have demonstrated that all three doses of triamcinolone were associated with sustained improvement in allergic rhinitis symptoms over the course of 1 year. No significant side effects were reported, and mean serum cortisol levels were not suppressed during long-term treatment. Similarly, Feiss et al. [118] have reported that 6 weeks of treatment with intranasal triamcinolone aerosol (220 or 440 µg daily) had no effect on adrenocortical function in adults with allergic rhinitis.

Moreover, Welch et al. [142] have demonstrated that triamcinolone aerosol (165 µg/day) was effective in controlling the symptoms of perennial rhinitis and in improving nasal airflow in peadiatric patients (ages 4–12 years). A lower dose (82.5 µg/day) was marginally effective. Both doses were, however, safe and well tolerated in the children studies.

7.2.3.5. Flunisolide. Flunisolide is a potent, poorly water-soluble topical corticosteroid with similar topical potency to triamcinolone but with greater systemic potency than triamcinolone, beclomethasone or budesonide. The half-life of flunisolide is very short, approximately 1–2 h, with a plasma elimination time of about 2 h. The recommended dose is 200–300 µg per day of a 0.025% aqueous flunisolide solution for adults. The dose is halved for children [93, 105, 115, 143].

No evidence of adrenal suppression has been reported in either children or adults [93]. The most common adverse effects observed with use of flunisolide nasal spray are transient nasal burning and stinging, after-taste and pharyngeal irritation [143].

7.3. Systemic Corticosteroids

To achieve systemic exposure, corticosteroids can be given orally or as a depot injection of a microcrystalline ester. A number of corticosteroids are available for systemic use, including short-acting cortisone and hydrocortisone, intermediate-acting preparations such as methylprednisolone, prednisolone, prednisone and triamcinolone, and long-acting preparations such as betamethasone and dexamethasone [144].

In some cases of severe allergic rhinitis, patients may require a short course of oral prednisolone prior to continuation with topical therapy. Prednisolone (30 mg o.m. for up to 2 weeks) may be required to treat severe seasonal allergic rhinitis, rhinitis medicamentosa, rhinitis in aspirin intolerant patients and nasal polyposis [144]. Whenever possible, other therapy should be given concomitantly upon decreasing the dosage of oral steroid. This will provide symptomatic control after the action of the short course of systemic steroid has ended. Intramuscular injection of depot steroid prior to, or early in, the pollen season has been shown to improve symptoms of seasonal allergic rhinitis for several weeks [145]. The depot preparations, although effective, should be discouraged, however, as they can produce severe side effects. Once these preparations are applied, they cannot be withdrawn from the body and may suppress adrenal cortex function for long periods [38]. Systemic corticosteroids should not be used for treatment of rhinitis in children or during pregnancy [38].

Systemic administration of corticosteroids is contraindicated in patients with peptic ulcer, osteoporosis, psychosis or severe psychoneurosis. Corticosteroids should be used only with great caution in the presence of congestive heart failure, hypertension, diabetes mellitus, epilepsy, glaucoma, infectious diseases, ocular herpes simplex infection, chronic renal failure, uraemia and in elderly persons. Side effects include ocular hypertension, posterior subcapsular cataracts, hyperglycaemia, menstrual irregularities, oedema, tachycardia, hypertension, gastrointestinal irritation, activation of peptic ulcer, muscle wasting, osteoporosis, aseptic necrosis of femoral head and mental aberration (from insomnia to mood changes and psychosis) [91].

8. Guidelines

The relative efficacies of the therapeutic agents used in the treatment of allergic rhinitis are outlined in Table 8. Seasonal and perennial rhinoconjunctivitis should be managed in a stepwise fashion depending on the severity of symptoms (Figure 1).

Underpinning the management of all cases of allergic rhinoconjunctivitis is allergen avoidance. Sometimes this can be sufficient itself to relieve symptoms.

Table 8. Treatment of allergic rhinitis

	Nasal decongestants	SCG/NS	Antihistamines	Topical corticosteroids
Nasal symptoms				
blockage	+++	–	+	++
impaired smell	–	–	–	+
itching	–	+	+++	+++
rhinorrhoea	–	+	++	+++
sneezing	–	+	+++	+++
Non-nasal symptoms				
eye itching	–	++	++	
eye redness	–	++	++	Not
eye tearing	+	++	++	advised
itching of ears	–	++	++	
–/+ palate				

NS/SCG: nedocromil sodium/sodium Cromoglycate; – none; + moderate; ++ good; +++ very good.

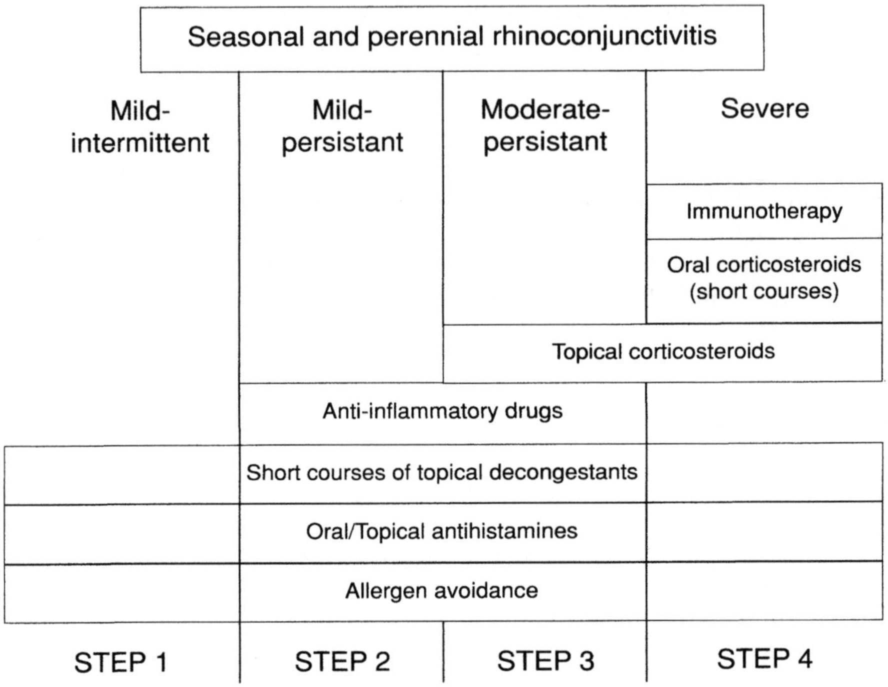

Figure 1. Stepwise treatment of seasonal and perennial rhinoconjunctivitis.

Step 1: Mild intermittent

The majority of sufferers from this very common disease experience mild intermittent symptoms. Oral or topical antihistamines are the mainstay of treatment. There is no rationale for the use of any of the first-generation antihistamines with their attendant unwanted effects. The treatment of this common non-life threatening disease demands the use of the safest therapy. On this basis the antihistamines of choice are those which do not have significant interactions with other drugs and are without life-threatening side effects when administration of antihistamines to the nose and eyes offers a very attractive alternative to orally administered therapy. When nasal blockage is the predominant symptom, intermittent topical application of decongestants remains the therapy of choice.

Step 2: Mild persistant

If allergen avoidance and intermittent use of antihistamines and decongestants is insufficient to control persisting symptoms, anti-inflammatory therapy should be started. SCG eye drops are very effective for controlling the symptoms of allergic conjunctivitis, whilst topically applied nedocromil sodium is very helpful in the management of mild persistant symptoms.

The advantage of these nonsteroidal anti-inflammatory drugs lies in their lack of any significant unwanted effects, and thus their safety for children and in pregnancy.

Step 3: Moderate persistant

Topical corticosteroids remain the most effective treatment for allergic rhinitis but should be reserved for patients who have not responded satisfactorily to the treatments outlined in steps 1 and 2. These therapeutic agents are effective for treatment of nasal blockage, which can be one of the most debilitating rhinitic symptoms. As with other anti-inflammatory drugs, treatment is best given on a regular basis, and the initial management of nasal blockage may require the use of topical decongestants. This ensures rapid relief of symptoms and enables the topically applied corticosteroids to reach the inflammed nasal mucosa. Patients who regularly suffer moderate to severe symptoms of allergic rhinitis during particular seasons, e.g. ragweed, grass and tree pollinosis, greatly benefit from topical corticosteroid therapy started just prior to the pollen season. This has been shown to prevent influx of inflammatory cells into the mucosa, abolishing nasal priming. Topical corticosteroids are also beneficial in the prevention of the recurrence of nasal polyps. The use of once-daily topical corticosteroids, particularly fluticasone propionate ANS, seems to be remarkably free of significant unwanted effects, but as with all corticosteroid therapy their use must be matched to the severity of clinical symptoms.

Step 4: Severe

Severe persistant rhinitis is disabling and requires urgent and effective treatment. In the short term the most effective therapy is the use of oral prednisolone at a dose of 30 mg daily for 2 weeks. Improvement can then usually be maintained with topical corticosteroids administered two or even three times daily. This should be followed by careful review of the therapeutic options, particularly immunotherapy.

References

1. Colloff MJ, Ayres J, Carswell F, Howarth PH, Merrett TG, Mitchell EB, et al. The control of allergens of dust mites and domestic pets: a position paper. Clin Exp Allergy 1992; 22(suppl 2): 1–28.
2. Howarth PH, Lunn A, Tomkins S. Bedding barrier intervention in house dust mite respiratory allergy. Clin Exp Allergy 1992; 22: 140.
3. Kniest FM, Young E, van Praag G, Vos H, Kort H, Koers WJ, et al. Clinical evaluation of a double-blind dust-mite avoidance trial with mite-allergic rhinitis patients. Clin Exp Allergy 1991; 21: 39–47.
4. Brown HM, Merrett TG. Effectiveness of an acaricide in management of house dust mite allergy. Ann Allergy 1991; 67(1): 25–31.
5. Reisman RE, Mauriello PM, Davies GB, Georgitis JW, DeMasi JM. A double-blind study of the effectiveness of a high-efficiency particulate air (HEPA) filter in the treatment of

patients with perennial allergic rhinitis and asthma. J Allergy Clin Immunol 1990; 85(6): 1050–57.

6. Devalia JL, Godfrey RWA, Sapsford RJ, Severs NJ, Jeffery PK, Davies RJ. No effect of histamine on human bronchial epithelial cell premeability and tight junctional integrity *in vitro*. Eur Respir J 1994; 7: 1958–65.
7. Persson CGA, Erjefalt I, Alkner U, Baumgarten C, Greiff L, Gustafsson B, et al. Plasma exudation as a first line respiratory mucosal defence. Clin Exp Allergy 1991; 21: 17–24.
8. Krause HF. Antihistamines and decongestants. Otolaryngol Head Neck Surg 1992; 107: 835–40.
9. McLoughlin JA, Nall M, Berla E. Effect of allergy medication on children's reading comprehension. Allergy Proc 1990; 11(5): 225–28.
10. Collins SL. The cervical sympathetic nerves in surgery of the neck. Otorlaryngol Head Neck Surg 1991; 105(4): 544–55.
11. Krause HF. Pharmacology of upper respiratory allergy [Review]. Otolaryngol Clin North Am 1992; 25(1): 134–50.
12. Corey JP. Advances in the pharmacotherapy of allergic rhinitis: second-generation H_1-receptor antagonists. Otolaryngol Head Neck Surg 1993; 109: 584–92.
13. Miadonna A, Milazzo N, Lorini M, Marchesi E, Tedeschi A. Inhibitory effect of the H_1 antagonist loratadine on histamine release from human basophils. Int Arch Allergy Immunol 1994; 105(1): 12–17.
14. Faraj BA, Jackson RT. The effect of astemizole on atigen-mediated histamine release from the blood op patients with allergic rhinitis. Allergy 1992; 47: 630–34.
15. Campbell AM, Chanez P, Marty-Ane C, Albat P, Bloom M, Michel FB, et al. Modulation of eicosanoid and histamine release from human dispersed lung cells by terfinadine. Allergy 1993; 48(2): 125–29.
16. Berthon B, Taudou G, Combettes L, Czarlewski W, Carmi-Leroy A, Marchand F, et al. *In vitro* inhibition, by loratadine and decarboxyethoxyloratadine, of histamine release from human basophils and of histamine release and intracellular calcium fluxes in rat basophilic leukaemia cells. Biochem Pharmacol 1994; 47(5): 789–94.
17. Kreutner W, Chapman RW, Gulbekian A, Siegel MI. Antiallergic activity of loratadine, a non-sedating antihistamine. Allergy 1987; 42(1): 57–63.
18. Katayama S, Tsunoda H, Sakuma Y, Kai H, Tanaka I, Katayama K. Effect of azelastine on the release and action of leukotriene C4 and D4. Int Arch Allergy Appl Immunol 1987; 83(3): 284–89.
19. Fadel R, Herpin-Richard M, Rihoux JP, Henocq E. Inhibitory effect of cetirizine 2HCL on eosinophil migration *in vivo*. Clin Allergy 1987; 17: 373–79.
20. Canonica GW, Ciprandi G, Buscaglia S, Pesce G, Bagnasco M. Adhesion molecules of allergic inflammation: recent insights into their functional roles. Allergy 1994; 49: 135–41.
21. Bousquet J, Lebel B, Chanal I, Morel A, Michel FB. Antiallergic activity of H_1 receptor antagonists assessed by nasal challenge. J Allergy Clin Immunol 1988; 82: 881–87.
22. Ciprandi G, Buscaglia S, Pesce GP, Marchesi E, Canonica GW. Protective effect of loratidine on specific conjunctival provocation test. Int Arch Allergy Appl Immunol 1991; 96: 344–47.
23. Ciprandi G, Buscaglia S, Marchesi E, Danzig M, Kuss F, Canonica GW. Protective effect of loratidine in late phase reaction induced by conjunctival provocation test. Int Arch Allergy Appl Immunol 1993; 100: 185–89.
24. Pazdrak K, Gorski P, Ruta U. Inhibitory effect of levocabastine on allergen-induced increase of nasal reactivity to histamine and cell influx. Allergy 1993; 48: 598–601.
25. Van Wauwe JP. Animal pharmacology of levocabastine: a new type of H_1-antihistamine well suited for topical application. In: Mygind N, Naclerio RM, editors. Rhinoconjunctivitis: new perspectives in topical treatment. Toronto: Hogrefe & Huber, 1989: 27–34.
26. Naclerio RM. Additional properties of cetirizine, a new H_1 antagonist. Allergy Proc 1991; 12(3): 187–91.
27. Chervinsky P, Georgitis J, Banov C, Boggs P, Vande-Stouwe R, Greenstein S. Once daily loratidine versus astemizole once daily. Ann Allergy 1994; 73: 109–13.
28. Boner AL, Richelli C, Castellani C, Marchesi E, Andreoli A. Comparison of the effects of loratadine and astemizole in the treatment of children with seasonal allergic rhinoconjunctivitis. Allergy 1992; 47: 98–102.

29. Businco L, Monteleone A, Ruggeri L, Cantani A, Chevallier P. New strategies for the prevention and treatment of allergic rhinitis in children [Review]. Rhinology 1992; 13(suppl): 51–60.
30. Lobaton P, Moreno F, Coulie P. Comparison of cetirizine with atemizole in the treatment of perennial allergic rhinitis and study of the concomitant effect on histamine and allergen-induced wheal responses. Ann Allergy 1990; 65(5): 401–5.
31. Dolovich J, Moote DW, Mazza JA, Clermont A, Petit C, Danzig M. Efficacy of loratidine versus placebo in the prophylactic treatment of seasonal allergic rhinitis. Ann Allergy 1994; 73: 235–39.
32. Simons FE. Loratidine, a non-sedating H_1-receptor antagonist [editorial]. J Allergy Clin Immunol 1989; 63(4): 266–68.
33. Bruttmann G, Charpin D, Germouty J, Horak F, Kunkel G, Wittmann G. Evaluation of the efficacy and safety of loratidine in perennial allergic rhinitis. J Allergy Clin Immunol 1989; 83: 411–16.
34. Frolund L, Etholm B, Irander K, Johannessen TA, Odkvist L, Ohlander B, et al. A multicentre study of loratidine, clemastine and placebo in patients with perennial allergic rhinitis. Allergy 1990; 45: 254–61.
35. Carlsen KH, Kramer J, Fagertun HE, Larsen S. Loratidine and terfenadine in perennial allergic rhinitis. Allergy 1993; 48: 431–36.
36. Bronsky E, Bogs P, Findlay S, Gawchik S, Georgitis J, Mansmann H, et al. Comparative efficacy and safety of a once-daily loratidine-pseudoephedrine combination versus its components alone and placebo in the management of seasonal allergic rhinitis. J Allergy Clin Immunol 1995; 96(2): 139–47.
37. Badhwar AK, Druce HM. Allergic rhinitis [Review]. Med Clin North Am 1992; 76(4): 789–803.
38. International rhinitis management working group: international consensus report on the diagnosis and management of rhinitis. Allergy 1994; 19(49) (suppl): 19–24.
39. Nielsen L, Johnsen CR, Bindslev-Jensen C, Poulson LK. Efficacy of acrivastine in the treatment of allergic rhinitis during natural pollen exposure: onset of action. Allergy 1994; 49: 630–36.
40. Mansmann HC Jr, Altman RA, Berman BA, Buchman E, Dockhorn RJ, Leese PT, et al. Efficacy and safety of cetirizine therapy in perennial allergic rhinitis. Ann Allergy 1992; 68(4): 348–53.
41. Jobst S, van den Wijngaart W, Schubert A, van de Venne H. Assessment of the efficacy and safety of three dose levels of cetirizine given once daily in children with perennial allergic rhinitis. Allergy 1994; 49: 598–604.
42. Berman BA. Perennial allergic rhinitis: clinical efficacy of a new antihistamine [Review]. J Allergy Clin Immunol 1990; 86: 1004–8.
43. Grant JA, Nicodemus CF, Findlay SR, Glovsky MM, Grossman J, Kaiser H, et al. Cetirizine in patients with seasonal rhinitis and concomitant asthma: prospective, randomized, placebo-controlled trial. J Allergy Clin Immunol 1995; 95: 923–32.
44. Clement P, Roovers MHW; Francillon C, Dodion P. Dose-ranging, placebo-controlled study of cetirizine nasal spray in adults with perennial allergic rhinitis. Allergy 1994; 49: 668–72.
45. Grossman J, Halverson PC, Meltzer EO, Shoenwetter WF, van Bavel JH, Woehler TR, et al. Double-blind assessment of azelastine in the treatment of perennial allergic rhinitis. Ann Allergy 1994; 73: 141–46.
46. Davies RJ, Lund VJ, Harten-Ash VJ. The effect of intranasal azelastine and beclomethasone on the symptoms and signs of nasal allergy in patients with perennial allergic rhinitis. Rhinology 1993; 31(4): 159–64.
47. Balzano G, Gallo C, Masi C, Cocco G, Ferrantu P, Melillo E, et al. Effect of azelastine on the seasonal increase in non-specific bronchial responsiveness to methacholine in pollen allergic patients. A randomized, double-blind placebo-controlled, crossover study. Clin Exp Allergy 1992; 22(3): 371–77.
48. Ratner PH, Findlay SR, Hampel F, van Bavel J, Widlitz MD, Freitag JJ. A double-blind, controlled trial to assess the safety and efficacy of azelastine nasal spray in seasonal allergic rhinitis. J Allergy Clin Immunol 1994; 94(5): 818–25.
49. Gastpar H, Nolte D, Aurich R, Brendt P, Enzmann H, Giesemann G, et al. Comparative efficacy of azelastine nasal spray and terfenadine in seasonal and perennial rhinitis. Allergy 1994; 49(3): 152–58.

50. Janssens MM, Vanden-Bussche G. Levocabastine: an effective topical treatment of allergic rhinoconjunctivitis [Review]. Clin Exp Allergy 1991; 21 (suppl 2): 29–36.
51. Ciprandi G, Cerqueti MP, Sacca S, Cilli P, Canonica GW. Levocabastine versus cromolyn sodium in the treatment of pollen-induced conjunctivitis. Annals Allergy 1990; 65: 156–58.
52. Schata M, Jorde W, Richarz-Barthauer U. Levocabastine nasal spray better than sodium cromoglycate and placebo in the topical treatment of seasonal allergic rhinitis. J Allergy Clin Immunol 1991; 87 (4): 873–78.
53. Frostad AB, Olsen AK. A comparison of topical levocabastine and sodium cromoglycate in the treatment of pollen-provoked allergic conjunctivitis. Clin Exp Allergy 1993; 23: 406–9.
54. Davies BH, Mullins J. Topical levocabastine is more effective than sodium cromoglycate for the prophylaxis and treatment of seasonal allergic conjunctivitis. Allergy 1993; 48 (7): 519–24.
55. Janssens MM. Levocabastine: a new topical approach for the treatment of paediatric allergic rhinoconjunctivitis [Review]. Rhinology 1992; 13 (suppl): 39–49.
56. Abelson MB, George MA, Schaefer K, Smith LM. Evaluation of the new ophthalmic antihistamine 0.05% levocabastine, in the clinical allergen challenge model of allergic conjunctivitis. J Allergy Clin Immunol 1994; 94: 458–64.
57. Bahmer FA, Ruprecht KW. Safety and efficacy of topical levocabastine compared with oral terfenadine. Ann Allergy 1994; 72: 429–34.
58. Sohoel P, Freng BA, Kramer J, Poppe S, Rebo R, Korsrud FR, et al. Topical levocabastine compared with orally administrated terfenadine for the prophylaxis and treatment of seasonal rhinoconjunctivitis. J Allergy Clin Immunol 1993; 92: 73–81.
59. Swedish GP Allergy Team. Topical levocabastine compared with oral loratidine for the treatment of seasonal allergic rhiniconjunctivitis. Allergy 1994; 49: 611–15.
60. Dechant KL, Goa KL. Levocabastine: a review of its pharmacological properties and therapeutic potential as a topical antihistamine in allergic rhinitis and conjunctivitis [Review]. Drugs 1991; 41 (2): 202–24.
61. Simons FE, Simons KJ. Optimum pharmacological management of chronic rhinitis. Drugs 1989; 38: 313–31.
62. Simons FE, Watson WT, Simons KJ. Pharmacokinetics and pharmacodynamics of ebastine in children. J Pediatrics 1993; 122 (4): 641–46.
63. Johnson DA, Hricik JG. The pharmacology of alpha-adrenergic decongestants [Review]. Pharmacotherapy 1993; 13: 110S–15S.
64. Kanfer I, Dowse R, Vuma V. Pharmacokinetics of oral decongestants [Review]. Pharmacotherapy 1993; 13: 116S–28S.
65. Hendeles L. Selecting a decongestants [Review]. Pharmacotherapy 1993; 13: 129S–34S.
66. Gardiner LJ. Decongestant, anticholinergics and saline in allergic rhinitis management. J Respir Dis 1991; 11 (suppl 3 A): S29.
67. Scadding GK. Rhinitis medicamentosa [editorial]. Clin Exp Allergy 1995; 25: 391–94.
68. Kobayashi RH, Kiechel F, Kobayashi AL, Mellion MB. Topical nasal sprays: treatment of allergic rhinitis [Review]. Am Family Physician 1994; 50 (1): 151–57.
69. Barrody FM, Majchel AM, Roecker MM, Roszko PJ, Zegarelli EC, Wood CC, et al. Ipratropium bromide (Atrovent nasal spray) reduces the nasal responce to methacholine. J Allergy Clin Immunol 1992; 89 (6): 1065–75.
70. Wagenmann M, Baroody FM, Jankowski R, Nadal JC, Roecker-Cooper M, Wood CC, et al. Onset and duration of inhibition of ipratropium bromide nasal spray on methacholine-induced nasal secretions. Clin Exp Allergy 1994; 24 (3): 288–90.
71. Meltzer EO, Orgel HA, Bronsky EA, Findlay SR, Georgitis JW, Grossman J, et al. Ipratropium bromide aqueous nasal spray for patients with perennial allergic rhinitis: a study of its effect on their symptoms, quality of life and nasal cytology. J Allergy Clin Immunol 1992; 90 (2): 242–49.
72. Lozewicz S, Gomez E, Clague J, Gatland D, Davies RJ. Allergen-induced changes in the nasal mucous membrane in seasonal allergic rhinitis: effect of nedocromil sodium: J Allergy Clin Immunol 1990; 85: 125–31.
73. Bruijnzeel PLB, Warringa RAJ, Kok PTM, Kreukniet J. Inhibition of neutrophil and eosinophil induced chemotaxis by nedocromil sodium and sodium cromoglycate. Br J Pharmacol 1990; 99: 798–802.

74. Eady RP. The pharmacology of nedocromil sodium. Eur J Respir Dis 1986; 69(suppl 147): 112–19.
75. Ciprandi G, Buscaglia S, Albano M, Bertolini C, Truffelli T, Catrullo A, et al. Nedocromil sodium and the immune responce. J Invest Allergol Clin Immunol 1993; 3(6): 311–14.
76. Kimata H, Fujimoto M, Mikawa H. Nedocromil sodium acts directly on human B cells to inhibit immunoglobulin production without affecting cell growth. Immunology 1994; 81(1): 47–52.
77. Kimata H, Mikawa H. Nedocromil sodium selectively inhibits IgE and IgG 4 production in human B cells stimulated with IL-4. J Immunology 1993; 151(12): 6723–32.
78. Paulmichl M, Norris AA, Rainey DK. Role of chloride channel modulation in the mechanism of action of nedocromil sodium. Int Arch Allergy Immunol 1995; 107: 416.
79. Donnelly A, Casale TB. Nedocromil sodium is rapidly effective in the therapy of seasonal allergic rhinitis. J Allergy Clin Immunol 1993; 91(5): 997–1004.
80. Mabry RL. Topical pharmacotherapy for allergic rhinitis: nedocromil [Review]. Am J Otolaryngology 1993; 14(6): 379–81.
81. King HC. Mast cell stabilizers. Otolaryngol Head Neck Surg 1992; 107: 841–44.
82. Businco L, Cantani A, DiFazio A, Bernardini L. A double-blind, placebo-controlled study to assess the efficacy of nedocromil sodium in the management of childhood grass-pollen asthma. Clin Exp Allergy 1990; 20: 683–88.
83. Corrado OJ, Gomez E, Baldwin DL, Clague JE, Davies RJ. The effect of nedocromil sodium on nasal provocation with allergen. J Allergy Clin Immunol 1987; 80(2): 218–22.
84. Schuller DE, Selcow JE, Joos TH, Hannaway PJ, Hirsch SR, Schwartz HJ, et al. A multicenter trial of nedocromil sodium, 1% nasal solution, compared with cromolyn sodium and placebo in ragweed seasonal allergic rhinitis. J Allergy Clin Immunol 1990; 86: 554–61.
85. Ruhno J, Denburg J, Dolovich J. Intranasal nedocromil sodium in the treatment of ragweed-allergic rhinitis. J Allergy Clin Immunol 1988; 81(3): 570–74.
86. Simons FE, Simons KJ. Optimum pharmacological management of chronic rhinitis. Drugs 1989; 38: 313–31.
87. Orgel HA, Meltzer EO, Kemp JP, Ostrom NK, Welch MJ. Comparison of intranasal cromolyn sodium, 4%, and oral terfenadine for allergic rhinitis: symptoms, nasal cytology, nasal ciliary clearance and rhinomanometry. Ann Allergy 1991; 66(3): 237–44.
88. Schwartz HJ. Cromolyn sodium and its effects on nasal disease. Am J Rhinol 1988; 2: 129–33.
89. Cohan RH, Bloom FL, Rhoades RB, Wittig HJ, Haugh LD. Treatment of perennial allergic rhinitis with cromolyn sodium. J Allergy Clin Immunol 1976; 58: 121–28.
90. Barnes PJ, Adcock IM. Transcription factors. Clin Exp Allergy 1995; 25(2): 46–49.
91. Mabry RL. Corticosteroids in the management of upper respiratory allergy: the emerging role of steroid nasal sprays. Otolaryngol Head Neck Surg 1992; 107: 885–60.
92. Pauwles R. Mode of action of corticosteroids in asthma and rhinitis. Clin Allergy 1986; 16(4): 281–88.
93. Siegel SC. Topical intranasal corticosteroid therapy in rhinitis. J Allergy Clin Immunol 1988; 81: 984–91.
94. Barnes PJ, Adcock IM. Anti-inflammatory actions of steroids: molecular mechanisms. Trends Pharmacol Sci 1993; 14: 436–41.
95. DeGraaf-in't Veld C, Garrelds IM, Jansen APH, Van Tootenengergen AW, Mulder PGH, et al. Effect of intranasal fluticasone proprionate on the immediate and late allergic reaction and nasal hyperreactivity in patients with a house dust mite allergy. Clin Exp Allergy 1995; 25: 966–73.
96. Meltzer EO, Orgel HA, Rogenes PR, Field EA. Nasal cytology in patients with allergic rhinitis: effects of intranasal fluticasone propionate. J Allergy Clin Immunol 1994; 94(4): 708–15.
97. Gomez E, Clague JE, Gatland D, Davies RJ. Effect of topical corticosteroids on seasonally induced increases in nasal mast cells. Br Med J 1988; 296: 1572–73.
98. Otsuka H, Denburg JA, Befus AD, Hitch D, Lapp P, Rajan RS, et al. Effect of beclomethasone dipropionate on nasal metachromatic cell sub-populations. Clin Allergy 1986; 16(6): 589–95.
99. Pipkorn U. Allergic rhinitis: diagnosis and treatment. In: Holgate S, Church MK, editors. Allergy. London: Gower Medical Publishing, 1993; 18.1–18.10.

100. Howarth PH. Allergic rhinitis: a rational choice of treatment. Respir Med 1989; 83: 179–88.
101. Gomez E, Clague JE, Gatland D, Davies RJ. Effect of topical corticosteroids on seasonally induced increases in nasal mast cells. Br Med J Clin Res 1988; 296(6636): 1572–73.
102. Lozewicz S, Wang J, Duddle J, Thomas K, Chalstrey S, Reilly G, et al. Topical glucocorticoids inhibit ativation by allergen in the upper respiratory tract. J Allergy Clin Immunol 1992; 89(5): 951–57.
103. Linder A, Venge P, Deuschl H. Eosinophil cationic protein and myeloperoxidase in nasal secretions as marker of inflammatory in allergic rhinitis. Allergy 1988; 42: 583–90.
104. Welch MJ. Topical nasal steroids for allergic rhinitis. Western J Med 1993; 158(6): 616–17.
105. Check WA, Kaliner MA. Pharmacology and pharmacokinetics of topical corticosteroids derivates used for asthma therapy. Am Rev Respir Dis 1990; 141: S 44–S 51.
106. van As A, Bronsky E, Grossman J, Meltzer E, Ratner P, Reed C. Dose tolerance study of fluticasone propionate aqueous nasal spray in patients with seasonal allergic rhinitis. Ann Allergy 1991; 67: 156–62.
107. Toogood HJ. Efficacy of topical steroids in the treatment of nasal and pulmonary diseases. Immunol Allergic Proc 13: 4, 1991; 321–29.
108. Studham JM, O'Connel F, Henderson J, Thomas VE, Fuller RW, Pride NB, et al. Effect of topical beclomethasone on histamine-induced increases in nasal airflow resistance and secretion in perennial rhinitis. Clin Otolaryngol 1993; 18: 285–90.
109. Naclerio RM, Adkinson NF, Creticos PS, Barrody FM, Hamilton RG, Norman PS. Intranasal steroids inhibit seasonal increases in ragweed-specific immunoglobulin E antibodies. J Allergy Clin Immunol 1993; 92(5): 717–21.
110. Gronborg H, Bisgaard H, Romeling F, Mygind N. Early and late nasal symptoms response to allergen challenge: Allergy 1993; 48: 87–93.
111. Juliusson S, Holmberg K, Karlsson G, Enerback L, Pipkorn U. Mast cells and mediators in the nasal mucosa after allergen challenge. Effects of four weeks' treatment with topical glucocorticoid. Clin Exp Allergy 1993; 23: 591–99.
112. Bisgaard H, Gronborg H, Mygind N, Dahl R, Lindqvist N, Venge P. Allergen-induced increase of eosinophil cationic protein in nasal lavage fluid: effect of the glucocorticoid budesonide. J Allergy Clin Immunol 1990; 85(5): 891–95.
113. Findlay S, Huber F, Garcia J, Huang L. Efficacy of once-a-day intranasal administration of triamcinolone acetonide in patients with seasonal allergic rhinitis. Ann Allergy 1992; 68: 228–32.
114. Bascom R, Wachs M, Naclerio R, Pipkorn U, Galli SJ, Lichtenstein LM. Basophil influx occurs after nasal antigen challenge: effects of topical corticosteroid pretreatment. J Allergy Clin Immunol 1988; 81: 580–89.
115. Mygind N. Glucocorticosteroids and rhinitis [Review]. Allergy 1993; 48: 476–90.
116. Ward MJ. Inhaled corticosteroids-effect on bone? Respir Med 1993; 87(suppl A): 33–36.
117. Mabry RL. Uses and misuses of intranasal corticosteroids and cromolyn. Am J Rhinol 1991; 5: 121–24.
118. Feiss G, Morris R, Rom D, Mansfield L, Dockhorn R, Ellis E, et al. A comparative study of the effects of intranasal triamcinolone acetonide aerosol (ITTA) and prednisone on adrenocortical function. J Allergy Clin Immunol 1992; 89: 1151–56.
119. Wolthers OD, Pedersen S. Short-term growth in children with allergic rhinitis treated with oral antihistamine, depot and intranasal glucocorticosteroids. Acta Paediatr 1993; 82: 635–40.
120. Banov CH, Woehler TR, LaForce C, Pearlman DS, Blumenthal MN, Morgan WF, et al. Once daily intranasal fluticasone propionate is effective for perennial allergic rhinitis. Ann Allergy 1994; 73: 240–46.
121. Dolovich J, Wong AG, Chodirker WB, Drouin MA, Hargreave FE, Herbert J, et al. Multicenter trial fluticasone propionate aqueous nasal spray in ragweed allergic rhinitis. Ann Allergy 1994; 73: 147–53.
122. van As A, Bronsky EA, Dockhorn RJ, Grossman J, Lumry W, Meltzer EO, et al. Once daily fluticasone propionate is as effective for perennial as twice daily beclomethasone dipproprionate. J Allergy Immunol 1993; 91(6): 1146–54.
123. Haye R, Gomez EG. A multicentre study to assess long-term use of fluticasone propionate aqueous nasal spray in comparison with beclomethasone dipropionate aqueous nasal spray in the treatment of perennial rhinitis. Rhinology 1993; 31(4): 169–74.

124. Meltzer EO, Orgel HA, Bronsky EA, Furukawa CT, Grossman J, LaForce CF, et al. A dose-ranging study of fluticasone propionate aqueous nasal spray for seasonal allergic rhinitis assessed by symptoms, rhinomanometry and nasal cytology. J Allergy Clin Immunol 1990; 86(2): 221–30.
125. Meltzer EO. Is the successful control of perennial rhinitis achievable? Eur Respir Rev 1994; 4(20): 266–70.
126. Ratner PH, Paull BR, Findlay SR, Hampel F, Martin B, Krai KM, et al. Fluticasone propionate given once daily is as effective for seasonal allergic rhinitis as beclomethasone dipropionate given twice daily. J Allergy Clin Immunol 1992; 90: 285–91.
127. Darnell R, Pecoud A, Richards DH. A double-blind comparison of fluticasone propionate aqueous nasal spray, terfenadine tablets and placebo in the treatment of patients with seasonal allergic rhinitis to grass pollen. Clin Exp Allergy 1994; 24: 1144–50.
128. Charpin D, Vervloet D. Treating seasonal rhinitis: antihistamines or intranasal corticosteroids? Eur Respir Rev 1994; 4(20): 256–59.
129. Grossman J, Banov C, Bronsky EA, Nathan RA, Pearlman D, Winder JA, et al. Fluticasone propionate aqueous nasal spray is safe and effective for children with seasonal allergic rhinitis. Pediatrics 1993; 92(4): 594–99.
130. Boner A, Sette L, Martinati L, Sharma RK, Richards DH. The efficacy and tolerability of fluticasone propionate aqueous nasal spray in children with seasonal allergic rhinitis. Allergy 1995; 50: 498–505.
131. Boner AL, Sette L. Rhinitis is children: efficacy and safety of a new intranasal corticosteroid. Eur Respir Rev 1994; 4(20): 271–73.
132. Harding SM. The human pharmacology of fluticasone propionate. Respir Med 1990; 84(suppl A): 25–29.
133. Phillipps GH. Structure-activity relationships of topically active steroids: the selection of fluticasone propionate. Respir Med 1990; 84(suppl A): 19–23.
134. Juniper EF, Guyatt GH, Archer B, Ferrie PJ. Aqueous beclomethasone dipropionate in the treatment of ragweed pollen-induced rhinitis: further exploration of "as needed" use. J Allergy Clin Immunol 1993; 92: 66–72.
135. Juniper EF, Kline PA, Hargreave FE, Dolovich J. Comparison of beclomethasone dipropionate aqueous nasal spray, astemizole, and the combination in the prophylactic treatment of ragweed-induced rhinoconjunctivitis. J Allergy Clin Immunol 1989; 83(3): 627–33.
136. Bunnag C, Jareoncharsri P, Wong EC. A double-blind comparison of nasal budesonide and oral astemizole for the treatment of perennial rhinitis. Allergy 1992; 47: 313–17.
137. Wight RG, Jones AS, Beckingham E, Andersson B, Ek L. A double-blind comparison of intranasal budesonide 400 micrograms and 800 micrograms in perennial rhinitis. Clin Otolaryngology 1992; 17(4): 354–58.
138. Agertoft L, Wolthers OD, Fuglsang G, Pedersen S. Nasal powder administration of budesonide for seasonal rhinitis in children and adolescents. Pediatr Allergy Immunol 1993; 4: 152–56.
139. Day JH, Andersson CB, Briscoe MP. Efficacy and safety of intranasal budesonide in the treatment of perennial rhinitis in adults and children. Ann Allergy 1990; 64(5): 445–50.
140. Storms W, Bronsky E, Findlay S, Pearlman D, Rosenberg S, Shapiro G, et al. Once daily triamcinolone acetonide nasal spray is effective for the treatment of perennial allergic rhinitis. Ann Allergy 1991; 66(4): 329–34.
141. Welch MJ, Bronsky E, Findlay S, Pearlman DS, Southern DL, Storms WW, et al. Long-term safety of triamcinolone acetonide nasal aerosol for the treatment of perennial allergic rhinitis. Clin Ther 1994; 16(2): 253–62.
142. Welch MJ, Bronsky EA, Grossman J, Shapiro GG, Tinkelman DG, Garcia JD, et al. Clinical evaluation or triamcinolone acetonide nasal aerosol in children with perennial allergic rhinitis. Ann Allergy 1991; 67(5): 493–98.
143. Conley SF. Comparative trial of acceptability of beclomethasone dipropionate and a new formulation of flunisolide. Ann Allergy 1994; 72: 529–32.
144. Mabry RL: Corticosteroids: general considerations of systemic therapy. In: Krause HF, editor. Otolaryngic allergy and immunology. Philadelphia: WB Saunders, 1989: 182–95.
145. Laursen LC, Faurschou P, Munch EP. Intramuscular betamethasone dipropionate vs. topical beclomethasone dipropionate and placebo in hay fever. Allergy 1988; 43: 420–24.

Rhinitis: Immunopathology
and Pharmacotherapy
ed. by D. Raeburn and M. A. Giembycz

CHAPTER 6
Vasomotor Rhinitis

Jane Krasnick * and Roy Patterson

Division of Allergy-Immunology and the Ernest S. Bazley Asthma and Allergic Diseases Center of the Department of Medicine of Northwestern Memorial Hospital and Northwestern University Medical School, Chicago, Illinois, USA

1. Introduction

The differential diagnosis of rhinitis is extensive (Table 1). Vasomotor rhinitis describes a noninfectious and nonallergic perennial form of chronic rhinitis or rhinopathy. The term "nonallergic rhinitis" (though often used

* Corresponding author.

Table 1. Differential diagnosis of rhinitis

Adenoidal hypertrophy
Allergic rhinitis (perennial, seasonal)
Atrophic rhinitis
Cerebral spinal fluid rhinorrhea
Chronic sinusitis (infectious, allergic)
Ciliary disorders (dyskinetic cilia syndrome, Kartagener's syndrome)
Congenital choanal atresia
Foreign body
Granulomatous disease (sarcoidosis, Wegener's granulomatosis)
Hypothyroidism
Infectious rhinitis (bacterial, viral, fungal)
Malignant nasopharyngeal tumors
Nasal polyposis
Rhinitis medicamentosa
Rhinitis of pregnancy
Septal deviation
Syphilis
Vasomotor rhinitis

interchangeably with "vasomotor rhinitis") is a more general term referring to rhinitis without an allergic component based on negative skin tests. Symptoms vary in intensity but consist mainly of nasal congestion, rhinorrhea, postnasal discharge and sometimes sneezing. Mygind reserved the diagnosis of perennial rhinitis to patients who suffer from nasal symptoms for greater than 1 h daily for most days [1]. Symptoms of vasomotor rhinitis can mimic allergic rhinitis, but skin tests are negative, there is no characteristic seasonal variation and patients almost always lack ocular symptoms. Even if some skin test are positive, they usually do not correlate well with the patient's clinical history, i.e. positive skin test to grass allergen, with lack of seasonal variation in symptoms during spring season. It is important to make a distinction between vasomotor rhinitis and allergic rhinitis so that the correct treatment can be determined.

Vasomotor rhinitis is not exacerbated by antigen exposure; instead, symptoms can worsen spontaneously or from irritant exposure. Examples of irritant triggers of vasomotor rhinitis are listed in Table 2. Following

Table 2. Triggers of vasomotor rhinitis

Alcoholic beverages
Change in barometric pressure
Cigarette smoke (active or passive)
Cold, dry air
Exercise
Hot, spicy foods
Newsprint
Strong odors and perfumes
Upper respiratory tract infections

irritant exposure, inflammatory mediators are released, causing the nasal mucosa to become edematous. The edema can be severe, causing obstruction, overgrowth of bacteria and subsequent sinusitis.

2. Neurovascular Physiology

2.1. Autonomic Nervous System

The nasal cavity contains a rich supply of venous sinusoids, capillaries and seromucous glands. These structures have dual innervation from the autonomic nervous system. Sympathetic stimulation causes dilation and emptying of venous sinusoids, effectively causing vasoconstriction, decrease in mucosal edema and improvement in nasal airway resistance. Parasympathetic stimulation causes the opposite effect of vasodilation of capacitance vessels and mucosal swelling, with resulting symptomatology of rhinorrhea and nasal congestion. A delicate balance between sympathetic and parasympathetic innervation is essential to maintain normal nasal homeostasis. Vasomotor rhinitis is felt to be a result of autonomic dysfunction with a relative parasympathetic predominance. Following exposure to irritant stimuli there is an overexaggerated response to stimuli with a decrease in vascular tone, vasodilation and increased mucous secretion. These changes lead to symptoms of rhinorrhea, nasal congestion and post-nasal discharge.

3. Therapy for Vasomotor Rhinitis

Once the diagnosis of vasomotor rhinitis is made and other medical conditions which can mascarade as vasomotor rhinitis are eliminated, several treatment options can be explored. If irritant stimuli can be identified by clinical history, appropriate avoidance techniques should be implemented. Overall vasomotor rhinitis symptoms can be refractory to treatment efforts, causing frustration to both the patient and physician and adding substantially to medical costs. The benefits and risks of various treatment options must be weighed when considering therapy. Chronic nasal obstruction is a very significant problem for many patients and can lead to infectious sinusitis and significant morbidity. The following is a review of the current therapeutic options available for the treatment of vasomotor rhinitis.

3.1. Corticosteroids

Corticosteroids have had a major impact on the treatment of allergic diseases, including allergic rhinitis and asthma. The introduction of topical inhaled corticosteroids has greatly decreased the untoward systemic side effects without compromising efficacy. Topical nasal steroids have also been effective in the treatment of nonallergic disorders such as nonallergic rhinitis and vasomotor rhinitis.

3.1.1. Immunologic effects of corticosteroids: Corticosteroids have several effects in patients with vasomotor rhinitis. Steroids cause a decrease in inflammatory mediators and in mucosal edema and help to decrease microvascular permeability. The basic premise for the use of corticosteroids in rhinitis is for the anti-inflammatory actions. Vasomotor rhinitis, although considered to be a nonallergic form of rhinitis, may be in part be caused by inflammatory mediators.

Although systemic steroids may not inhibit the early-phase response, topical inhaled steroids have been shown to inhibit both early- and late-phase responses. After antigen challenge, treatment with corticosteroids decreases mediators such as *p*-tosyl arginine methyl ester (TAME)-esterase, histamine and kinins in patients with allergic rhinitis [2].

3.1.2. Role of corticosteroids in nonantigenic, non-IgE-mediated inflammation: Nonantigenic stimuli, such as cold, dry air, can elicit vasomotor rhinitis symptoms which correlate with a rise in inflammatory mediators such as histamine, prostaglandin D2, kinins and TAME-esterase. The release of these mediators is consistent with mast cell activation [3–7]. Nasal challenges with cold, dry air induce both an early- and late-phase reaction which correlates positively with nasal symptoms and local inflammatory mediator release [6]. Cruz et al. showed that 1 week of intranasal steroids (beclomethasone dipropionate) could inhibit the histamine induced by cold, dry air challenge but did not alter TAME-esterase levels, albumin level or symptoms. This suggested that mast cell activation was not the only mechanism involved in inflammatory mediator release secondary to nonantigenic stimulation [7].

3.1.3. Mechanism of action of corticosteroids: The lipophilic structure of corticosteroids allows rapid absorption across mucosal surfaces. After intranasal administration, unbound glucocorticoid molecules diffuse into the cell cytoplasm and bind to class-specific steroid receptors. The steroid receptor undergoes a conformational change and is translocated into the cell nucleus. Here this complex binds to a specific site called a glucocorticoid response element (GRE) which is located next to a promotor region on the cell's DNA. New specific DNA is transcribed, and subsequently new protein products are translated.

Steroid protein products have various effects, including inhibiting inflammatory mediators from basophils and mast cells and decreasing the number of lymphocytes, eosinophils, monocytes and basophils [8]. They also decrease kinins, prostaglandins and leukotrienes. Corticosteroids also decrease the sensitivity of irritant receptors and secretory responses to muscarinic cholinoceptors [9].

Steroids have also been shown to decrease mediators that cause increased microvascular permeability, which leads to exudation of protein and fluid causing nasal congestion and rhinorrhea [10]. This may be accomplished by the ability of steroids to inhibit the response of the endothelial cells to permeability-increasing mediators seen *in vivo* [11].

Glucocorticoids are known to have a vasoconstrictor effect. Topically applied glucocorticoids cause pallor or blanching of the skin. This vasoconstrictor effect is, however, questionable in patients with vasomotor rhinitis. A study by Lindqvist et al. showed that topically applied budesonide had no vasoconstrictor effect on nasal capacitance vessels and caused no change in sensitivity to α- or β-adrenoceptor stimulation [12].

The vasodilating properties of prostaglandins may also play a role in nasal congestion. Another mechanism by which corticosteroids may exert their effect is through inhibition of prostaglandin precursors. Lipocortin is a steroid protein product which inhibits release of arachidonic acid by inhibiting the enzyme phospholipase A_2. A block in the arachidonic acid pathway results in a decrease in formation of prostaglandins and leukotrienes. Recombinant lipocortin has been shown to inhibit eicosanoid-dependent edema [13, 14]. This reduction in edema may be the important effector function in relieving the nasal congestion of rhinitis.

3.1.4. Topical inhaled corticosteroids: Topical dexamethasone, a potent and long-acting steroid, was the earliest topical steroid used to treat rhinitis. Dexamethasone, however, had significant side effects, such as adrenal suppression and nasal septal perforation [15]. With the development of newer glucocorticoids (budesonide, triamcinolone, flunisolide, beclomethasone dipropionate and fluticasone) side effects have been minimized. A list of the newer inhaled topical steroids is shown in Table 3. These agents have a much lower side-effect profile due to a shorter half-life and rapid first-pass hepatic metabolism. The chemical structures of the topical steroids are shown in Figure 1.

Table 3. Topical nasal steroids

Generic name	Trade name	Dose/spray	Dose*
Beclomethasone dipropionate	Beconase, Vancenase	42 µg	1–4 sprays/day
Budesonide	Rhinocort	32 µg	4 sprays/day
Dexamethasone	Dexacort	84 µg	4–6 sprays/day
Flunisolide	Nasalide	25 µg	4–6 sprays/day
Triamcinolone	Nasacort	55 µg	1–4 sprays/day

* Recommended total daily starting dose based per each nostril.

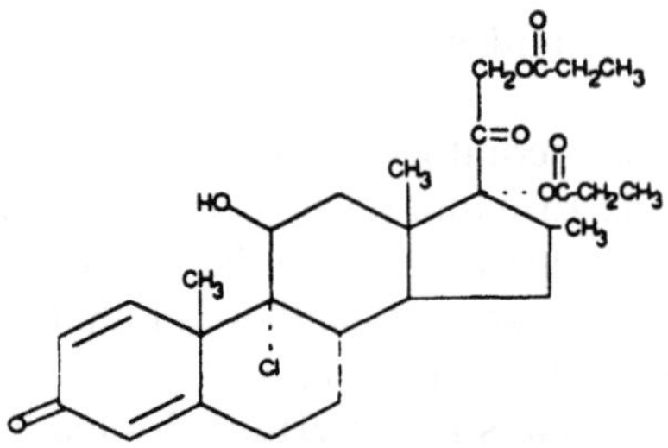

BECLOMETHASONE DIPROPIONATE

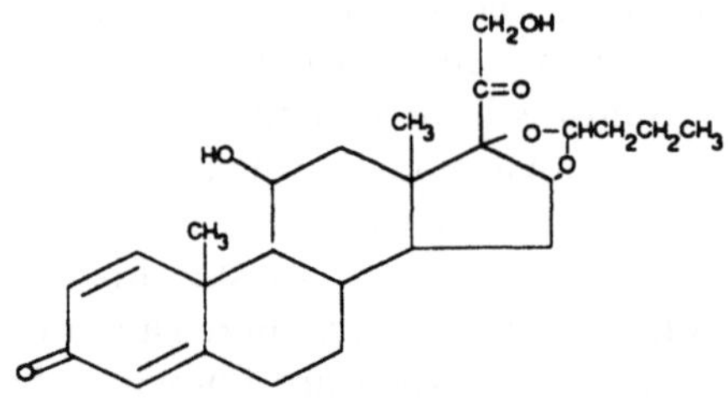

BUDESONIDE

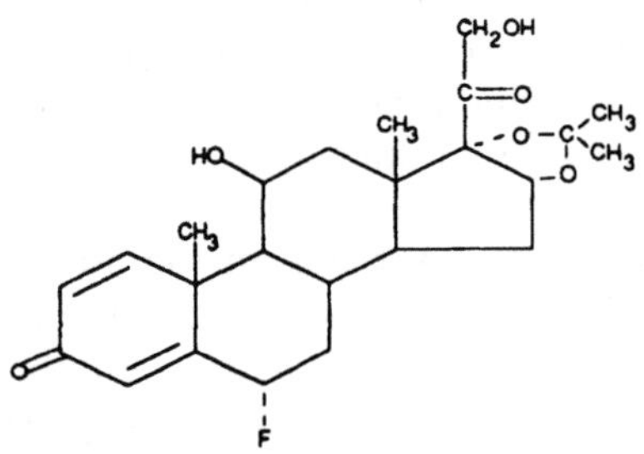

FLUNISOLIDE

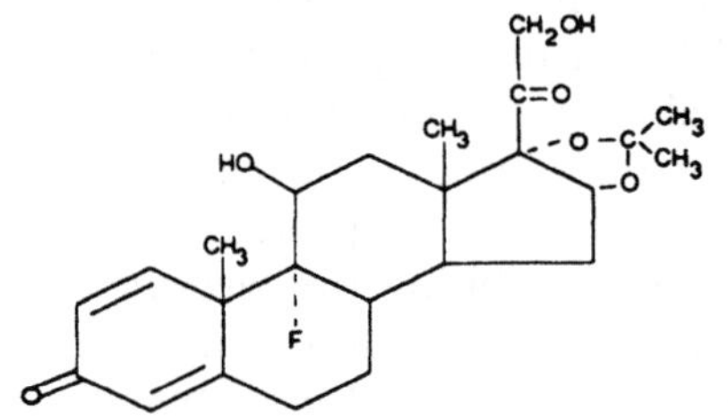

TRIAMCINOLONE ACETONIDE

Figure 1. Chemical structures of intranasal corticosteroids. Reprinted with permission from [16].

3.1.4.1. Beclomethasone dipropionate. Beclomethasone dipropionate (9-chloro-11,β,17,21-trihydroxy-16β-methylprega-1,4-diene-3,20-dione,17,21-dipropionate) was the earliest of the new synthetic topical glucocorticoids to be used for the treatment of rhinitis. It has far more glucocorticoid than mineralocorticoid activity. Two standard preparations are available, a pressurized nasal spray in a freon-propelled metered dose inhaler form (Beconase, Vancencase) which delivers 42 µg per spray and an aqueous suspension of 0.05% (Beconase AQ, Vancencase AQ). A study on patients with seasonal allergic rhinitis found that both the conventional pressurized spray and the aqueous spray were equally effective in relieving symptoms with a similar low incidence of side effects [17]. After intranasal application, the drug is absorbed rapidly and hydrolyzed to a *B*17 monopropionate moiety. This is further metabolized to free beclomethasone and finally an inactive metabolite before being excreted into the bile. The elimination half life is approximately 15 hours. Any amount of drug that is swallowed after administration is metabolized by the liver and excreted in the bile and urine. When beclomethasone dipropionate or its metabolites do appear in the systemic circulation, they are highly protein bound and have minimal systemic effect.

One of the earlier double-blind crossover studies using intranasal beclomethasone dipropionate done on patients with vasomotor rhinitis showed that 74% of patients considered themselves free of symptoms or improved after use of the drug compared with 30% of placebo users. No significant side effects such a *Candida* infection or suppression of the hypothalamic-pituitary axis were noted [18]. A study by Tarlo et al. showed that in 26 patients beclomethasone dipropionate was effective in decreasing symptoms of nasal congestion, sneezing and nasal airway resistance by 53% after 3 weeks and 73% after 6 months of therapy. Twenty-three of these patients had no evidence of allergy [19].

A double-blind trial comparing 200 μg and 400 μg of beclomethasone dipropionate versus placebo in patients with perennial rhinitis (half without evidence of allergy) after being treated for 12 months showed both doses to be effective, though some patients showed more improvement in nasal and conjunctival symptoms with the 400-μg dose. Four of the 108 patients had to reduce the dose of beclomethasone dipropionate due to epistaxis [20]. Currently, the recommended dose is one spray (42 μg) in each nostril, up to four times per day.

Overall beclomethasone dipropionate has been shown to be safe. Long-term studies performed on patients with perennial allergic rhinitis showed no evidence of mucosal damage on nasal biopsies, no evidence of *Candida* infection and only mild epistaxis [21, 22]. Others have shown that there was no evidence of atrophic rhinitis or squamous metaplasia after 1 year of therapy [23]. Although adrenal suppression from inhaled steroids has been reported for beclomethasone dipropionate, these are rare case reports [24]. Rarely, nasal septal perforation has also been reported [25]. Inhaled oral beclomethasone was shown to be used safely in the treatment of 45 pregnant asthmatics and is therefore safe for use in pregnant rhinitis patients [26].

3.1.4.2. Budesonide. Budesonide (16α,17β-butyldiene-dioxypregna-1,4-diene-11β,21-diol-3,20-dione) is a nonhalogenated corticosteroid that is metabolized rapidly in the liver after absorption. Approximately 20% of the drug reaches the systemic circulation. It is available in a freon-propelled metered dose inhaler form which delivers 32 μg per spray. The half-life is 2 h and the recommended dose is two sprays 1–2 times daily.

Pipkorn et al. evaluated 12 patients treated for 12 months with budesonide. They found that all patients ha a significant decrease in symptoms, no *Candida* infections and no change in the hypothalamic-pituitary axis by measuring cortisol levels after adrenal cortisol tropic hormone (ACTH) stimulation test. There were also no significant morphological changes in nasal mucosa before and after 1 year of therapy [27]. Twenty-four patients evaluated for up to 5.5 years showed no significant change in nasal biopsies and no adrenal suppression, and all had a decrease in symptoms of both allergic rhinitis and nonallergic rhinitis [28].

Varying doses of budesonide have been compared, and studies showed both the 400-μg and 800-μg doses of budesonide to be effective in decreasing nasal obstruction, sneezing and lacrimation, but without a difference between the doses [29]. Neither dose had a significant effect on postnasal discharge.

Mucociliary clearance has been assessed using the saccharine test, in which saccharine particles are placed on the nasal mucosa and the time for the subject to taste the saccharine is measured. In one study, after 1 week of therapy with budesonide there was a 30% decrease in mucociliary activity [30]. A similar study on beclomethasone did not show any decrease after 1 week of therapy [31].

3.1.4.3. Flunisolide. Flunisolide (6α-fluro-11β,16α,17,21 tetrahydroxy pregna-1,4-diene-3,20-dione cyclic, 16,17 acetal) is a flurodinated steroid preparation in aqueous solution (0.25%) delivered by a pump spray which gives 25 μg per spray. It is in a vehicle of 20% propylene glycol and 15% polyethylene glycol with extensive first-pass hepatic metabolism, and a half-life of 1 to 2 h [32]. Approximately 20% of the drug reaches the systemic circulation when given orally. Side effects include mild transient nasal burning. In one study of nonallergic rhinitis patients no significant decrease in total symptom score was found, and yet a substantial number of patients chose to continue flunisolide because of subjective improvement in nasal symptoms [33]. The recommended dose is two sprays each nostril up to three times per day.

3.1.4.4. Triamcinolone. Triamcinolone is (9-fluro-11β,16α 17,21-tetrahydroxypregna-1,4-diene-3,20 dione cyclic 16,17 acetal) a water-soluble halogenated corticosterioid preparation which is eight times more potent than prednisone. Peak plasma concentrations occur at 3–4 h and the half-life is approximately 4 (1–7) h long. Triamcinolone has an efficacy and side-effect profile similar to those of the other inhaled nasal steroids mentioned. The starting dose is 220 μg per day up to 440 μg per day.

3.1.5. Complications of topical nasal corticosteroids: Serial examinations of patients taking nasal steroids chronically are necessary in order to evaluate for thinning of the nasal mucosa and development of nasal septal perforation. Although these are rare side effects, Schoelzel and Menzel reported seeing eight patients within 2 years with perforated nasal septums [25]. Four patients were using beclomethasone dipropionate, one was using flunisolide, and one used a decongestant spray. Interestingly, two patients had no history of using nasal sprays. Nasal septal perforation was also reported in a 9-year-old girl who had used flunisolide for several months [34]. The perforation was preceded by crusting and ulcerations of the septum. Other reports of septal perforation from dexamethasone have been reported [35]. Our experience is that nasal septal perforation is an extremely uncommon complication, usually explained by concomitant drug abuse such as intranasal cocaine use.

3.2. Anticholinergic Therapy

Patients with vasomotor rhinitis have a hypersecreting nasal mucosa. One potential explanation is that these patients have an imbalance in their autonomic innervation of the nasal cavity with a dominance of parasympathetic over sympathetic drive. Theoretically, a drug with anticholinergic properties would be helpful for alleviating symptoms by blocking the action of acetylcholine at nerve end terminals.

3.2.1. Muscarinic cholinoceptors: The nasal cavity contains both M1 and M3 postganglionic muscarinic cholinoceptors. These receptors are responsible for the parasympathetic effects on blood vessels and seromucous glands which lead to an increase in secretions [36]. Muscarinic cholinoceptor antagonists have been beneficial, but mainly as bronchodilators in the treatment of chronic obstructive pulmonary disease.

3.2.2. Ipratropium bromide: Ipratropium bromide (Atrovent), a parasympathomimetic, is a quaternary ammonium compound derived from, *N*-isopropyl atropine. Its molecular structure is shown in Figure 2. It is available as an intranasal spray by a manual pump which delivers 70 µg per spray. Depending on the concentration 0.03 % and 0.06 %, it delivers 21 or 42 µg of ipratropium bromide per spray, respectively.

3.2.3. Metabolism of ipratropium bromide: Topical intranasal ipratropium bromide has limited central nervous system penetration and is poorly

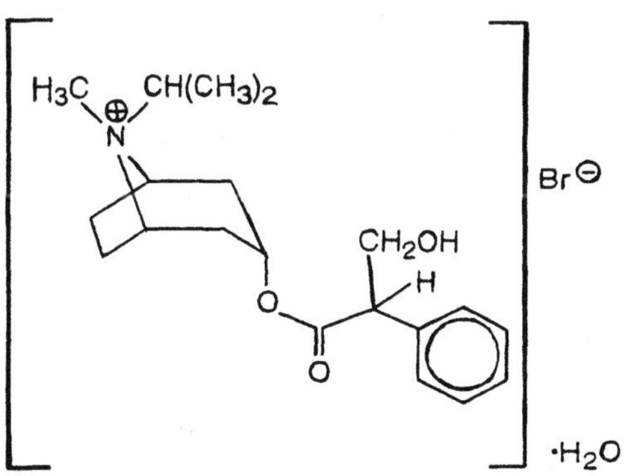

Figure 2. Chemical structure of ipratropium bromide. Reprinted with permission [37].

absorbed from the gastrointestinal mucosa. Once absorbed it is rapidly metabolized by ester hydrolysis to tropic acid and *N*-isopropylmethyl nortropium, which are both inactive. Approximately 10% of the drug reaches the systemic circulation after topical intranasal administration [37]. In one study, there was a small (10%) decrease in salivation rate, but this was felt to be of little clinical significance [38].

3.2.4. Methacholine studies: Metacholine, a muscarinic cholinoceptor agonist, usually induces bronchoconstriction at lower concentrations in patients with reactive airways disease than in normal patients. In a double-blind placebo-controlled trial, Borum was the first to show that topically applied intranasal ipratropium bromide could inhibit methacholine-induced nasal hypersecretion in normal subjects as well as patients with perennial rhinitis [39]. This effect occurred without local or systemic side effects. Serial dilutions of methacholine given by intranasal administration to both healthy volunteers and patients with nonallergic perennial rhinitis produced measurable amounts of increased nasal secretions in both groups, but significantly more secretions in patients with perennial nonallergic rhinitis [40]. Others induced increasing amounts of nasal secretions with incremental doses of intranasal methacholine (7.5, 15, 30, 60 and 120 mg/ml). When patients were pretreated with different doses of ipratropium bromide (40 µg, 100 µg and 200 µg), the volumes of secretions were significantly decreased. Each dose was effective in decreasing the volumes of secretions but the 200-µg dose was the most effective [41]. In another model of nonallergic rhinitis, Naclerio et al. showed that ipratropium bromide significantly reduced the nasal secretions stimulated by cold, dry air challenge by 60 to 70% [42].

Ipratropium bromide as been shown to be more effective than placebo in reducing the amount of rhinorrhea in patients with perennial rhinitis compared with controls [43]. Bronsky et al. [44] studied 233 patients with perennial rhinitis in an 8-week, multicenter, double-blind, randomized control group study using intranasal ipratropium bromide. They showed a 30% reduction in rhinorrhea. Ipratropium bromide was well tolerated with no evidence of nasal rebound with discontinuation of the drug. Epistaxis was seen in 9.4% of patients but was mild and did not require stopping therapy. Five percent of patients had nasal dryness. There was no evidence of an adverse effect on nasal cytology [44].

A long-term study of 285 patients treated for 1 year with an 0.03% solution of ipratropium bromide, two sprays, three times daily showed significant improvement in rhinorrhea. Approximately 10% of patients had adverse side effects of nasal dryness and epistaxis. There was only a 6% (17 patients) failure rate. There was also significant improvement in quality-of-life measurements as indicated by changes in physical activity, mental work, fatigue, irritability, sleeping, reading, depression and anxiety. The need for other rhinitis medications was also decreased from 26 to 13% [45].

A similar study using the 0.06% of ipratropium bromide dosage also provided patients with improvement in rhinorrhea. None of the above-mentioned studies showed any statistically significant improvement in other symptoms of rhinitis such as sneezing, postnasal discharge or nasal congestion [46].

Multiple studies have been conducted to determine the most effective and safest dose of ipratropium bromide [47–49]. Dolovich et al. studied 25 patients with vasomotor rhinitis treated with 20 μg in each nostril, four times daily for 3 weeks. Forty percent of patients had a decrease in severity and duration of nasal discharge. The most common side effects were nasal dryness, burning and epistaxis. They reported a higher proportion of side effects (84%) of patients than other authors [50]. In patients with vasomotor rhinitis treated with 20 and 40 μg, four times daily, both doses decreased rhinorrhea, but the 40 μg group had a slightly higher incidence of increased nasal congestion. Subsequently, the investigators recommended ipratropium bromide be given in a dose of 20 μg, four times daily [47].

Very high dose ipratropium bromide has also been studied [48]. In a double-blind crossover design trial, 80 and 400 μg, four times daily, were compared. Both doses were effective in reducing rhinorrhea, with a slightly greater effect with the 400 μg dose. Most of the side effects were confined to the nose and consisted of dryness and epistaxis. A few cases of systemic reactions occurred with the 400 μg dose. Neither dose had any effect on the number of times the patients sneezed, on nasal blockage or on nasal mucociliary transport. In addition, after cessation of therapy, no rebound of symptoms was observed with either dose.

Druce et al. studied lower dosages of ipratropium bromide. They compared 21 and 42 μg per day in 140 patients. Both doses were effective in decreasing severity and duration of rhinorrhea with no significant difference between the two doses, although there was a trend toward more improvement with the 42 μg dose. There was no change in sneezing, postnasal discharge or congestion. Sixty percent of both patients and physicians judged ipratropium bromide to be either excellent or good at controlling rhinorrhea. This study reported a higher incidence of headache (23% of patients) than did other studies [49].

The effect of ipratropium bromide in elderly patients has also been evaluated. Patients over age 60 who had watery rhinorrhea and had already failed to respond to topical nasal steroids and antihistamines were treated with ipratropium bromide. A significant decrease in the amount of nose blowing and a decrease in nasal secretions after methacholine challenge in these patients were seen [51].

Overall, ipratropium bromide is a well-tolerated drug, and is safe and effective in reducing rhinorrhea but not nasal congestion or sneezing in patients with nonallergic rhinitis [46, 52]). Side effects are mild and usually do not require discontinuation of the drug [46]. No effect on mucociliary transport has been detected with intranasal use of ipratropium bromide [53]. Patients can be safely started at a dose of 21 μg, from three to four times per day, and increased up to 84 μg, four times per day, depending on symptom control and side effects.

3.3. Decongestants

The nasal mucosa contains a rich vascular supply. Vascular tone and blood flow is regulated by adrenergic influence via α- and β-adrenoceptors. The amount of blood flow (from resistance vessels) and subsequent blood content influences nasal patency and nasal resistance. Decongestants, both oral and topical forms, have been used to vasoconstrict nasal vessels and decrease nasal resistance via action on α-adrenoceptors. Decongestants are used to improve the nasal airway for different types of rhinitis, including allergic rhinitis and rhinitis secondary to upper respiratory tract infections. Decongestants have also shown to be effective in decreasing nasal congestion in patients with nonallergic perennial rhinitis [54].

3.3.1. α_1 Adrenoceptor agonists: There are two types of vasoconstrictors, α_1 and α_2 adrenoceptor agonists.

α_1-Receptor agonists are sympathomimetic amines exemplified by ephedrine sulphate, pseudoephedrine hydrochloride and phenylpropanolamine hydrochloride. These sympathomimetic amines have both α_1 and α_2 activity except for phenylpropanolamine hydrochloride, which is α_1 selective.

3.3.2. α_2 Adrenoceptor agonists: Pure α_2 agonists are imidazole derivatives and include oxymetazoline hydrochloride, xylometazoline hydrochloride and naphazoline hydrochloride. Although α-adrenoceptor agonist vasoconstrictors are effective in decreasing nasal congestion, they have little effect on sneezing and rhinorrhea.

3.3.3. α-Adrenoceptor agonists: β-Adrenoceptors have been found in nasal mucosa but are not felt to be important in determining nasal vascular tone. Ephedrine sulphate and pseudoephedrine hydrochloride both have β_1 and β_2 activity, which may influence the physician's choice in drug selection when considering patients' coexisting medial problems and potential β-agonist side effects. An absolute contraindication to use of sympathomimetic agents is the concomitant use of monoamine oxidase inhibitors.

3.3.4. Topical nasal decongestants: In one study, a topically applied α_2 agonist (oxymetazoline) caused a rapid decrease in nasal blood flow to the nasal mucosa assessed by the xenon-washout technique. A topical α_1 agonist (phenylephrine), however, did not cause a similar decrease in blood flow. The investigators concluded that α_2 agonists were more effective in regulating resistance vessels, but an α_1 agonist preparation may be preferred to decongest the nose without reduction blood flow [55].

Bende et al. have shown that topical phenylephrine produces a dose-dependent decongestant effect as measured by rhinometric techniques [56]. A correlation of decrease in nasal airway resistance and decrease in nasal blood flow which lasted up to 6 h has been demonstrated with topical oxymetazoline [57].

3.3.5. Rhinitis medicamentosa and other adverse side effects: Topical decongestants provide excellent initial relief of nasal congestion, but prolonged use as early as 4–6 days can cause rebound nasal congestion and worsening of symptoms. Rebounded nasal congestion causes the patient to increase the use of the drug to obtain the same decongestion results. One possibility is that the vasoconstriction caused by α-adrenoceptor stimulation causes nasal mucosa hypoxia and resultant vasodilation. This rebound effect is known as rhinitis medicamentosa or rhinitis caused by medications [58].

Topical nasal decongestants also can cause histologically confirmed damage to the nasal mucosa and decrease in mucociliary clearance. A study of 30 patients using topical nasal decongestants for various reasons including allergic rhinitis, nonallergic rhinitis, upper respiratory tract infections, deviated septum and hypertrophic rhinitis, revealed histopathological changes after use ranging from 2 weeks to 10 years. These changes included increased friability of nasal mucosa with destruction and edema of epithelial lining, dilated blood vessels, abnormal cilia, hyperplastic changes in capillaries, and irregular and dystrophic columnar epithelial cells. After stopping the nasal decongestants and substituting nasal steroids, the epithelium returned to normal. Mucociliary clearance was also shown to be decreased by the saccharine test [59].

Treatment for rhinitis medicamentosa due to α-adrenoceptor agonist exposure consists of discontinuation of the drug and substitution with nasal steroids. Sometimes, in severe cases, a short course of oral corticosteroids (20–30 mg of prednisone daily for 3 days) may be necessary to act as bridge for the patient until the effects of rebound vasodilation subside and the effects of the nasal steroid takes effect.

The β-adrenoceptor agonist-associated side effects of decongestants (listed in Table 4) must be considered in those patients with other coexisting medical problems such as hypertension, tachyarrythmias and glaucoma [60]. Horowitz et al. demonstrated the hypertensive effects of a single capsule of phenylpropanolamine in normal subjects. In 37 subjects, all had some elevation of supine diastolic blood pressure within 1 h of ingestion of 85 mg of the decongestant drug, with a mean rise of 24 mmHg in diastolic

Table 4. Side effects of decongestants

Bladder outlet obstruction
Glaucoma
Hypertension
Impaired gastrointestinal mobility
Insomnia
Nervousness
Palpitations
Tachycardia
Tremulousness

blood pressure [61]. Severe hypertension following ingestion of 170 mg of phenylpropanolamine, causing an intracerebral hemorrhage, has also been reported in one patient [62].

3.4. Antihistamines

Antihistamines (histamine receptor antagonists) have been used for many years in treating patients with allergic rhinitis, chronic urticaria and atopic dermatitis. Few studies looked at the role of antihistamines in vasomotor rhinitis. Antihistamines for nasal therapy are specifically H_1-receptor antagonists. Wihl et al. compared the effect of astemizole, a nonsedating selective H_1-receptor antagonist in both patients with allergic and nonallergic rhinitis. He found that astemizole had a statistically significant effect in decreasing the amount of sneezing and nose blowing with a marginal effect on nasal blockage in both groups. When a nasal steroid (beclomethasone dipropionate) was added to the antihistamine, nasal blockage improved and the number of sneezes and nose blowing dropped further [63]. Antihistamines may be helpful in treating patients with vasomotor rhinitis, especially when rhinorrhea is the predominating symptom secondary to the anticholingergic, drying effect on the nasal mucosa.

3.5. Capsaicin

Capsaicin is a peptide derived from *Capsicum* plants which has been shown to decrease symptoms of chronic nonallergic rhinitis. Its molecular structure is shown in Figure 3. Although capsaicin is not currently marketed for the treatment of vasomotor rhinitis, its effect on sensory neurones is interesting. The mechanism of action of capsaicin on neurones is believed to be twofold. First an excitatory phase occurs with depolarization of nerve endings and transmitter release causing generation of the neural efferent impulse. Subsequently, the sensory neurone action is blocked, possibly by

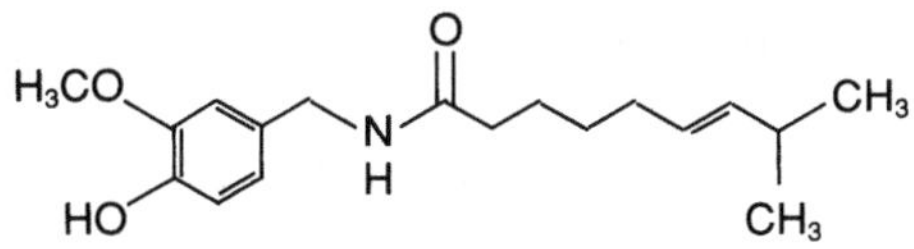

Figure 3. Chemical structure of capsaicin.

neuropeptide depletion, with the nerve terminal becoming refractory to capsaicin and other stimuli.

In one study of 20 patients with vasomotor rhinitis treated with nine doses of capsaicin (15 µg per dose) over 3 days, the patients initially complained of painful burning, nasal obstruction and occasional sneezing. By the ninth application, the patients demonstrated tachyphylaxis with 100% decrease in rhinorrhea and nasal congestion and 80% decrease in local pain. All patients showed a 50% decrease in symptom score after 1 month follow-up. Patients also showed no gross changes on rhinoscopy, and the drug was well tolerated [64].

Lacroix studied patients with vasomotor rhinitis treated with capsaicin (25 µg intranasal) weekly for 5 weeks. Symptom scores were recorded, and nasal biopsies were performed before and 6 months after treatment. Levels of calcitonin gene-related peptide (CGRP), a neuropeptide with vasodilator properties present in sensory nerves, were also measured. Patients with vasomotor rhinitis had more discomfort and vascular responses than did controls, yet showed marked reduction of symptoms even after 6 months of follow-up. Radioimmunoassay of nasal biopsies showed a 50% reduction of CGRP, supporting the hypothesis that capsaicin desesitization is associated with depletion of peptides from sensory nerves [65].

4. Rhinitis in Pregnancy

Rhinitis symptoms occur in up to 30% of pregnant women [66]. The differential diagnosis of rhinitis includes new onset allergic rhinitis, nasal polyps, infectious sinusitis and rhinitis of pregnancy. It is not surprising that patients may present with rhinitis for the first time, as allergic rhinitis may occur in up to 20% of women of child-bearing age [67].

Rhinitis of pregnancy is a form of rhinitis that usually occurs in the second trimester and continues until parturition. Symptoms can vary but usually consist of nasal congestion. Congestion can be severe, causing disturbance in sleep, increased sense of dyspnea and bacterial sinusitis.

The cause of rhinitis during pregnancy is in part secondary to the effects of increased sex hormones acting locally in the nasal mucosa. The increased circulating blood volume also contributes to increased vascular pooling and mucosal edema.

4.1. Histochemical Changes in the Nasal Mucosa during Pregnancy

Toppozada et al. studied the ultrastructure and histochemical changes seen in the nasal mucosa in both nonpregnant women receiving estrogen and in pregnant women [68, 69]. He found that asymptomatic women in both groups had glandular hyperactivity, increased acid mucopolysaccharide content of the ground substance and increased phagocytic activity. Symptomatic women, however, had glandular hyperactivity along with vascular congestion, dilation and increased extracellular fluid. Evidence of increased secretory activity of the seromucinous glands was shown by the increase in succinic dehydrogenase enzyme activity and increased α-esterase and alkaline phosphatase enzyme activity. These changes were similar to changes seen in nasal biopsies obtained from patients with chronic hypertrophic nonallergic rhinitis [70]. In symptomatic pregnant patients, there was also an increase in choline esterase enzyme activity, indicating that an increased parasympathetic influence was present causing an increase in secretions and vasodilation.

4.2. Medications in Pregnancy

The risk and benefits of the various treatment options must be weighed before deciding on specific medications in any pregnant patient. The benefits of decreasing nasal obstruction to provide improved sleep and prevent infectious sinusitis must be considered and discussed with the patient and the patient's obstetrician. In patients who have worsening of their asthma symptoms secondary to sinusitis, therapy should be strongly considered.

The use of nasal steroids is first-line therapy for the rhinitis of pregnancy. Beclomethasone dipropionate has been used safely in pregnancy in treatment of pregnant asthmatics [26, 71, 72]. Greenberger et al. reported use of inhaled beclomethasone during 45 pregnancies without direct evidence of teratogenic effect or neonatal adrenal insufficiency [26].

Data from the Collaborative Perinatal Project (CPP) of the National Institute of Neurologic and Communicative Disorders and Stroke showed that in 3082 mother-child exposures during 4 lunar months of pregnancy exposed to all sympathomimetic drugs, there were 249 malformed children with a hospital standardized relative risk of 1.19. There were 39 exposures to pseudoephedrine with only 1 malformed child and a relative risk of 0.35 [73]. Although many institutions use decongestants, the authors do not use vasoconstrictors because of the potential vasoconstricting effects on the uterine vessels. Ipratropium bromide is not currently indicated for the treatment of rhinitis during pregnancy.

5. Nonallergic Rhinitis with Eosinophils (NARES)

Nonallergic rhinitis with eosinophils or NARES syndrome includes patients with vasomotor rhinitis with 25 % nasal eosinophilia on nasal smears. They are unique in that they have a higher incidence of nasal polyps and higher response to therapy. Mullarkey et al. compared patients with NARES to patients with seasonal allergic rhinitis, perennial allergic rhinitis and vasomotor rhinitis without eosinophils. NARES patients had the highest response rate to antihistamines (83 %). In those patients that had failed antihistamine therapy, 93 % responded to a course of oral followed by intranasal steroids. Although treatment recommendations are the same regardless of the presence of eosinophils, the detection of eosinophils may help predict a patient's response to therapy [74].

6. Treatment Recommendations

Selecting medications in the treatment of patients with vasomotor rhinitis depends on the predominant symptom. An initial trial of intranasal steroids and oral decongestants is safe and effective and reasonable for patients, and most patients will have satisfactory control. Patients with mixed rhinitis (both an allergic and nonallergic component) may benefit from nasal steroids as well as an antihistamine-decongestant combination preparation. In patients with rhinorrhea as a predominant symptom who have failed intranasal steroids and oral decongestants, a trial of intranasal ipratropium bromide should be considered. Chronic use of topical intranasal vasoconstrictors and oral steroids is not recommended.

7. Anosmia

Special attention should be given to patients who present with olfactory loss. Patients with anosmia, in the setting of allergic rhinitis, may have olfactory loss due to inflammatory effects on the olfactory epithelium [75–76]. Mechanical obstruction from either congestion or nasal polyps can occur from both allergic or nonallergic rhinitis. When obstruction is the cause of olfactory loss, a short course of oral corticosteroids is used to decrease obstruction, followed by intranasal corticosteroids. Olfactory loss secondary to rhinitis should be reversible. The short course of oral prednisone can sometimes serve as both a diagnostic and therapeutic trial. If olfaction does not return with appropriate treatment for rhinitis, then other causes of anosmia should be investigated.

8. Treatment Failures

As mentioned previously, patients with vasomotor rhinitis do not respond as well as patients with seasonal allergic rhinitis. Patients are often frustrated because they cannot identify "an allergen" which they can avoid to relieve their symptoms. Often a combination of nasal steroids and decongestants is used to abate symptoms, but patients continue to have symptoms despite maximal medial therapy.

When patients present with bilateral nasal obstruction, a short course of prednisone (20–30 mg daily for 3–5 days) can be helpful to relieve obstruction as topical nasal steroids take effect. Chronic oral steroid use, however, is not appropriate therapy for a non-life-threatening disorder.

When patients present with refractory symptoms of vasomotor rhinitis, it is important to reassess the patient for other factors that may be contributing to the symptoms. A thorough history should be obtained inquiring about any new medications the patient may be taking that may exacerbate rhinitis, such as certain antihypertensive medications (Table 5). The patient should be asked if any changes in the environment have occurred. If the patient has acquired a new pet, consider repeat skin testing to rule out the possibility of the development an new IgE-mediated allergy.

In patients who complain of a change in their usual symptomatology, such as foul odor or bloody discharge, the physician is obligated to look for

Table 5. Antihypertensive drugs that cause rhinitis

Trade name	Generic name	Symptoms
Aldomet	Methyldopa	Nasal stuffiness
Apresoline	Hydralazine	Nasal congestion, dyspnea
Catapres	Clonidine	Dryness of nasal mucosa
Corgard	Nadalol	Nasal stuffiness, bronchospasm, cough
Harmonyl	Deserpidene	Bronchospasm in asthmatics, nasal congestion, dyspnea
Ismelin	Guanethidine	Dyspnea, asthma in susceptible individuals, nasal congestion
Minipress	Prazosin	Nasal congestion
Normodyne	Labetalol	Nasal stuffiness, wheezing
Raudixin	Rauwolfia Serpentina	Nasal congestion, dyspnea
Regroton	Chlorthalidone and reserpine	Nasal congestion, dyspnea
Serpasil	Reserpine	Nasal congestion, dyspnea
Trandate	Labetolol	Nasal stuffiness, dyspnea, bronchospasm
Wytensis	Guanabenz acetate	Nasal stuffiness, dyspnea

Reprinted with permission from Dr. G. A. Settipane [77].

a coexisting infection, foreign body (especially in children), a malignant tumor or the development of obstructing nasal polyps. Diagnostic modalities that may be appropriate in such circumstances include rhinoscopic exam, biopsy and possible radiographic imaging of the sinuses.

9. Nasal Neurosis

Patients with vasomotor rhinitis often have symptoms refractory to treatment. Unfortunately, in some patients after re-evaluating with a thorough history (including assessing compliance) and physical examination, no alternative diagnosis can be given to explain continued symptoms, and the patient must accept the chronic nature of the disease. Other patients often are fixated on their nasal symptoms and have subjective complaints out of proportion to objective findings. We refer to these patients as having a nasal neurosis. It is important to identify this subpopulation of patients in order to avoid the prescription of unnecessary medications and diagnostic tests. Some patients with nasal neurosis may benefit from psychiatric counseling. Others will totally resist any implications that their problem is not organic and not due to an allergen in their environment. Limiting therapy to the use of safe medications, avoidance of unnecessary nasal surgery and reassurance is the best that can be offered to these patients, but a successful outcome is not often seen.

Acknowledgements

This work was supported by a grant from Rhône-Poulenc Rorer, Inc.

References

1. Mygind N. Perennial rhinitis. In: Nasal allergy, 2nd ed., Oxford: Blackwell Scientific Publications, 1979: 224–32.
2. Pipkorn U, Proud D, Lichtenstein LM, Kagey-Sobotka A, Norman PS, Naclerio RM. Inhibition of mediator release in allergic rhinitis by pretreatment with topical glucocorticoids. N Engl J Med 1987; 316: 1506–10.
3. Togias A, Naclerio RM, Proud D, Pipkorn U, Bascom R, Iliopoulos, et al. Studies on the allergic and nonallergic nasal inflammation. J Allergy Clin Immunol 1988; 81: 782–90.
4. Togias AG, Proud D, Lichtenstein LM, Adams III GK, Norman PS, Kagey-Sobotka A, et al. The osmolality of nasal secretions increases when inflammatory mediators are released in response to inhalation of cold, dry air. Am Rev Respir Dis 1988; 137: 625–29.
5. Togias AG, Naclerio RM, Proud D, Fish JE, Adkinson JR NF, Kagey-Sobotka A, et al. Nasal challenge with cold, dry air results in release of inflammatory mediators: possible mast cell involvement. J Clin Invest 1985; 76: 1375–81.
6. Iliopoulos O, Proud D, Norman PS, Lichtenstein LM, Kagey-Sobotka A, Naclerio RM. Nasal challenge with cold, dry air induces a late-phase reaction. Am Rev Respir Dis 1988; 138: 400–5.
7. Cruz AA, Togias AG, Lichtenstein LM, Kagey-Sobotka A, Proud D, Naclerio RM. Steroid-induced reduction of histamine release does not alter the clinical nasal response to cold, dry air. Am Rev Respir Dis 1991; 143: 761–65.

8. Saavedra-Delgado AMP, Mathews KP, Pan PM, Kay DR, Muilenberg ML. Dose-response studies of the suppression of whole blood histamine and basophil counts by prednisone. J Allergy Clin Immunol 1980; 66: 464–71.
9. Malm L, Wihl JA, Lamm CJ, Lindquist N. Reduction of methacholine-induced nasal secretion by treatment with a new inhaled topical steroid in perennial non-allergic rhinitis. Allergy 1981; 36: 209–14.
10. Williams TJ, Yarwood H. Effect of glucocorticoids on microvascular permeability. Am Rev Respir Dis 1990; 141: S39–S43.
11. Tsurufuji S, Sugio K, Takemasa F. The role of glucocorticoid receptor and gene expression in the anti-inflammatory action of dexamethasone. Nature 1979; 280: 408–10.
12. Lindqvist N, Holmberg K, Pipkorn U. Intranasally administered budesonide, a glucocorticoid, does not exert its clinical effect through vasoconstriction. Clin Otolaryngol 1989; 14: 519–23.
13. Peers SH, Flower RJ. The role of lipocortin in corticosteroid actions. Am Rev Respir Dis 1990; 141: S18–S21.
14. Flower RJ. Lipocortin and the mechanism of action of the glucocorticoid. Br J Pharmacol 1988; 94: 987–1015.
15. Norman PS, Winkenwerder WL, Agbayni BF, Migeon CJ, et al. Adrenal function during the use of dexamethasone aerosols in the treatment of ragweed hay fever. J Allergy 1967; 40: 57–61.
16. Schleimer RP. Glucocorticoids. In: Middleton E Jr, Reed CE, Ellis EF, Adkins NF Jr, Yuninger JW, Busse WW, editors. Allergy principles and practice. St Louis: Mosby, 1993: 896.
17. Sidwell S. A comparison of the efficacy and tolerance of an aqueous beclomethasone dipropionate nasal spray with the conventional pressurized spray. Curr Med Res Opin 1983; 8: 659–64.
18. Lofkvist T, Svensson G. Treatment of vasomotor rhinitis with intranasal beclomethasone dipropionate (Bectide). Acta Allergologica 1976; 31: 227–38.
19. Tarlo SM, Cockcroft DW, Dolovich J, Hargreave FE. Beclomethasone dipropionate aerosol in perennial rhinitis. J Allergy Clin Immunol 1976; 59: 232–36.
20. Bromptom Hospital Medical Research Council Collaborative Trial. Double-blind trial comparing two dosage schedules of beclomethasone dipropionate aerosol with a placebo in the treatment of perennial rhinitis for twelve months. Clin Allergy 1980; 10: 239–51.
21. Brown HM, Storey G, Jackson FA. Beclomethasone dipropionate aerosol in treatment of perennial and seasonal rhinitis: A review of five years experience. Br J Clin Pharmacol 1977; 4: 283S–86S.
22. Holopainen E, Malmberg H, Binder E. Long-term follow-up of intra-nasal beclomethasone treatment: a clinical and historic study. Acta Otolaryngol 1982; S386: 270–73.
23. Mygind N. Effects of beclomethasone dipropionate aerosol on nasal mucosa. Br J Clin Pharacol 1977; 4: 287S–91S.
24. Sorkin S, Warren D. Probable adrenal suppression from intranasal beclomethasone. J Fam Pract 1986; 22: 449–50.
25. Schoelzel EP, Menzel ML. Nasal sprays and perforation of the nasal septum. J Am Med Assoc 1985; 252: 2046.
26. Greenberger PA, Patterson R. Beclomethasone dipropionate for severe asthma during pregnancy. Ann Intern Med 1983; 98: 478–80.
27. Pipkorn U, Berge T. Long-term treatment with budesonide in vasomotor rhinitis. Acta Otolaryngol 1983; 95: 167–71.
28. Pipkorn U, Pukander J, Suonpaa J, Makinens J, Lindqvist N. Long-term safety of budesonide nasal aerosol: a 5.5-year follow-up study. Clin Allergy 1988; 18: 253–59.
29. Wight RG, Jones AS, Beckingham E, Andersson B, Ek L. A double blind comparison of intranasal budesonide 400 µg and 800 µg in perennial rhinitis. Clin Otolaryngol 1992; 17: 354–58.
30. Holmberg K, Pipkorn U. Mucociliary transport in the human nose: effect of topical glucocorticoid treatment. Rhinology 1985; 23: 181–85.
31. Holmberg K, Pipkorn U. Influence of topical beclomethasone dipropionate suspension on human nasal mucociliary activity. Eur J Clin Pharmacol 1986; 30: 625–27.
32. Chaplin MD, Rooks II W, Swenson EW, Cooper WC, Nerenberg C, Chu NI, Flunisolide metabolism and dynamics of a metabolite. Clin Pharmacol Ther 1980; 27: 402–13.
33. Turkeltaub PC, Norman PS, Johnson JD, Crepea S. Treatment of seasonal and perennial rhinitis with intranasal flunisolide. Allergy 1982; 37: 303–11.

34. Soderberg-Warner ML. Nasal septal perforation associated with topical corticosteroid therapy. J Pediatr 1984; 105: 840–41.
35. Miller FF. Occurrence of nasal septal perforation with use of intranasal dexamethasone aerosol. Ann Allergy 1975:34: 107–9.
36. White MV. Muscarinic receptors in human airways. J Allergy Clin Immunol 1995; 95: 1065–68.
37. Wood CC, Fireman P, Grossman J, Wecker M, MacGregor T. Product characteristics and pharmacokinetics of intranasal ipratropium bromide. J Allergy Clin Immunol 1995; 95: 1111–16.
38. Kaila T, Suonpaa J, Grenman R, Iisalo E. Vasomotor rhinitis and the systemic absorption of ipratropium bromide. Rhinology 1990; 28: 83–89.
39. Borum P. Intranasal ipratropium: inhibition of methacholine-induced hypersecretion. Rhinology 1978; 16: 225–33.
40. Borum P. Nasal methacholine challenge: a test for the measurement of nasal reactivity. J Allergy Clin Immunol 1979; 63: 253–57.
41. Sjogren I, Jonsson L, Koling A, Jansson C, Osterman K, Hakansson B. The effect of ipratropium bromide on nasal hypersecretion induced by methacholine in patients with vasomotor rhinitis. Acta Otolaryngol 1988; 106: 453–59.
42. Naclerio RM, Baroody FM. *In vivo* human models for the study of anticholinergic drugs. J Alergy Clin Immunol 1995; 95: 1069–79.
43. Borum P, Mygind N, Larsen FS. Intranasal ipratropium: a new treatment for perennial rhinitis. Clin Otolaryngol 1979; 4: 407–11.
44. Bronsky EA, Druce H, Findlay SR, Hampel FC, Kaiser HK, Ratner P, et al. A clinical trial of ipratropium bromide nasal spray in patients with perennial nonallergic rhinitis. J Allergy Clin Immunol 1995; 95: 1117–22.
45. Grossman J, Banov C, Boggs P, Bronsky EA, Dockhorn RJ, Druce H, et al. Use of ipratropium bromide nasal spray in chronic treatment of nonallergic perennial rhinitis, alone and in combination with other perennial rhinitis medications. J Allergy Clin Immunol 1995; 95: 1123–27.
46. Kaiser HB, Findlay SR, Georgitis JW, Grossman J, Ratner PH, Tinkelman DG, et al. Long-term treatment of perennial allergic rhinitis with ipratropium bromide nasal spray 0.06%. J Allergy Clin Immunol 1995; 95: 1128–32.
47. Dolovich J, Mukherjee J, Salvatori VA. Intranasal ipratropium bromide to control the hypersecretion of vasomotor rhinitis: a dose-response study. Am J Rhinology 1989; 3: 221–24.
48. Kirkegaard J, Mygind N, Molgaard F, Grahne B, Holopainen E, Malberg H, et al. Ordinary and high-dose ipratropium in perennial nonallergic rhinitis. J Allergy Clin Immunol 1987; 79: 585–90.
49. Druce HM, Spector SL, Fireman P, Kaiser H, Meltzer EO, Boggs P, et al. Double-blind study of intranasal ipratropium bromide in nonallergic perennial rhinitis. Ann Allergy 1992; 69: 53–60.
50. Dolovich J, Kennedy L, Vickerson F, Kazim F. Control of the hypersecretion of vasomotor rhinitis by topical ipratropium bromide. J Allergy Clin Immunol 1987; 80: 274–78.
51. Malmberg H, Grahne B, Holopainen E, Binder E. Ipratropium (Atrovent) in the treatment of vasomotor rhinitis of elderly patients. Clin Otolaryngol 1983; 8: 273–76.
52. Milford CA, Mugliston TA, Lund VJ, Mackay, IS. Long-term safety and efficacy study of intranasal ipratropium bromide. J Laryngol Otol 1990; 104: 123–25.
53. Ohi M, Sakakura Y, Murai S, Miyoshi Y. Effect of ipratropium bromide on nasal mucociliary transport. Rhinology 1984; 22: 241–46.
54. Broms P, Malm L. Oral vasoconstrictors in perennial non allergic rhinitis. Allergy 1982; 32: 67–74.
55. Andersson KE, Bende M. Adrenoreceptors in the control of human nasal mucosal blood flow. Ann Otol Rhinol Laqryngol 1984; 93: 179–82.
56. Bende M, Andersson KE; Johansson CJ, Sjogren C, Svensson G. Dose-response relationship of a topical nasal decongestant: phenylpropanolamine. Acta Otolaryngol 1984; 98: 543–47.
57. Bende M, Loth S. Vascular effects of topical oxymetazoline on human nasal ucosa. J Laryngol Otol 1986; 100: 285–88.
58. Black MJ, Remsen KA. Rhinitis medicamentosa. Can Med Assoc J 1980; 122: 881–84.

59. Jing-ging W, Guo-xuan B. Studies of rhinitis medicamentosa. Chinese Med J 1991; 104: 60–63.
60. Pontel P. Toxicity of the over-the-counter stimulants. J Am Med Assoc 1984; 252: 1898–1903.
61. Horowitz JD, Howes LG, Christophidis N, Lang WJ, Fennessy MR, Rand MJ, et al. Hypertensive responses induced by phenylpropanolamine in anorectic and decongestant preparations. Lancet 1980; 1: 60–61.
62. King J. Hypertension and cerebral haemorrhage after trimolets ingestion. Med J Aust 1979; 2: 258.
63. Wihl JA, Petersen BN, Petersen LN, Gundersen G, Bresson K, Mygind N. Effect of the nonsedative H_1-receptor antagonist astemizole in perennial allergic an nonallergic rhinitis. J Allergy Clin Imunol 1985; 75: 720–27.
64. Marabini S, Ciabatti PG, Polli G, Fusco BM, Geppetti P. Beneficial effects of intranasal applications of capsaicin in patients with vasomotor rhinitis. Eur Arch Otorhinolaryngol 1991; 248: 191–94.
65. Lacroix JS, Buvelot JM, Polla BS, Lundberg JM. Improvement of symptoms on non-allergic chronic rhinitis by local treatment with capsaicin. Clin Exp Allergy 1991; 21: 595–600.
66. Mabry RL. Intranasal steroid injection during pregnancy. South Med J 1980; 73: 1176–79.
67. Hagy GW, Settipane GA. Bronchial asthma, allergic rhinitis and allergy skin tests among college students. J Allergy 1969; 18: 323–32.
68. Toppozada H, Michaels L, Toppozada M, El-Ghazzawi I, Talaat M, Elwany S. The human respiratory nasal mucosa in pregnancy. J Laryngol Otol 1982; 96: 613–26.
69. Toppozada H, Toppozada M, El-Ghazzawi I, Elwany S. The human respiratory nasal mucosa in females using contraceptive pills. J Laryngol Otol 1984; 98: 43–51.
70. Toppozada H, El-Mansour A, El-Ghazzawi I, Mandour M. Chronic non-allergic hypertrophic rhinitis. Acta Otolaryngol 1979; 87: 324–29.
71. Apter AJ, Greenberger PA, Patterson R. Outcomes of pregnancy in adolescents with severe asthma. Arch Int Med 1989; 149: 2571–75.
72. Greenberger PA, Patterson R. The outcome of pregnancy complicated by severe asthma. Allergy Proc 1988; 9: 539–43.
73. Heinonen OP, Slone D, Shapiro S. Drugs affecting the autonomic nervous system. In: Kaufman B, editor. Birth defects and drugs in pregnancy. Littelton: Publishing Sciences Group Inc., 1977: 345–49.
74. Mullarkey MF, Hill JS, Webb DR. Allergic and nonallergic rhinitis: their characterization and attention to the meaning of nasal eosinophilia. J Allergy Clin Immunol 1979; 65: 122–26.
75. Apter AJ, Mott AE, Cain WS, Spiro JD, Barwick MC. Olfactory loss and allergic rhinitis. J Allergy Clin Immunol 1992; 90: 670–80.
76. Apter AJ, Mott AE, Frank ME, Clive JM. Allergic rhinitis and olfactory loss. Ann Allergy 1995; 75: 311–16.
77. Settipane GA. Rhinitis, 2nd ed. Providence: Oceanside, 1991.

Rhinitis: Immunopathology
and Pharmacotherapy
ed. by D. Raeburn and M.A. Giembycz

CHAPTER 7
Infectious Agent-Induced Rhinitis

S. Criscione* and E. Porro

Department of Experimental Medicine, University of Aquila, Aquila, Italy

1. Introduction

Little is known about the epidemiology of nonallergic infectious agent-induced rhinitis. This is not completely surprising, as the diagnosis of infectious rhinitis relies on the recognition of signs and symptoms of varying severity, while a doubt about allergic underlying conditions is always present. In a recent study [1] the estimated minimum prevalence of rhinitis in the general population was 24%, of these, 3% had seasonal symptoms only (of whom 78% were atopic), 13 had perennial symptoms only (of whom 50% were atopic) and 8% had perennial symptoms with seasonal exacerbations (of whom 68% were atopic).

Underestimating the prevalence of rhinitis may also be due to the many people who do not seek medical attention for mild symptoms. For example, Sibbald [2] reported that 40% of normal subjects had experienced nasal symptoms the previous day, although these subjects did not consider that they were suffering from rhinitis. Sibbald [1] also calculated a minimum

* Address for correspondence: Via G. Mussi 5, 00139 Rome, Italy.

prevalence of rhinitis in adults (16–65 years old) in London of 16% of whom 8% had perennial symptoms, 6% both perennial and seasonal and 2% only seasonal symptoms.

We can of course argue that in all studies a large overlap between allergy- and infectious-induced symptoms exists, and, as in allergic rhinitis, it is conceivable that geographic differences due to climate exist, as environmental, socioeconomical and even ethnic factors.

2. Infectious Agent-Induced Rhinitis

Accurate differentiation between infectious agent-induced rhinitis (IAIR) and allergic rhinitis (AR) is often difficult unless nasal secretions, obtained by different means such as nasal lavage, are examined for microbial culture, eosinophil count and for specific allergens. These, supported by history taking, are performed to confirm an infectious or allergic aetiology. This approach applies most of all to recurrent or seasonal rhinitis; however acute events may be seen in infectious and in allergic rhinitic patients.

This may explain that although rhinitis is common, most studies have focussed on AR rather than IAIR, which remains relatively unstudied epidemiologically.

Finding a common definition of IAIR is still a matter of concern, the simplest diagnosis being the "common cold". The common cold is a frequent disease in humans, which many authors have studied experimentally by inducing it in volunteers [3–8]. The mean frequency of the common cold in children 2–6 years old is six cases per year [9].

Most information regarding the mechanisms of rhinitis concern allergy, while few studies have focussed on nonallergic aspects. Rhinitis is characterized by nasal mucosal exudation of bulk blood plasma involving "flooding" of the lamina propria with mucosal exudation of plasma-derived proteins [6]. Akerlund [4] proposed that the nasal exudation reflects the degree of subepithelial inflammation and suggested that plasma bulk exudate may be involved in the resolution of acute viral rhinitis.

2.1. Diagnosis

The differential diagnosis of rhinitis includes nonallergic rhinitis with eosinophils, vasomotor and hormonal rhinitis, the rebound congestion associated with overuse of topical adrenergic agents, cold-induced rhinorrhea, which may affect allergic as well as nonallergic individuals describing similar degrees of rhinorrhea, and less frequently nasal congestion and sneezing [10].

Diagnostic tools are often misleading since an allergic component always has to be excluded even in clearly defined infectious aetiologies. Sneezing, itching and diurnal variation in symptoms [1] as well as a family history of atopy, most of all in seasonal symptoms, are likely to point towards atopy, whereas a personal history of eczema or migraine, past or current wheezing, and a family history of nose troubles other than hay fever seems to suggest perennial rhinitis.

The only easily available diagnostic features we have found to differentiate an infectious- from an allergy-induced rhinitis are the reddening of the mucosa in infectious rhinitis coupled with the presence of bacteria and/or polymorphonuclear leukocytes in nasal smears. Interestingly, a positive eosinophil count may be found both in allergic and nonallergic rhinitis with eosinophilia syndrome [9]. Many tests, such as release of mediators from peripheral blood cells, nasal secretions or urine, and nasal challenge for allergens, are research tools only, limited by the potential danger, especially in asthmatics. This is also true of methacoline and histamine challenges used to check for enhanced nonspecific reactivity. The latter seem to be restricted to patients with atopic rhinitis [11].

Among the diagnostic means, other than history taking, used to find predisposing factors (see Section 3) we may underscore the widespread used total immunoglobulin (Ig)E count, which could be useful in a first screening for allergy if supported by history, and suggest a wider use of the evaluation of nasal mucociliary clearance by saccharin [12] or by a coloured tracer in younger, noncooperating subjects.

Chronic bacterial IAIR is often associated with sinusitis and otitis. In fact, once a bacterial infection is established, a middle ear and/or sinus involvement must always be suspected. An overuse of topical decongestants and steroid sprays seems [13] to be a predisposing factor, while the commonest bacterial pathogens are *Streptococcus pneumoniae, Haemophilus influenzae* and – in our as well as in the experience of others [14] – *Staphylococcus aureus*, which can frequently be isolated in nasal discharge, mainly when sinuses are involved.

There may again be an age discriminant; in a series of 101 patients with purulent nasal discharge, Yaniv et al. [15] found that the condition was much more common in children under the age of 6 years. Furthermore, when patients were treated randomly with either an antihistamine or an antibiotic, irrespective of the nature of the nasal discharge, different results were seen according to age: 49% of children over the age of 6 years showed a resolution of symptoms, but only 14% in the group under 6 years did. Conversely, antibiotic treatment led to a resolution of symptoms in 58% of subjects under 6 years compared with 35% of those over 6 years. These data concur with our epidemiological data [16] where we demonstrated that skin-negative rhinitis was more frequent during the first years of age (when normalizing the population for normal values of IgE) and were also more frequent during winter (when viral infections giving rise to common cold are more frequent).

2.2. *Chronic Rhinitis*

Chronic rhinitis affects about 20 million Americans, and its estimated prevalence is as high as 18%. It is extraordinarily common in children of all ages and is often accompanied by conjunctivitis. A wide variety of conditions may lead to persistent blocked nose or rhinorrhea, although this symptom is most commonly caused by allergy.

Patient history, physical examination, scores for symptoms, scores for signs, rhinomanometry, nasal cytology, along with skin tests and other laboratory tests, can help to differentiate various rhinopathies more precisely [9]. When symptoms persist, with concomitant sinusitis, a chronic situation is deemed to exist after 8 to 12 weeks [9]. The symptoms are mainly cough, nasal congestion, mucopurulent nasal discharge, with facial pain and pressure and olfactory disturbance, suggesting an involvement of the sinuses. Chronic purulent rhinitis, often with sinus involvement, may hide a cell-mediated immunity [17] or severe defects in the mucociliary system. Fungal infection (see later) has the same suspicion value, while allergic responses to fungi may be elicited at the same time [18]. In children, there is evidence of spontaneous recovery from chronic, therapy-resistant, purulent rhinitis [19]. In a series of 40 children with 6 years follow-up, Otten et al. [19] found that the condition resolved spontaneously in 95% of the children, usually after reaching the age of 7 years.

2.3. *Viral Rhinitis*

Most cases of IAIR are in fact acute events with a viral aetiology. However, it seems likely that many mechanisms are involved in IAIR. For example, cytokines such as interleukin (IL)-1 β, IL-6 and IL-8 seem to be involved in the pathophysiology of common cold [20]. Additionally, interferon (IFN)γ was increased [6] in subjects whose common colds were induced by corona virus. Secretory leukocyte protease inhibitor of granulocyte elastase was found in an active form in virus-induced nasal secretions [21]. Impaired olfactory ability often accompanies the common cold, due to nasal congestion, as is the case with allergic rhinitis [1].

Infectious rhinitis is usually one of the first diseases in life, and it becomes more frequent with exposure to other children. Recently, Monto and Sullivan [22] explored the epidemiology of upper respiratory infection (URI) in children by examining throat and nasal specimens taken within 2 days of disease onset. Age was found to be a discriminating factor, as children in the first 6 months of life were relatively spared. The peak incidence was found in the 1- to 2-year-old group. The mean number of episodes was 4.9 per year in the 0- to 4-year-old group, dropping down to 2.8 episodes per year in the 5- to 19-year-old group. The recent estimation by Wald et al. confirms these yearly means [23].

In the survey cited [22], rhinoviruses were the most frequently isolated agents (39%) in children 0 to 4 years. Respiratory syncytial virus (RSV) and parainfluenza virus were the next most common and accounted for 19 and 18%, respectively. Adenoviruses (11%) and influenza A virus (8%) were next in terms of frequency, while other viruses accounted for 4%.

Many recent studies [4, 6, 7] utilize coronavirus in experimentally induced rhinitis. As the authors of the cited study [22] suggest, there may have been an underestimation of this virus because of difficulties in viral isolation.

2.4. Bacterial Rhinitis

Bacterial rhinitis has been poorly studied in recent years. IAIR, primarly viral in aetiology, may nevertheless be followed by secondary bacterial infection [15]. The latter is often characterized by purulent nasal discharge and occurs more frequently in preschool children, in whom it may be the "cause" of chronic rhinitis and may interfere with antiallergic therapies in AR. This may explain why preschool children seem to recover more frequently with antibiotic treatment than do older children [15]. It is difficult to conceive a bacteria-induced acute rhinitis, i.e. the initial event. It is more likely that viruses open the way to secondary bacterial infection by lessening host defences (especially local) and by damaging the mucosa of the upper respiratory tract. Secondary bacterial rhinitis may prolong an acute infection from a few days to several weeks.

In children, more than in adults, inflammation of the nasal cavity can easily produce rhinosinusitis [9]. The ethmoidal sinuses are well developed at birth, while the maxillary sinuses gradually increase and are well developed at the age of 3 Frontal sinuses, on the contrary can only be well visualized, from about 8 up to 14 years.

2.5. Fungal Rhinitis

The reported incidence of fungal infections varies widely and has been studied mainly in subjects with maxillary sinusitis (81 of 600 cases of this latter disease were found to have a fungal infection) [24]. *Aspergillus fumigatus* is the main fungal agent involved. In another study Laskownick et al. [25] reported 22 fungal and 97 mixed fungal and bacterial infections among 414 children with maxillary sinusitis, giving an incidence of about 28%. The most common aetiology was by *Penicillium* (49 cases), *Aspergillus* (30 cases), *Candida* (20 cases) and *Dematium* (12 cases).

Factors favouring fungal infection were found to be mainly a history of diabetes and prolonged antibiotic therapy [26]. A conversion from saprophytic to pathogenic organisms seems [21] to be due to sinus obstruction (as in chronic rhinitis), with impaired ventilation in both normal individuals and those with impairment of local or systemic defences. As cited previously, climate appears to be a factor influencing the development of fungal infections, as there are geographic areas such as North India [28], Sudan [29], the southwestern United States [30] and Hawaii [31] where fungal sinusitis is endemic.

Allergy may again be considered a predisposing factor by mucosal thickening [27] and, of course, an immunodeficiency status must always be suspected, although in this latter case the nasal and sinus fungal infection cannot reasonably be the most outstanding feature.

In the last decade a new entity allergic fungal sinusitis, has been elucidated [32, 33], reported to have a wide similarity to allergic bronchopulmonary aspergillosis. We believe that in the future this field of investigation exploring allergic entities in the respiratory airways with a sensitization to moulds might expand to clarify the relative roles of allergy and infection to the same agent.

A special consideration is justified for IAIR in the elderly, in whom an allergic mechanism is very difficult to conceive, although a genuine AR may occur at any age. Infectious rhinitis in the elderly is often the sequelae of earlier nasal disorders and their treatment [9]. A physiological impairment of host defences must always be taken in account.

3. Predisposing Factors

In children, (see Figure 1) anatomical features such as narrowing of the upper respiratory airways [34], increased by physiological hypertrophy of

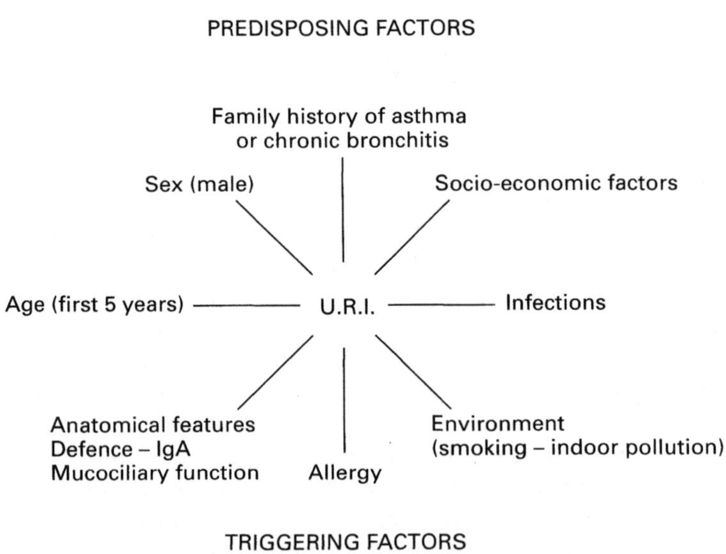

Figure 1. Factors that predispose to IAIR.

the adenoid tissue [35], may be considered as factors that predispose to IAIR, but functional factors may also be involved, such as rheologic characteristics of the mucous lining and clearing by ciliary movements. The latter is maximally compromised in Kartagener's syndrome [36]. Young's syndrome [37] and in cystic fibrosis [9]. While these syndromes represent the most severe alteration of ciliary function, other transient failures (secondary to infection) are also important causes whose incidence is underestimated [38].

Amongst immunological factors, the transient deficit of secretory IgA in children [39], lowering the surface defence mechanisms, should be considered, as well as other (congenital or acquired) immune deficiencies.

3.1. Atopy and Environmental Factors

A relationship between AR and URI has not been fully established, and some authors [40] have reported that allergic individuals do not have more frequent or more long-lasting URIs than nonallergic subjects. Nevertheless, other groups [41] have demonstrated that children with physician-diagnosed allergic rhinitis (PDAR) are most likely to have rhinitis as an early (within the first year of life) manifestation of an atopic predisposition. We can suggest that first episodes of rhinitis even in allergic subjects are mostly viral, and no attempt has been made do determine whether there is an enhanced susceptibility to viral infection in PDAR sufferers who had an onset of rhinitis in the first year of life. Furthermore, most authors [42–45] agree that there are many factors such as beginning foods other than breast milk in the first months of life or being born to "heavy-smoking" mothers that facilitate the onset of rhinitis. We may add that as the nose is the major pathway to the lungs, upper airways, sinuses and middle ears, it can react to all the factors, such as indoor and outdoor pollution, known to affect the lower respiratory tract.

In fact, in our previous preliminary study [16], the higher incidence of winter rhinitis in skin-negative subjects, as well as the highest frequency of epidemic peaks for viruses which can cause a rhinitis, led us to propose the underlying influence of viral as well as atopic factors. When we further examined our data, we found that children living in polluted areas or in indoor pollution environments had an earlier onset of recurrent rhinitis (unpublished observation).

An impaired function of nasal mucociliary clearance has been detected [11] in patients with positive skin reactions and positive methacholine challenge as well as in smokers [46]. Although the cited authors [11] were unable to show any consistent effect on nasal mucociliary clearance induced by passive smoking, and we do not know the time course of the alterations of this defence mechanism in smokers, a relationship between IAIR and impaired function of the mucociliary mechanism may exist both in passive and in active smokers.

3.2. Asthma and Lower Respiratory Tract Infections

While the common cold in normal subjects seems to be a self-limiting process which has no influence on the overall respiratory airways, most authors [8, 47, 48] agree that changes may be seen in affected allergic patients in whom enhanced release of histamine, persistent histamine leak several hours after the infection and greater recruitment of eosinophils to the airways can occur [8].

In fact, as reported previously [19, 20], viral respiratory infections are capable of inducing the release of mediators which can be involved in the immediate- and late-phase asthmatic reaction. An increased responsiveness of the nasal mucosa to intranasal histamine and cold air challenge has been found in both allergic and nonallergic subjects after experimentally induced rhinovirus infection [5]. Because the nasal response to the challenges was measured as symptom scores for rhinorrhea and congestion, counts of sneezing, weight of secretion and inspiratory conductance – all symptoms and signs common to IAIR – the question can arise whether an altered response of the nasal mucosa may indicate any variation in the lower respiratory tract in normal subjects as well, as suggested by Martinez et al. [49] in their study of infants.

The same viruses that precipitate attacks in patients with asthma who already have hyperresponsive airways may cause otherwise healthy persons to respond abnormally to challenges for several months after infections [47]. On the other hand, different viruses seems to have different "asthmogenic" properties, this observation being furthermore complicated by the influence of age. Duff et al. [50] found viral agents in 70% of wheezing children less than 2 years of age presenting to an emergency room, but in only 31% of children older than 2 years. The predominant virus associated with wheezing in the first group was RSV, whereas rhinovirus was the leading wheezing inducer in the older group. These findings have been confirmed by other groups [51]. Furthermore, and similar to our findings [16], IgE antibodies to inhaled allergens were found in only 9% of wheezers under the age of 2 years but in 72% in the older group [52].

These findings suggest that in the very first years of life the relationship between wheezing and virus infection is more important than allergy even in subjects who are expected to become openly allergic. Whether the infection itself and/or the wheezing-inducing properties of the different kinds of viruses are selected by age or by intrinsic characteristics of the virus involved is still not resolved [52].

The importance of the nose in contributing to the "whole respiratory problem" has been highlighted by our data (Table 1). In our sample of 2035 schoolchildren we found 261 subjects with respiratory troubles. We reported any "diagnosis" as being an isolated illness. Cases added up in this way to 530, due to overlapping. In the data presented in Table 1 this overlap is clearly evident.

Table 1.

Diagnosis	Asthma Otitis Rhinitis	Bronchitis Otitis Rhinitis	Asthma Rhinitis	Bronchitis Rhinitis	Asthma	Otitis Rhinitis	Otitis	Rhinitis	Total
Cases	16	70	49	4	64	44	7	7	261
Prick +	14	22	40	–	44	3	–	5	128

Diagnosis (530)
Asthma = 129
Bronchitis = 74
Otitis = 137
Rhinitis = 190

Among 190 diagnoses of recurrent rhinitis, only 7 were an isolated illness (5 being allergic). Most cases of recurrent skin-negative rhinitis were associated to recurrent otitis alone or found in recurrent bronchitis subjects. Most cases of recurrent skin-positive rhinitis were associated with the diagnosis of asthma. Our data fit with those of Taussig on PDAR [41] and add to the latter on nonallergic recurrent rhinitis occurring mostly in winter, when the incidence of viral infections is the highest.

On the other hand, we feel our data clarify the view that recurrent IAIRs are not an isolated problem but only a part of a more generalized respiratory illness involving the middle ear and/or the bronchi and often the sinuses, whereas allergic rhinitis is the actual additional symptom in asthma.

Indoor (passive smoking included) and outdoor pollution are factors that can influence the natural history of these cases, implying an earlier onset of symptoms [53, 54]. Furthermore, an early onset of rhinitis may be the marker of furhter respiratory troubles.

4. Therapy

Chronic rhinitis is a frustrating condition for patients and physicians alike. A comprehensive flow chart about managing the condition can be found in the *International Consensus Report on the Diagnosis and Management of Rhinitis* published by the International Rhinitis Management Working Group [9].

Few other illnesses can be so poorly altered [56] in their course as the most ubiquitous of human infection, the common cold.

Regardless of the virus involved (e.g. rhinovirus, coronavirus, RSV) the symptoms – cough, congestion, sneezing and sore throat – are always the same.

4.1. Cough and Cold Remedies

Use of cough and cold medicines is widespread except in infants under 6 month of age [55] and seems due more to parental pressure than to their true effectiveness. Scientific review on the efficacy of these remedies over

40 years (1950–91) [56] showed poor results in modifying the course of the common cold. This was particularly true in preschool children. In older children a combination antihistamine-decongestant medicine that included an analgesic [57] showed reduction in cough, sore throat and ache. When adolescents and adults are concerned, antihistamines and perhaps even better decongestants, produced relief of cold symptoms [56]. Expectorants were not found to be useful in reducing cough frequency, while cough remedies (codeine and dextromethorphan) were useless in controlling cough associated with URIs in adolescent and adults and in suppressing cough of acute onset during the night in younger children [58]. Cough seems to improve along with the nasal symptoms regardless of the therapy used.

4.2. *Antihistamines*

Because many cases of IAIR can involve allergy, we feel that therapy with antihistamines (histamine receptor antagonists) could be of value since an allergic component of the symptoms can be removed, and antihistamines will reduce symptoms potentiated by concurrent allergy [59]. Although recently a meta-analysis of studies on antibiotic treatment in children with URIs [60] showed that neither the course of URIs was shortened nor pneumonia was prevented, we believe that antibiotic treatment can be useful in preschool children, according to previously noted experiences [14], mostly when a nasal discharge grey to yellow-green is present in a with fever of at least 3 days' duration child or a blocked nose with fever, also of at least 3 days' duration.

4.3. *Ipratropium Bromide*

Recently, ipratropium bromide, a muscarinic cholinoceptor antagonist has shown good effectiveness in the management of nonallergic (vasomotor) rhinitis [61]. It has subsequently been tested in the symptomatic relief of rhinorrhea in adults with cold with fairly good alleviation of symptoms compared with placebo [62].

4.4. *Corticosteroids*

While there is no indication for use of systemic corticosteroids, topical delivery to the nose of rapidly deactivated forms such as beclomethasone dipropionate and flunisolide could effectively be used in the same indications as antihistamines.

4.5. *Non-pharmacological Treatments*

Among simpler remedies the efficacy of heated vapour on symptoms of common cold has been tested [63, 64] owing to the known action of high temperatures on viruses. Patients with coryza have shown benefit from steam inhalation. No benefit, however, was demonstrable either in naturally occurring or in experimentally induced rhinovirus infections.

Nevertheless, inhalation of humidified air is in our opinion very useful during the acute phase to hydrate the nasal secretions, especially in winter when internal environmental air is hot and dry. Recent work [65] on circadian rhythms in symptomatology in persons suffering from virus-induced rhinorrhea suggests, remarkably, that symptoms are more prominent during the daytime, especially during the morning hours after awakening from sleep. As the treatment for these diseases is normally scheduled as equal-interval, equal-dose medication, a change in the timing of therapy according to the temporal pattern of symptoms could optimize (and better control) doses of drugs given.

4.6. Prophylaxis

Prophylaxis of IAIR is now being attempted in some western countries by means of so-called immunostimulating agents [66]. Most of these agents are a mixture of bacterial extracts that purportedly enhance nonspecific immunity, acting as nonspecific antigens mainly on secretion of IgAs. We feel that no convincing evidence exists that significant results have been obtained with this technique. However, in still-developing immune systems (i.e. in children under 6 years of age) it is possible that an enhanced, nonspecific immunological "experience" may help the child to boost its defences. Intranasal IFNα and monoclonal antibodies may be regarded as future therapies, whereas effective vaccines are still limited by the wide variety of viral serotypes involved [52].

5. Conclusion

Because the lack of a clear aetiology can make the diagnosis of rhinitis, based on patient history and physical examination difficult, the common practice in therapy is to try a variety of treatments until one is found which works. This, incidentally, also assists in making a more definitive diagnosis.

As noted previously [14], antihistamines and antibiotics are the most commonly used drugs, as bacterial infection and allergy are the most common cause of chronic rhinitis in preschool and older subjects, respectively, once a sinusitis has been radiographically excluded and significant adenoidal obstruction evaluated. Furthermore, a bacterial infection may complicate allergy in older subjects.

Chronic rhinitis therapy relies on patients understanding that strict compliance will contribute greatly to overall treatment effectiveness [9].

This requires more from the clinician, especially understanding the noted frustrating conditions of the diseases and the need to personalize and self-manage the therapy than simply prescribing appropriate medication. Chronic, as well as acute, rhinitis impacts heavily on health-related quality of life due to its negative impact on everyday activities. The social cost of rhinitis may be high, although few patients require hospitalization, due to impaired work ability and the frequency and number of persons affected. Since the cost of medication may not always be available through national health or personal insurance schemes, personal income can be negatively impacted. Ironically, modest disorders such as rhinorrhea require more prescribing than do life-threatening conditions [67]; the therapeutic continuum of quality and cost becomes foreshortened, and safety is an additional concern.

We can conclude by agreeing with Meltzer et al. [67] that "choosing the appropriate medication for rhinorrhea, can pose a challenge to the clinician, just as choosing a vital medication can".

References

1. Sibbald B, Ring E. Epidemiology of seasonal and perennial rhinitis: clinical presentation and medical history. Thorax 1991; 46: 895–901.
2. Sibbald B. Epidemiology of allergic rhinitis. In: Burr ML, editor. Epidemiology of clinical allergy. Monographs in allergy. Basel: Karger, 1993: 61–79.
3. Calhoun WJ, Swenson CA, Dick EC, Schwartz LB, Lemanske RF Jr, Busse WW. Experimental rhinovirus 16 infection potentiates histamine release after antigen bronchoprovocation in allergic subjects. Am Rev Respir Dis 1991; 144: 1267–73.
4. Akerlund A, Greiff L, Andersson M, Bende M, Alkner U, Persson CG. Mucosal exudation of fibrinogen in coronavirus-induced common colds. Acta Otolaryngol 1993; 113: 642–48.
5. Doyle WJ, Skoner DP, Seroky JT, Fireman P, Gwaltney JM. Effect of experimental rhinovirus 39 infection on the nasal response to histamine and cold air challenges in allergic and nonallergic subjects. J Allergy Clin Immunol 1994; 93: 534–42.
6. Linden M, Greiff L, Andersson M, Svensson C, Akerlund A, Bende M, et al. Nasal cytokines in common cold and allergic rhinitis. Clin Exp Allergy 1995; 25: 166–72.
7. Akerlund A, Bende M, Murphy C. Olfactory threshold and nasal mucosal changes in experimentally induced common cold. Acta Otolaryngol 1995; 115: 88–92.
8. Calhoun WJ, Dick EC, Schwartz LB, Busse WW. A common cold virus, rhinovirus 16, potentiates airway inflammation after segmental antigen bronchoprovocation in allergic subjects. J Clin Invest 1994; 94: 2200–2208.
9. International Consensus Report on the diagnosis and management of rhinitis. International Rhinitis Management Working Group. Allergy 1994; 49(19 suppl): 1–34.
10. Silvers WS. The skier's nose: a model of cold-induced rhinorrhea. Ann Allergy 1991; 67: 32–63.
11. Gerth van Wijk R, Dieges PH. Nasal hyper-responsiveness to histamine, methacholine and phentolamine in patients with perennial non-allergic rhinitis and in patients with infectious rhinitis. Clin Otolaryngol 1991; 16: 133–37.
12. Corbo GM, Foresi A, Bonfitto P, Mugnano A, Agabiti N, Cole PJ. Measurement of nasal mucociliary clearance. Arch Dis Child 1989; 64: 546–50.
13. Gwaltney JM, Scheld M, Sande MA, Sydnor A. The microbial etiology and antimicrobial therapy of adults with acute community-acquired sinusitis: a fifteen-year experience at the University of Virginia and review of other selected studies. J Allergy Clin Immunol 1992; 90: 457–62.

14. Gittelman PD, Jacobs JB, Lebowitz AS, Tierno PM Jr. *Staphylococcus aureus* nasal carriage in patients with rhinosinusitis. Laryngoscope 1991; 101: 733–73.
15. Yaniv E, Oppenheim D, Fuchs C. Chronic rhinitis in children. Int J Pediatr Otorhinolaryngol 1992; 23: 51–57.
16. Porro E, Calamita P, Rana I, Montini L, Criscione S. Atopy and environmental factors in upper respiratory infections: an epidemiological survey on 2304 school children. Int J Pediatr Otorhinolaryngol 1992; 24: 111–20.
17. Scheeren RA, Keehnen RM, Meijer CJ, van der Baan S. Defects in cellular immunity in chronic upper airway infections are associated with immunosuppressive retroviral p15E-like proteins. Arch Otolaryngol Head Neck Surg 1993; 119: 439–43.
18. Kivity S, Schwarz Y, Fireman E. The association of perennial rhinitis with *Trichophyton* infection. Clin Exp Allergy 1992; 22: 498–500.
19. Otten FW, Van Aarem A, Grote JJ. Long-term follow-up of chronic therapy resistant purulent rhinitis in Long-term follow-up of chronic therapy resistant purulent rhinitis in children. Clin Otolarnygol 1992; 17: 32–33.
20. Roseler S, Holtappels G, Wagenmann M, Bachert C. Elevated levels of interleukins IL-1 beta, IL-6 and IL-8 in naturally acquired viral rhinitis. Eur Arch Otorhinolaryngol (suppl) 1995; 1: 61–63.
21. Fryksmark U, Jannert M, Ohlsson K, Tegner H, Wihl JA. Secretory leukocyte protease inhibitor in normal, allergic and virus induced nasal secretions. Rhinology 1989; 27: 97–103.
22. Monto AS, Sullivan KM. Acute respiratory illness in the community: frequency of illness and the agent involved. Epidemiol Infect 1993; 110: 145–60.
23. Wald ER, Guerra N, Beyers C. Upper respiratory tract infections in young children: duration of and frequency of complications. Pediatrics 1991; 87: 129–33.
24. Grigoriu D, Brambule J, Delacretaz J, Savary M. La sinusite maxillaire fungique. Dermatologica 1979; 159: 180–86.
25. Laskownick AA, Kurdzielewicz J, Macura A, Okrasinkska-Cholewa B. Mycotic sinusitis in children. Mykosen 1978; 21: 407–11.
26. Stammberger H. Endoscopic surgery for mycotic and chronic recurring sinusitis. Ann Otol Rhinol Laryngol 1985; 94(suppl 119): 1–11.
27. Blitzer A, Lawson W. Fungal infections of the nose and paranasal sinuses. Part 1. Otolaryngol Clin North Am 1993; 26: 1007–35.
28. Chakrabarti A, Sharma SC, Chander J. Epidemiology and pathogenesis of paranasal sinus mycoses. Otholaryngol Head Neck Surg 1992; 107: 745–50.
29. Milosev B, Margoub ES, Abdel A, Hassan AM. Primary aspergilloma of the paranasal sinus in the Sudan – a review of seventeen cases. Br J Surg 1969; 56: 132–37.
30. Ence BK, Gourley DS, Jorgensen NL. Allergic fungal sinusitis. Am J Rhinol 1990; 4: 169–78.
31. Zieske LA, Kopke RD, Hamill A. Dematiaceous fungal sinusitis. Otholaringol Head Neck Surg 1991; 105: 567–77.
32. Millar JW, Johnston A, Lamb D. Allergic aspergillosis of the maxillary sinuses. Thorax 1981; 36: 710.
33. Katzenstein AA, Sale SR, Greenberger PA. Allergic *Aspergillus* sinusitis: a newly recognized form of sinusitis. J Allergy Clin Immunol 1983; 72: 89–93.
34. Tos M, Stangerup SE. Secretory otitis and pneumatization of the mastoid process: sexual differences in the size of mastoid cell system. Am J Otholaringol 1985; 6: 199–205.
35. Battistini A, Grzincich GL. L'ipertrofia adenotonsillare. Rivista Italiana di Pediatria 1979; 5: 561–68.
36. Umeki S. Primary mucociliary transport failure. Respiration 1988; 54: 220–25.
37. Young D. Surgical treatment of male interfertility. J Reprod Fertil 1970; 23: 541–42.
38. Carson JL, Collier AM, Hu SS. Acquired ciliary defects in nasal epithelium of children with acute viral upper respiratory infections. N Engl J Med 1985; 312: 463–67.
39. Taylor B, Norman AP, Orgel HA, Stokes CR, Turner MW, Soothill JF. Transient IgA deficiency and pathogenesis of infantile atopy. Lancet 1973; 3: 2–6.
40. Hinriksdottir I, Melen I. Allergic rhinitis and upper respiratory tract infections. Acta Otolaryngol Suppl 1994; 515: 30–32.
41. Wright AL, Holberg CJ, Martinez FD, Halonen M, Morgan W, Taussig LM. Epidem iology of physician-diagnosed allergic rhinitis in childhood. Pediatrics 1994; 94: 895–901.

42. Bock SA. Prospective appraisal of complaints of adverse reactions to foods in children during the first 3 years of life. Pediatrics 1987; 79: 683–88.
43. Kramer MS, Moroz BL. Do breastfeeding and delayed introduction of solid foods protect against subsequent atopic eczema? J Pediat 1981; 98: 546–50.
44. Wright AL, Holberg CJ, Martinez FD. Breastfeeding and lower respiratory tract illness in the first year of life. Br Med J 1989; 299: 946–49.
45. Holberg CJ, O'Rourke MK, Lebowitz MD. Multivariate analysis of ambient environmental factors and respiratory effects. Int J Epidemiol 1987; 16: 399–410.
46. National Research Council, Environmental tobacco smoke: measuring exposure and assessing health effects. Washington, DC: National Academy Press 1989: 188–212.
47. Eggleston PA. Upper airway inflammatory diseases and bronchial hyperresponsiveness. J Allergy Clin Immunol 1988; 81: 1036–41.
48. Korppi M. Viruses and airborne allergens as precipitants of obstructive respiratory difficulties in children. Ann Clin Res 1988; 20: 417–22.
49. Martinez FD, Taussig LM, Morgan WJ. Infants with upper respiratory illnesses have significant reductions in maximal expiratory flow. Pediatr Pulmonol 1990; 9: 91–95.
50. Duff AL, Pomeranz ES, Gelber LE, Price GW, Farris H, Hyden FG, et al. Risk factors for acute wheezing in infant and children: viruses, passive smoke, and IgE antibodies to inhalant allergens. Pediatrics 1993; 92: 535–40.
51. Johnston S, Pattemore P, South S. Viral infections in exacerbations in schoolchildren with cough or wheeze: a longitudinal study. Am Rev Respir Dis 1992; 145: A546.
52. Johnston S, Bardin PG, Pattemore PK. Viruses as precipitants of asthma symptoms III: rhinoviruses: molecular biology and prospects for future intervention. Clin Exp Allergy 1993; 23: 237–46.
53. Etzel R, Pattishall E, Haley N, Fletcher RH, Henderson F. Passive smoking and middle ear effusion among children in day care. Pediatrics 1992; 90: 228–32.
54. Doyle WJ, Skoner DP, Fireman P, Seroky JT, Green I, Ruben F, et al. Rhinovirus 39 infection in allergic and nonallergic subject. J Allergy Clin Immunol 1992; 89: 968–78.
55. Gadomski AM, Rubin JD. Cough and cold medicine use in young children: a survey of Maryland pediatricians. Maryland Med J 1993; 42: 647–50.
56. Smith MBH, Feldman W. Over-the-counter cold medications: a critical review of clinical trials between 1950 and 1991. J Am Med Assoc 1993; 269: 2258–63.
57. Jaffe G, Grimshaw JJ. Randomized single-blind trial in general practice comparing the efficacy and palatability of two cough Linctus preparations, "Pholcolix" and "Actifed" compound, in children with acute cough. Curr Med Res Opin 1983; 8: 594–99.
58. Taylor JA, Novack AH, Almquist JR, Roger JE. Efficacy of cough suppressants in children. J Pediatr 1993; 122: 799–802.
59. Middleton DB. An approach to pediatric upper respiratory infections. Am Fam Physician 1991; 44(5 suppl): 33–40.
60. Gadomski AM. Potential interventions for preventing pneumonia among young children: lack of effect on antibiotic treatment for upper respiratory infections. Pediatr Infect Dis J 1993; 12: 115–20.
61. Dolovich J, Mukherjee J, Salvatori VA. Intranasal ipratropium bromide to control the hypersecretion of vasomotor rhinitis: a dose response study. Am J Rhinol 1989; 3: 221–24.
62. Dockhorn R, Grossman J, Posner M, Zinny M, Tinkelman D. A double-blind, placebo-controlled study of the safety and efficacy of ipratropium bromide nasal spray versus placebo in patients with common cold. J Allergy Clin Immunol 1992; 90: 1076–82.
63. Forstall GJ, Macknin ML, Yen-Lieberman BR, Medendorp SV. Effect of inhaling heated vapor on symptoms of the common cold. J Am Med Assoc 1994; 271: 1109–11.
64. Hendley JO, Abbott RD, Beasley PP, Gwaltney JM. Effect of inhalation of hot humidified air on experimental rhinovirus infection. J Am Med Assoc 1994; 271: 1112–14.
65. Smolensky MH, Reinberg A, Labrecque G. Twenty-four hour pattern in symptom intensity of viral and allergic rhinitis: treatment implications. J Allergy Clin Immunol 1995; 95: 1084–96.
66. Collet JP, Decruet T, Kramer MS, Haggerty J, Floret D, Chomel JJ, et al. Stimulation of nonspecific immunity to reduce the risk of recurrent infections in children attending day-care centers. Pediat Infect Dis J 1993; 12: 648–52.
67. Meltzer EO, Tyrell RJ Jr, Rich D, Wood CC. A pharmacologic continuum in the treatment of rhinorrhea: the clinician as economist. J Allergy Clin Immunol 1995; 95: 1147–52.

Rhinitis: Immunopathology
and Pharmacotherapy
ed. by D. Raeburn and M. A. Giembycz

CHAPTER 8
Specific Immunotherapy in Allergic Rhinitis

Jean Bousquet, Pascal Demoly and François-B. Michel

*Clinique des Maladies Respiratoires, Hôpital Arnaud de Villeneuve,
Centre Hospitalier Universitaire, Montpellier, France*

1. Introduction

Specific immunotherapy (SIT) was introduced in 1911 for the treatment of pollinosis by Noon and Freeman [1]. Immunotherapy is still controversial since many protocols have been devised empirically, some allergens are still poorly defined, the mechanisms of action are not yet clear, the duration is poorly characterized and the therapeutic index of SIT has been contested for many years. In the 1970s, SIT was found to be ineffective, especially in asthma [2]. In the 1980s, it was found that SIT was effective under optimal conditions including a demonstrated immunoglobulin (Ig)E-mediated disease, a high-quality extract, an optimal allergen dose and a correct indication [3], but its safety was questioned as systemic reactions that may exceptionally become life-threatening were noticed [4–7]. It is possible that the use of potent extracts may have resulted in a greater number of systemic reactions and possibly of deaths, especially in asthmatics. Thus, the value of SIT was again contested and its use threatened with some decline for pneumoallergens. However, SIT is still one of the most common treatments in children and adolescents in many parts of the world. In this current decade, pharmacoeconomic considerations may also cause problems, since the costs for SIT may be greater than that of pharmacotherapy. However, SIT is the only treatment that can affect the natural course of the disease, and it may prevent the onset of asthma. New routes of administration of SIT are currently being explored, and nasal, sublingual or oral SIT, using high-allergen doses, may represent interesting ways of administering allergens. Moreover in the future new technologies and the improvement of our knowledge of the basic mechanisms of allergic diseases may completely change the scope of immunotherapy.

2. Mechanisms

The allergic reaction mediated by IgE manifests itself as an inflammation which develops in several stages. The allergens react with cells present at the mucosal surfaces via the membrane-bound IgE molecules. Mast cells are the first cells activated and start a chain reaction resulting in an allergic inflammation or involving several other cell types and factors including eosinophils, the vasoactive mediators (histamine, platelet activating factor (PAF), leukotrienes (LT), prostaglandins (PG), cytokines such as interleukin (IL)-3, IL-4, IL-5, granulocyte macrophage colony stimulating factor (GM-CSF)), adhesion molecules and cytotoxic mediators derived particularly from eosinophils. The allergic reaction is therefore initiated by IgE but rapidly results in a much more widespread inflammation which may last for several days following a single allergic contact. Furthermore, repeated allergic stimulation results in a persistent inflammation and is the foundation of nonspecific hyperreactivity of the airways.

Desensitization mechanisms cannot therefore be explained solely on the basis of a reduction in the synthesis of IgE, as has been proposed by some researchers, but must involve a number of other factors in which modulation of the synthesis of IgE is perhaps not the major mechanism. It is probable that several mechanisms play a sequential role in the process, these mechanisms being perhaps different for SIT to pneumoallergens and those for SIT to *Hymenoptera* venoms.

2.1. Reduction of Inflammation in Cells and Tissues

When it is effective, SIT is accompanied by a reduction in cutaneous [8, 9], bronchial [10, 11] nasal [11–13] or ocular [14] reactivity with respect to the allergen during skin and provocation tests. In nasal provocation tests not only is the quantity of allergen necessary to provoke a reaction in the target organ increased, but also mediators of anaphylaxis (such as histamine) are released in lower amounts [15, 16] and there is a reduction in cellular recruitment during provocation [17, 18]. It is, therefore, a phenomenon, involving a hyposensitization of the tissue and is specific to the allergen. At the end of SIT treatment, after a period of several months or a few years, particularly for subjects having a perennial allergy, the tissue reactivity reoccurs, often to the same extent as before, suggesting the importance of continuing SIT.

Tissue hyposensitization appears rapidly when the dose is sufficient and does not correlate with levels of immunoglobulins in serum or secreted which are specific to the allergen (IgE or IgG) [19]. On the other hand, it is often correlated with clinical improvements [20]. This mechanism seems to occupy an important place in understanding the efficacy of SIT to pneumoallergens.

Moreover, a reduction in cellular reactivity to the allergen has been shown in studies involving the degrenulation of blood basophils or on platelet cytotoxicity [21]. Rak et al. have conducted several elegant studies in which they investigated the activation of eosinophils and measured the levels of chemotactic factors in serum or in the bronchi during the pollen season [22, 23]. In patients who have not received SIT, an increase in the levels of ECP (eosinophil cationic protein) in the serum [24] as well as a chemotactic activity towards eosinophils is seen [25], these two events being blocked in desensitized subjects. The same author has also demonstrated the reduction of pulmonary inflammation during desensitization to extracts of birch pollen [26]. Therefore, an associated cellular hyposensitization would appear to exist.

The mechanisms underlying this cellular and tissue hyposensitization are poorly understood at present, but may well involve cytokines and histamine-releasing factors [27], despite the fact that the direct specificity of the reaction would tend to suggest another mechanism.

2.2. Modification of Serum Immunoglobulins

For a long time, attempts have been made to demonstrate the clinical advantages of desensitization by measuring the reduction of IgE and the increase of IgG levels or the variations of subclasses of IgG known as blocking antibodies [28].

During SIT, one frequently observes an increase in the initial levels of specific IgE in serum, which, curiously, accompanies a clinical improvement. After several months or even years of treatment, the levels of IgE diminish but rarely become lower than their starting value, except in subjects allergic to *Hymenoptera* venom. In pollen allergy, one observes no elevation of specific IgE titre in desensitized subjects during the pollen season [29]. Thus, the variation in the levels of specific IgE certainly does not explain the benefits of SIT for subjects with allergy to inhaled pneumoallergens.

The great theory of SIT mechanisms developed over many years was based on blocking antibodies [30]. The supporters of this theory explain that allergens are "captured" by IgG before reaching the mast cell-bound IgE, hence the name "blocking antibodies". However, the theory of blocking antibodies does not seem to have been demonstrated in the case of allergy to pneumoallergens. This has led to attempts to explain the efficacy of desensitization by the development of subtypes of IgG [31] or via increases in IgA or IgG secretion, but to date no precise correlation has been found [32]. IgG may, however, modulate the immune reaction via an intermediary of the network idiotype-anti-idiotype [33].

2.3. Modulation of the Lymphocyte Subclass

The synthesis of IgE is governed by the powerful action of T lymphocytes (helper (Th) and suppressor) on the B lymphocytes carrying the membrane IgE. Over the past few years, studies on cytokines have radically changed our understanding of the synthesis of IgE. IL-4, IL-13 and IL-5 facilitate the synthesis of IgE, whilst interferon (IFN)γ and IFN-α inhibit it. At the same time, there is a modulation of proinflammatory cytokines released by lymphocytes and perhaps also mast cells. At least in mice, two types of T-lymphocyte ancillary cells exist: Th_1 and Th_2. Of these, Th_2 favours the synthesis of IgE (synthesis of IL-4, IL-13, IL-5, IL-6, IL-3, GM-CSF, IL-10), whilst Th_1 (synthesis of IFN-γ, IL-2, IL-3) inhibits it. Certainly in humans, the concept of Th_1-Th_2 is not as simple as in the mouse; the subclasses of lymphocytes are relatively differentiated and synthesize proinflammatory mediators which modulate the synthesis of IgE and allergic reactions [34, 35]. The Th_1 lymphocytes suppress the allergic and inflammatory reactions, whilst the Th_2 lymphocytes increase the synthesis of IgE (IL-4 and IL-13) and in the inflammatory reaction (IL-5 in particular, an important cytokine in tissue eosinophilia).

Despite the small number of studies that have been conducted to date, it seems that specific desensitization is associated with a switch Th_2-Th_0 [36] or Th_2-Th_1 [37; Pène unpublished results].

Lymphocytes are not the only cells which synthesize cytokines. Macrophages and mast cells (at least in animal studies) also exhibit this potential. It is tempting to suggest a theory to unify the mechanisms of desensitization which modulates the reactivity of lymphocytes and that of cells carrying membrane IgE at both high affinity (mast cells and basophils) and low affinity (eosinophils, monocyte-macrophage) to account for cellular hyposensitization.

3. General Considerations

3.1. Immunotherapy as a Curative Treatment

The treatment of allergic diseases combines immunological and pharmacological treatments. In many patients, drugs can relieve nasal and ocular symptoms without side effects. In these patients, SIT is not indicated, but in a subset of patients for whom drugs are not sufficiently effective or induce side effects, SIT may be started.

However, differences between the pharmacological and immunological treatments of rhinitis may not be restricted to safety and efficacy. Drugs only offer symptomatic treatment, whereas SIT is the only treatment that might cure the disease (if it is shown that the effects of SIT last after its cessation) [38].

Before starting SIT it is essential to consider several factors to appreciate the respective value of allergen avoidance, pharmacotherapy and SIT [39]:

- Is the disease due to an IgE-mediated allergy and are high-quality extracts available?
- Are attempts being made to avoid allergens?
- What is the potential severity of the affection to be treated?
- What is the efficacy of available treatments, including the quality of allergen extracts that are used?
- What is the cost and duration of each type of treatment?
- What are the risks to the patient both of the allergic disease and of the treatments?

In patients receiving SIT, both SIT and pharmacotherapy should be used in combination, since few patients will be completely free of symptoms when treated with SIT; on the other hand, SIT reduced the need for medication in severely affected patients. Moreover, allergen avoidance should always be attempted even if it cannot be complete.

Specific immunotherapy needs to be prescribed by specialists and carried out by physicians who are trained to use emergency techniques if anaphylaxis occurs. Before starting SIT, each patient should be carefully informed of risks, duration and effectiveness of this treatment; cooperation and compliance with treatment are absolute requirements before starting it.

3.2. *Immunotherapy as a Preventative Treatment*

Specific immunotherapy has principally been used for the curative treatment of allergic diseases, but there are some suggestions indicating that SIT may also have a preventive efficacy. It has been proposed, but not yet confirmed, that SIT may prevent the onset of asthma in patients with rhinitis. Recently, it has been shown that about 50% of young children (age 2–6 years) sensitized to a single allergen species and who received SIT did not develop new allergenic sensitivities over a period of 3 years, whereas all of these who did not receive SIT developed new sensitivities during the same period of time. This study needs confirmation but suggests that SIT can alter the natural course of allergy (DesRoches, Bousquet, unpublished).

3.3. *The Need for Beginning SIT in Young Children*

Allergic sensitization usually begins early in life, and symptoms often start within the first decade. It has been shown that SIT was less effective in older patients than in children and that inflammation and remodelling of the airways in asthma offer a poor prognosis for an effective SIT. Moreover, if SIT is used as a preventive treatment, it should be started as soon as allergy has been diagnosed.

3.4. *Compliance with Treatment*

Compliance with SIT is rarely optimal [40], and many patients stop SIT after some months, leading to incomplete effectiveness. Reasons for poor compliance include the time spent in the physician's office during the course of the treatment, the duration of the treatment required to achieve efficacy and, for young children, the fear of injections.

4. Pollen Allergy

4.1. *Subcutaneuous Immunotherapy*

4.1.1. Efficacy: The efficacy of pollen-SIT is suggested by the decrease of target organ sensitivity during nasal and/or conjunctival allergen challenge [16, 18–20, 41–46]. It has been widely documented in optimally designed double-blind placebo-controlled trials which usually, but not always, demonstrated efficacy in rhinitis due to grass [16, 20, 41, 48–58], ragweed [59–73], *Parietaria* [46, 74], mountain cedar [75] and coconut tree pollen [76] (Tables 1 and 2). Grass and ragweed pollen extracts are effective in conjunctivitis [41, 47, 48, 77]. However, although studies comparing the

Table 1. Results of double-blind placebo-controlled studies in grass pollen allergy

Author	Species	Patient number A	Patient number P	Extract	Dose	Protocol schedule	Duration	Skin	Symptom-medication tests	Symptom-medication scores
Bousquet	grass	15		standardized	rush	pre- + co-season	1 yr	$p < 0.01$	N:	$P < 0.01$
	grass	16	11	formald. allergoid	rush	pre- + co-season	1 yr	$p < 0.02$	N:	$P < 0.05$
Bousquet	grass	15	10	formald. allergoid	clustered	pre- + co-season	1 yr	$p < 0.001$	N:	$P < 0.005$
Bousquet	grass	18		standardized	rush	pre- + co-season	1 yr	$p < 0.01$	N, O, B:	$P < 0.01$
	grass	15	14	formald. allergoid	clustered	pre- + co-season	1 yr	$p < 0.04$	O, B:	$< 0.05 < P < 0.01$
	grass	13		HMW-allergoid	clustered	pre- + co-season	1 yr	$p < 0.005$	N, O, B:	$P < 0.01$
Bousquet	grass	39	18	HMW-allergoid	clustered	pre- + co-season	1 yr	$p < 0.05$	N, B:	$0.005 < P < 0.01$
Bousquet	grass	16	17	standardized	rush	pre- + co-season	1 yr	$p < 0.02$	N:	$P < 0.02$
	multiple	16	17	standardized	rush	pre- + co-season	1 yr	NS	N:	NS
Frankland	grass	50	50	"pollaccine"	classical		1 yr		N:	$P < 0.001$
		50	50	purified antigen	classical				N:	$P < 0.001$
Grammer	grass	18	18	polymer. glutarald.	classical	12 injections	12 wk		N:	$P < 0.02$
Grammer	grass	22	22	polymer. glutarald.	accelerated	13 injections	9 wk		N:	$P < 0.05$
McAllen	grass	47	23	Allpyral	classical	?	1 yr		NB:	NS
		40		depot preparation	classical	?	1 yr		NB:	$P < 0.05$
Machiels	grass	7]	8]	Ag-Ab complexes	classical	pre- + co-season	3 mo		N:	NS
Machiels	grass	37	12	Ag-Ab complexes	classical	pre- + co-season	3 mo		NB:	$P < 0.03$ & $P < 0.001$
Ortolani	grass	8]	8]	standardized	classical	pre-season	1 yr		N:	$P < 0.001$
Starr	grass	42	10	alum-pyridine	classical	pre-season	1 yr		N:	79% improved
Varney	grass	20	20	standardized, alum	classical	pre- + co-season	1 yr		NB	$P < 0.01$
Weyer	grass	17	16	aqueous then $Al(OH)^3$	classical	pre-season	1 yr		N:	peak of season, $P < 0.03$

N: nasal; O: ocular, B: bronchial; HWM; high molecular weight; Ag-Ab: antigen-antibody.
Reprinted with permission from [3].

Table 2. Results of double-blind placebo-controlled studies in ragweed pollen rhinitis

Author	Number P	Number A	Extract	Schedule	Protocol	Dose	Duration	Symtom-medication scores
Arbesman	19	19	repository	12 injections	pre-season	M: 4000 PNU	2 yr	NS vs placebo
		22	aqueous	12 injections	pre-season	M: 10000 PNU	2 yr	improved
Cockroft	21	22	Pollinex	4 injections	pre-season	M: 4000 Noon U	1 yr	improved: A: 67%, P: 38%
Grammer	19	21	polymer. glutarald.	classical	15 injections	M: 6250 PNU, C: 50000 PNU	15 wk	$P < 0.02$
Hirsch	74	81	aqueous	Rinkel	pre- + co-season	M: 27–41 PNU, 0.1–0.15 µg AgE	2 yr	NS for ragweed
Lichtenstein	24	24	AgE	classical	pre-season	C: 17–800 µg	1 yr	$P < 0.01$
Lichtenstein	30	18	AE	classical	pre-season	1.0 mg	1 yr	$P < 0.01$
		21	AE + K	classical	pre-season	1.4 mg	1 yr	$P < 0.01$
		19	crude Rw, aqueous	classical	pre-season	C: 8800 PNU	1 yr	$P < 0.01$
Lowell	12	12	aqueous	classical	pre-season	not stated	1 yr	$P < 0.01$
Meriney	10	10	formald. allergoid	classical	pre-season	C: 10,710 PNU	20 wk	$P < 0.01$
Van Metre	12	12	aqueous	Rinkel	pre- + co-season	C: 94 ng AgE	3 mo	NS
Van Metre	17	15	aqueous	classical	pre- + co-season	C: 70 µg AgE	1 yr	$P < 0.01$
		18	aqueous	clustered	pre- + co-season	C: 17.5 µg AgE	1 yr	$P < 0.01$
Norman	21	21	aqueous whole rw	classical	pre-season	C: 9483 PNU per yr	4 yr	3rd, 4th yr: $P < 0.02$
		21	AgE	classical	pre-season	C: 195,530 PNU per yr	4 yr	3rd, 4th yr: $P < 0.04$
Norman	21	20	alum-precipitate	classical	pre-season	C: 13,746 PNU (yr 1)	3 yr	$P < 0.006$
Norman		22	formald. allergoid	cluster	pre-season	C: 63,600 PNU (yr 1)	2 yr	$P < 0.01$
		22	aqueous	classical	pre-season	C: 2,000 PNU (yr 1)	2 yr	$P < 0.01$

Dose: M: maximal doses; C: cumulative dose.
Reprinted with permission from [3].

efficacy of immunotherapy and pharmacotherapy are urgently required, as yet only one such study has been performed. Juniper et al. [78] compared the efficacy of budesonide, a highly effective topical corticosteroid, with Pollinex in the treatment of ragweed hay fever and observed that the pharmacological treatment was superior in efficacy and safety. However, the findings of this study cannot be extended, owing to the known low efficacy of Pollinex in ragweed pollen allergy [60]. In a recent, elegant double-blind placebo-controlled study, Varney et al. [57] evaluated the efficacy and safety of immunotherapy in patients with severe grass pollen allergy, not controlled by standard antiallergic drugs, and showed that SIT was effective in reducing symptoms and the need for medication, including the use of systemic corticosteroids. The efficacy of the treatment was further found in subsequent years [79]. Double-blind placebo-controlled trials have not been published yet for other pollen species, and although it is postulated that SIT is effective [80], proper trials remain to be done. Moreover, although it is postulated that SIT is effective [80], proper trials remain to be done. Moreover, although SIT has been shown to be effective in optimal conditions, this treatment fails completely when inappropriately used, and SIT is not equally effective in all patients. There are several parameters which have therefore to be examined, among which the quality of the extracts used, the SIT schedule, cross-reactivities between and the sensitization of patients are critical.

4.1.1.1. Extracts used. Standardized extracts are now available for many pollen species [81] but are still lacking for important regional allergens such as cypress pollen. Many different extracts have been proposed since the introduction of SIT. Aqueous extracts are effective, especially when standardized, but they expose patients to a high rate of systemic reactions, so attempts have been made to prepare extracts having a decreased allergenicity (reduction of side effects) without modification of immunogenicity (similar efficacy). Among the various preparations, adsorbed extracts on aluminium, tyrosine or calcium phosphate are commercially available and have been shown to decrease the incidence of side reactions. However, they only represent a first attempt, and their efficacy has only been reported in a placebo-controlled study with unstandardized extracts [56]. Extracts polymerized by formaldehyde [20, 41, 47, 48, 66], ragweed [59–65, 71–73, 82] or glutaraldehyde [50, 51, 60, 61, 83] are effective, but only high molecular weight preparations are safer and as effective as the aqueous extracts or the low molecular weight ones. Polyethyleneglycol (PEG)-modified extracts represent another interesting approach, but the high expectations which followed animal studies have, unfortunately not been realized in humans [84].

4.1.1.2. Maintenance dose. The maintenance dose is critical for the efficacy of SIT, but it is still a matter of debate. Initially, propositions suggested giving a high dose to patients, but owing to severe reactions, other investigators following the concept of Rinkel [85] proposed low doses after the so-called skin test titration. However, this technique has been found ineffective during placebo-controlled studies [62, 68, 86] and should no longer be used. It was then suggested that patients should be given the "highest tolerated dose" with potent extracts [87, 88], but again, severe systemic reactions were observed in many patients. We (Bousquet et al. [11, 89]) proposed an *optimal maintenance dose* (a dose inducing a change in cell reactivity but giving a low and acceptable rate of mild systemic reactions) and by serially studying skin tests after SIT, defined a dose inducing a decrease in the skin test end-point in over 80% of patients treated. This "optimal" dose was able to increase the provocative allergen dose during nasal challenge and achieved a significant protection in patients suffering from grass pollen-induced rhinoconjunctivitis and asthma [16, 20, 41, 47, 48]. With a ten fold greater dose, the number of systemic side reactions was increased without major changes in efficacy. However, although a much greater increase might have enhanced the effectiveness of SIT, it is likely that side reactions would be greater in number and unacceptable in severity. Turkeltaub et al. have used a similar approach for ragweed pollens [90].

4.1.1.3. Cross-reactivities between allergens. Many related or unrelated allergens share common epitopes leading to cross-reactivities that complicate the diagnosis and the treatment of allergic diseases. Important cross-reactivities exist among pollens of grasses or *Oleaceae* or some of the *Ambrosiaceae* or deciduous trees or, to a lesser extent, *Compositeae* [91, 92]. Patients allergic to grass pollens usually have positive skin tests and serum-specific IgE towards many if not most species. Thus, it should be determined whether patients need to be treated by all the relevant species or only a few of them or even only one. During the early years of SIT in Europe, timothy (*Phleum pratense*) was commonly used, as it was supposed to have a broad allergen content. In the middle of the century it was proposed that a mixture of five to six common grasses, including timothy, would improve the efficacy of SIT. During the last decade, the use of a single allergen species has tended to be favoured in northern Europe; however, this may not reflect a worldwide trend, since pollens of some species such as Bermuda grass (*Cynodon dactylon*) or cereals do not completely cross-react with timothy. Allergen mixtures present many defects. They may be less stable in an aqueous extract than single species, since interactions between allergens exist and enzymatic degradation of allergens has already been demonstrated. It is more difficult to standardize mixtures, and the dilution of major epitopes in mixtures may lead to a low-dose SIT regimen. On the other hand, single allergen species may be less effective because some relevant epitopes may be lacking. Using cross-immunoelectrophoresis, Løwenstein et al. [93] proposed that perennial rye grass possesses epitopes that might be relevant for most other grass pollen species and that SIT with single allergens may be effective. This was, at least partly, confirmed by Frostad et al. [94] and Bousquet et al. (unpublished observations), who observed that SIT with a single allergen species (perennial rye grass or orchard grass) was as effective as SIT with four or five species. Similar findings were observed with birch and deciduous tree pollens [95, 96].

Patients sensitized to birch pollen often present cross-reactive epitopes with many raw fruits and vegetables. Thus in theory, birch pollen SIT might reduce fruit allergy. Møller [97] examined the efficacy of birch pollen SIT in apple sensitivity but failed to observe any efficacy for fruit allergy. However, a recent study reported a single case where birch-pollen immunotherapy induced the loss of oral food allergy syndrome [98].

4.1.1.4. Polysensitized patients. The IgE immune response to environmental allergens depends both on genetic and environmental factors and is highly heterogeneous. It has been shown that patients allergic only to grass pollens differ only clinically and immunologically [99, 100] from those allergic to many pollen species. A controlled study and a double-blind placebo-controlled study compared the efficacy of SIT in these two groups of patients [16]. Grass pollen allergic patients were treated with an optimal maintenance dose of a standardized orchard grass pollen extract, whereas those allergic to multiple pollen species received the same biologically equivalent dose of all standardized allergens to which they were sensitized. The results of the study indicated that grass pollen allergic patients but not polysensitized patients were significantly protected. Using a higher allergen dose, it might have been possible to show efficacy in the polysensitized group, but the rate of systemic reactions using standardized extracts would have been unacceptable.

4.1.1.5. Age of the patients. For theoretical reasons, based on the mechanisms of the immune response, it is usually recommended to start SIT in children and adults and to avoid it in elderly subjects. In a study of ragweed pollen allergy, Hedlin et al. [101] compared the results of allergen immunotherapy in paediatric and adult populations. Biological responses were measured by nasal challenges, skin tests and the evolution of serum-specific immunoglobulins. They observed that ragweed immunotherapy leads to immunological and biological consequences that are comparable in children and adults. However, this study does not give clear information on elderly patients, who usually improve spontaneously.

SIT may be started in children under 5 years of age, but it is desirable to carefully evaluate the benefits, since SIT leads to a greater number of systemic reactions in this age group. Systemic reactions, especially asthma, may be more severe, and most young children have not fully developed their allergenic sensitization. On the other hand, a retrospective study has suggested that SIT in pollen-allergic patients may prevent the onset of asthma.

During pregnancy, when the severity of allergic diseases is often modified, SIT should not be started, but it may be continued in patients when it is effective [102].

4.1.2. Safety: Life-threatening reactions are not uncommon, even with high-quality extracts, and deaths have been reported. The rate of systemic reactions is greater with standardized pollen extracts than with either non-standardized extracts or high molecular weight preparations but does not differ from SIT performed with standardized extracts of other allergen species [7, 57, 89, 103, 104]. The occurrence of systemic reactions has been studied in over 500 grass pollen allergic individuals who received the same rush SIT protocol with the same standardized extracts [89]. It was observed that the rate of systemic reactions was higher in patients who had presented asthma (and rhino-conjunctivitis) during the previous pollen season than in those who had rhinoconjunctivitis alone. The incidence of generalized urticaria and anaphylaxis was similar in both groups, but bronchial symptoms occurred mostly in asthmatic patients. This study indicates that asthmatic patients are at higher risk during SIT. Rush immunotherapy may expose to a high risk of systemic reactions, and attempts have been made to reduce the incidence of reactions. With premedication, exclusion of asthmatic patients with FEV_1 (forced expiratory volume in 1 second) under 70% of predicted values at the time of the injection and stopping the rush schedule if large local reactions were noticed, systemic reactions were decreased to an acceptable rate, and the severity of these reactions was always mild. Step protocols decrease even further the rate and severity of systemic reactions [7]. Polymerized high molecular weight preparations have been consistently shown to induce few systemic reactions in grass, ragweed and tree pollen allergy [41, 48, 50, 51, 61, 83].

4.1.3. Duration: Duration of SIT is another matter of debate. In the case of inhalant allergy in atopic individuals, data are lacking to support any definite conclusion, but it appears, that long-term treatment, at least 3 years, is required. For nasal symptoms, Mosbech et al. [105] observed in a retrospective study that the effect of grass pollen SIT lasted several years after its cessation. Using high molecular weight polymerized extracts, Grammer et al. reached similar conclusions [106]. However, prospective controlled studies are lacking, and no definite conclusion can be made.

4.2. Other Routes of Allergen Administration

4.2.1. Efficacy: The usual route of administration of SIT is subcutaneous injection. However, recent studies have shown that alternative routes may be effective in reducing symptoms of rhinitis and medication needs. It must be stressed that only high-allergen doses should be given (about 500 times greater than those achieving efficacy with the subcutaneous route).

Nasal immunotherapy was effective in grass, ragweed and *Parietaria* pollen allergy in some but not all studies [107–121].

Oral SIT was ineffective in most trials in grass pollen allergy, possibly because these allergens can be destroyed by digestive enzymes [122]. In ragweed and birch pollen allergy, oral SIT was effective if high-allergen doses were administered [123–127]. Sublingual SIT was effective in grass and *Parietaria* pollen allergy [128, 129].

More studies are needed to establish fully the efficacy of local SIT using high doses of standardized allergen extracts. The magnitude of efficacy of SIT using local routes also needs to the better studied, and in particular it should be compared with subcutaneous and local SIT. It may be anticipated that local SIT will be less effective than subcutaneous SIT for a similar duration of treatment and a similar cumulative dose of allergen. On the other hand, the efficacy of prolonged treatment may be similar. The addition of oral SIT to boost parenteral SIT may be effective, but more data are required since negative studies have been published [130–132].

4.2.2. Safety: Systemic or focal reactions are uncommon with local administration of extracts. During nasal SIT, some patients complain of rhinitis symptoms during allergen insufflation, but using modified extracts adverse reactions become rare. High-dose oral SIT is also associated with focal reactions in the form of gastrointestinal symptoms. Sublingual SIT has been used in thousands of patients, and it is apparently well tolerated.

4.3. Compliance

The compliance of patients during SIT is a prerequisite for achieving efficacy. It has been known for years that compliance in subcutaneous SIT is poor. Compliance in local SIT is still unknown, but physicians who routinely use sublingual SIT estimate that it is far better than that seen in subcutaneous SIT.

5. House Dust Mite Allergy

House dust mites of the species *Dermatophagoides* are among the most prevalent perennial allergens throughout the world and have been shown to cause rhinitis and asthma, especially in childhood. Few double-blind placebo-controlled studies have been performed with house dust mites that have shown SIT to be effective [133–141], and house dust immunotherapy should no longer be used. With mite allergens, the indications of

SIT are still vague but can be envisaged, especially if the patient presents asthma. In rhinitis, a course of topical steroids is often required at the beginning of SIT, since symptoms are due to both allergy and inflammation.

Nasal and sublingual SIT have been carried out using high-allergen doses, and efficacy has been observed [142, 143]. Moreover, two studies using low-dose sublingual SIT have shown some efficacy. However, serious flaws in the design of the study and in the interpretation of the data do not make it possible to conclude that such a regimen is effective [144, 145].

6. Immunotherapy to Animal Proteins

Although it has been recommended by the Position Papers of the European Academy of Allergy and Clinical Immunology [146] and WHO/IUIS [147] that allergen avoidance be preferred to SIT in animal dander allergy, SIT may be envisaged. There are studies showing that SIT is effective in improving the threshold dose inducing positive bronchial challenges with cat or dog dander extract in asthmatic subjects, and that in a few studies asthma symptoms and pulmonary function were improved (for review see [148]). However, the clinical efficacy of cat or dog SIT remains to be ascertained in rhinitis, since only one study has been carried out [149].

Oral and sublingual SIT have been tried in cat allergic patients [150, 151]. It was claimed that sublingual SIT was not effective because symptoms were improved both in the active and placebo groups, although the improvement was greater in the active group [151]. Moreover, the only objective parameter of efficacy (nasal blockage index) was highly significantly improved in the treated group, whereas it was unchanged in the placebo group [152].

The cloning and the characterization of the structure of major allergens made it possible to synthesize peptides having the structure of the native allergens. Among them, two *Felis domesticus* (cat) allergen (Fel d1) peptides of 27 amino acids have been synthesized (Allervax Cat) [153]. These peptides stimulated cat-specific T cells *in vitro* but were unable to bind to cat allergen-specific IgE. A few clinical trials have been performed, and these two peptides have been found to protect patients against a cat room challenge in which nasal and bronchial symptoms were examined (Norman et al., unpublished data).

7. Immunotherapy to Moulds

Moulds are major allergens in asthma, but they often induce polysensitizations. The quality of extracts available in the early 80s was far from adequate, so that mould SIT was not recommended. However, efforts have been made to standardize extracts of some molds such as *Alternaria* and *Cladosporium*, and good-quality allergen extracts are now available [154]. SIT with standardized *Cladosporium* [155–157] and *Alternaria* extracts [158] has been attempted, but variable results have been obtained. In Nordic countries, patients treated with a standardized *Cladosporium* extract were polysensitized, and SIT was effective in challenges with the specific allergen; but symptom-medication scores were only minimally improved. On the other hand, in the double-blind placebo-controlled study of Horst et al. [158], performed over 1 year in 24 highly selected patients allergic only to *Alternaria*, both nasal challenges and symptom-medication scores were improved in the treated group and remained unchanged in the placebo group.

SIT with *Cladosporium* induced a high number of systemic reactions [155–157], whereas SIT with *Alternaria* was better tolerated, possibly because Horst et al. [158] attempted to define an "optimal maintenance dose" before starting SIT. Long-term safety of mould SIT has also been questioned, and type III allergic reactions have been described [159].

These studies suggest that mould SIT may be effective, but they do not favour SIT with many mould species or with extracts of unknown quality.

8. Immunotherapy with Other Extracts

Although SIT may be administered by oral or sublingual routes, there is no controlled study showing that it is effective in rhinitis or asthma with perennial allergens. SIT with extracts of undefined allergens (bacteria, foods, *Candida albicans*, insect dusts) should not be used anymore in clinical practice, but controlled trials may be started [39, 146, 147, 160].

9. Indications for SIT

9.1. General Considerations

Guidelines for the indication of SIT have largely been published within the past 5 or 6 years. The European Academy of Allergy and Clinical Immunology and the British Society for Allergy and Clinical Immunology [39, 146, 147, 160, 161] have proposed recommendations for the use of SIT. In all these recommendations the quality of the extract to be administered was stressed. Optimally, these extracts should be standardized, using the most modern techniques [81]. The indication of SIT should be carefully proposed in highly selected patients [162] and the length and cost of the treatment should be discussed with patients, since compliance with SIT is often poor [163].

Double-blind placebo-controlled studies have confirmed the efficacy of SIT, but clinical efficacy does not mean clinical indication, especially since controlled trials of SIT are optimally designed and may not always be applicable to daily medical practice and a safe and effective pharmacological treatment is also available for the treatment of allergic diseases. Thus, before starting SIT it is essential to consider several factors to appreciate the respective value of allergen avoidance, pharmacotherapy and SIT.

In patients receiving SIT, both SIT and pharmacotherapy should be used in combination, since very few patients will be completely free of symptoms when treated with SIT; on the other hand, SIT does reduce the need for medication in severely affected patients. Moreover, allergen avoidance should always be attempted even if it cannot be complete.

Specific immunotherapy needs to be prescribed by specialists and carried out by physicians who are trained to use emergency techniques if anaphylaxis occurs. Before starting SIT each patient should be carefully informed of risks, duration and effectiveness of this treatment; cooperation and compliance with the treatment are absolute requirements before starting it.

Absolute contraindication to SIT include patients with other serious immunopathological conditions, malignancies, poor compliance, severe psychological disorders and/or treatment by β-adrenoceptor antagonists, even if administered topically.

Before initiating SIT, avoidance of exposure to the provoking allergen(s) should always be attempted. Except in the case of animal dander, however, most common aeroallergens cannot be avoided completely, and this is particularly true for patients allergic to house dust mites and those who are allergic to multiple allergens.

9.2. Pollen Allergy

It is commonly accepted that SIT is indicated in severe rhinoconjunctivitis [146, 147] where pharmacotherapy insufficiently controls symptoms or produces undesirable side effects. On the other hand, SIT should not be started in mild to moderately severe pollinosis responding favorably to antihistamines and topical drugs, except if the pollen season is long-lasting, as is the case in southern Europe, South Africa and California.

Since rhinoconjunctivitis is present in most, if not all, patients suffering from pollen allergy, and asthma occurs generally in the most severely affected patients, it is impossible to propose indications without considering all symptoms. It also appears that SIT is indicated when asthma during the pollen season complicates rhinoconjunctivitis, although this recommendation is not accepted by all investigators because of the increased risk of systemic reactions. British recommendations have proposed that patients with asthma should be specifically excluded [164], but this recommendation appears to be important only if asthma is moderately severe or severe.

9.3. House Dust Mite Allergy

The indication of SIT in mite allergy is not easy to propose, and definite indications will not be available until the NIH-sponsored study on mite allergy has been published. From the current studies the following recommendations may be proposed [39]. (*1*) Only patients with house dust mites as perennial allergens should be treated. (*2*) Patients with aspirin intolerance or nonspecific triggers of asthma such as chronic sinusitis should not receive SIT. (*3*) The age of the patients should also be considered. On the one hand, children and young adults usually respond more efficiently to SIT; on the other hand, children under 5 years of age may not receive SIT because of an increased risk of systemic reactions, increased severity of the systemic reactions and also because the sensitivity of young patients may vary.

9.4. Immunotherapy with Other Allergens

In animal dander allergy allergen avoidance is the best choice, but SIT to cat or dog allergens may occasionally be an alternative in occupational allergy and in some children to whom the eviction of the animal may be a great shock.

In mould allergy, the elimination of indoor allergen is favoured, and SIT may be restricted to patients allergic only to *Alternaria* and/or *Cladosporium*.

10. Monitoring

After the first pollen season or after 6 months for perennial allergens, patients receiving SIT should be reassessed, and the treatment stopped if not effective. *In vivo* and *in vitro* methods have been proposed to evaluate the efficacy of SIT. The evolution of IgG, IgG subclasses or IgE against whole allergens or purified antigens does not give any valuable information [20, 165]. Provocation challenges are often correlated with the efficacy of SIT, but only when a group of patients is considered [16, 18–20, 41, 42]. They are less predictive for individual patients and are difficult to carry out routinely in clinical practice. The evolution of the cutaneous late-phase reaction may also be considered, since relationships between late cutaneous responses and specific antibody responses have been positively correlated with outcome of immunotherapy for seasonal allergic rhinitis [166].

Acknowledgements

The authors thank Dr W. Becker, A. Des Roches, H. Dhivert, F. Djoukhadar, A. Dotte, E. Frank, P. Godard, B. Guérin, A. Hejjaoui, B. Hewett, J. Knani, L. Paradis, H. J. Maasch, L. Martinot, J. L. Ménardo, W. Skassa-Brociek, R. Wahl, and Mrs M. Deltour for their help.

References

1. Noon L. Prophylactic inoculation against hay fever. lancet 1911; i: 1572–23.
2. Lichtenstein LM. An evaluation of the role of immunotherapy in asthma. Am Rev Respir Dis 1978; 117: 191–97.
3. Bousquet J, Michel F. Specific immunotherapy in allergic rhinitis and asthma. In: Busse W, Holgate S, editors. Asthma and rhinitis. Oxford: Blackwell Scientific Publications, 1995: 1309–24.
4. Committee on Syfety of Medicines. Desensitizing vaccines. Br Med J 1986; 293: 948.
5. Lockey RF, Benedict LM, Turkeltaub PC, Bukantz SC. Fatalities from immunotherapy (IT) and skin testing (ST). J Allergy Clin Immunol 1987; 79: 660–77.
6. Norman PS. Safety of allergen immunotherapy [editorial]. J Allergy Clin Immunol 1989; 84: 438–39.
7. Bousquet J, Michel FB. Safety considerations in assessing the role of immunotherapy in allergic disorders. Drug Safety 1994; 10: 5–17
8. Bousquet J, Guerin B, Dotte A. Comparison between rush immunotherapy with a standardized allergen and an alum adjuved pyridine extracted material in grass pollen allergy. Clin Allergy 1985; 15: 179–93.
9. Van-Metre Te J, Marsh DG, Adkinson N Jr. Immunotherapy decreases skin sensitivity to cat extract. J Allergy Clin Immunol 1989; 83: 888–99.
10. Warner JO, Price JF. Southill JF, Hey EN. Controlled trial of hyposensitisation to *Dermatophagoides pteronyssinus* in children with asthma. Lancet 1978; 2: 912–15.
11. Bousquet J, Calvayrac P, Guerin B. Immunotherapy with a standardized *Dermatophagoides pteronyssinus* extract. 1. *In vivo* and *in vitro* parameters after a short course of treatment. J Allergy Clin Immunol 1985; 76: 734–44.
12. Bousquet J, Lebel B, Dhivert H, Bataille Y, Martinot B, Michel FB. Nasal challenge with pollen grains, skin-prick tests and specific IgE in patients with grass pollen allergy. Clin Allergy 1987; 17: 529–36.
13. Frostad AB, Grimmer O, Sandvik L, Aas K. Hyposensitization; comparing a purified (refined) allergen preparation and a crude aqueous extract from timothy pollen. Allergy 1980; 35: 81–95.
14. Moller C, Dreborg S, Lanner A, Bjorksten B. Oral immunotherapy of children with rhinoconjunctivitis due to birch pollen allergy; a double blind study. Allergy 1986; 41: 271–79.
15. Creticos PS, Adkinson N Jr, Kagey-Sobotka A, Proud D, Meier HL, Naclerio RM, et al. Nasal challenge with ragweed pollen in hay fever patients; effect of immunotherapy. J Clin Invest 1985; 76: 2247–53.
16. Bousquet J, Becker WM, Hejjaoui A, Chandal I, Lebel B, Dhivert H, et al. Differences in clinical and immunologic reactivity of patients allergic to grass pollens and to multiple-pollen species. 2. Efficacy of a double-blind, placebo-controlled, specific immunotherapy with standardized extracts. J Allergy Clin Immunol 1991; 88: 43–53.
17. Furin MJ, Norman PS, Creticos PS, Proud D, Kagey-Sobotka A, Lichtenstein LM, et al. Immunotherapy decreases antigen-induced eosinophil cell migration into the nasal cavity. J Allergy Clin Immunol 1991; 88: 27–32.
18. Iliopoulos O, Proud D, Adkinson N, Jr. Effects of immunotherapy on the early, late and rechallenge nasal reaction to provocation with allergen: changes in inflammatory mediators and cells. J Allergy Clin Immunol 1991; 87: 855–66.
19. Hedlin G, Silber G, Naclerio R, Proud D, Eggleson P, Adkinson NF. Attenuation of allergen sensitivity early in the course of ragweed immunotherapy. J Allergy Clin Immunol 1989; 84: 390–99.

20. Bousquet J, Maasch H, Martinot B, Hejjaoui A, Wahl R, Michel FB. Double-blind, placebo-controlled immunotherapy with mixed grass-pollen allergoids. 2. Comparison between parameters assessing the efficacy of immunotherapy. J Allergy Clin Immunol 1988; 82: 439–46.
21. Tsicopoulos A, Tonnel AB, Wallaert B, Joseph M, Ramon P, Capron A. A circulating suppressive factor of platelet cytotoxic functions after rush immunotherapy in *Hymenoptera* venom hypersensitivity. J Immunol 1989; 142: 2683–88.
22. Rak S. Effects of immunotherapy on the inflammation pollen asthma. Allergy 1993; 48: 125–28.
23. Nagata M. Shibasaki M, Sakamoto Y, Fukuda T, Makino S, Yamamoto K, et al. Specific immunotherapy reduces the antigen-dependent production of eosinophil chemotactic activity from mononuclear cells in patients with atopic asthma. J Allergy Clin Immunol 1994; 94: 160–66.
24. Rak S, Lowhagen O, Venge P. The effect of immunotherapy on bronchial hyperresponsiveness and eosinophil cationic protein in pollen-allergic patients. J Allergy Clin Immunol 1988; 82: 470–80.
25. Rak S, Bjornson A, Hakanson L, Sorenson S, Venge P. The effect of immunotherapy on eosinophil accumulation and production of eosinophil chemotactic activity in the lung of subjects with asthma during natural pollen exposure. J Allergy Clin Immunol 1991; 88: 878–88.
26. Rak S, Hallden G, Sorenson S, Margari V, Scheynius A. The effect of immunotherapy on T-cell subsets in peripheral blood and bronchoalveolar lavage fluid in pollen-allergic patients. Allergy 1993; 48: 460–65.
27. Kuna P, Alam R, Kuzminska B, Rozniecki J. The effect of preseasonal immunotherapy on the production of histamine-releasing factor (HRF) by mononuclear cells from patients with seasonal asthma: results of a double-blind, placebo-controlled, randomized study. J Allergy Clin Immunol 1989; 83: 816–24.
28. Lichtenstein L, Norman P, Kagey-Sobotka A, Adkinson N Jr, Golden D. The immunologic basis for the efficacy of immunotherapy. In: Kerr J, Ganderton J, editors. Proceedings of the XI Congress of Allergology and Clinical Immunology. Chester, UK: McMillan Press Ldt, 1983: 285–88.
29. Gleich GJ, Zimmermann EM, Henderson LL, Yunginger JW. Effect of immunotherapy on immunoglobulin E and immunoglobulin G antibodies to ragweed antigens: a six-year prospective study. J Allergy Clin Immunol 1982; 70: 261–71.
30. Leynadier F, Abuaf N, Halpern GM, Murrieta M, Garcia-Duarte C, Dry J. Blocking IgG antibodies after rush immunotherapy with mites. Ann Allergy 1986; 57: 325–29.
31. Djurup R, Osterballe O. IgG subclass antibody response in grass pollen-allergic patients undergoing specific immunotherapy: prognostic value of serum IgG subclass antibody levels early in immunotherapy. Allergy 1984; 39: 433–41.
32. Xiao SF, Okuda M, Ohnishi M, Okubo K. Specific IgA and IgG antibodies to house dust mite *Dermatophagoides farinae* in nasal secretions. Arerugi 1994; 43: 634–44.
33. Hebert J, Bernier D, Mourad W. Detection of auto-anti-idiotypic antaibodies to Lol p I (rye I) IgE antibodies in human sera by the use of murine idiotypes: levels in atopic and non-atopic subjects and effects of immunotherapy. Clin Exp Immunol 1990; 80: 413–19.
34. Pene J, Rousset F, Briere F, Chrétien I, Paliard X, Banchereau J, et al. IgE production by normal human B cells induced by alloreactive T cell clones is mediated by IL-4 and suppressed by IFN-gamma. J Immunol 1988; 141: 1218–24.
35. Romagnani S. Human TH1 and TH2 subsets: doubt no more. Immunol Today 1991; 12: 256–57.
36. Varney VA, Hamid QA, Gaga M, Ying S, Jacobson M, Frew AJ, et al. Influence of grass pollen immunotherapy on cellular infiltration and cytokine mRNA expression during allergen-induced late-phase cutaneous responses. J Clin Invest 1993; 92: 644–51.
37. Secrist H, Chelen CJ, Wen Y, Marshall JD, Umetsu DT. Allergen immunotherapy decreases interleukin 4 production in CD4+ T cells from allergic individuals. J Exp Med 1993; 178: 2123–30.
38. Bousquet J, Dhivert H, Michel FB. Current trends in the management of allergic diseases. Allergy 1994; 49: 31–35.
39. International Consensus Report on Diagnosis and Management of Asthma. International Asthma Management Project. Allergy 1992; 47: 1–61.

40. Rudd S. Immunotherapy compliance – a shot in the dark. Ann Allergy Asthma Immunol 1995; 74: 195–98.
41. Bousquet J, Hejjaoui A, Soussana M, Michel FB. Double-blind, placebo-controlled immunotherapy with mixed grass-pollen allergoids. 4. Comparison of the safety and efficacy of two dosages of a high-molecular-weight allergoid. J Allergy Clin Immunol 1990; 85: 490–97.
42. Creticos PS, Marsh DG, Proud D, Kagey-Sobotka A, Adkinson NF, Friedhoff L, et al. Responses to ragweed-pollen nasal challenge before and after immunotherapy. J Allergy Clin Immunol 1989; 84: 197–205.
43. Frostad A, Bolle R, Grimmer Ø, Aas K. A new, well characterized, purified allergen preparation from timothy pollen. 2. Allergenic *in vivo* and *in vitro* properties. Int Arch Allergy Appl Immunol 1978; 55: 35–40.
44. Osterballe O. Immunotherapy in hay fever with two major allergens 19, 25 and partially purified extract of timothy grass pollen: a controlled double blind study. *In vivo* variables, season. I. Allergy 1980; 35: 473–89.
45. Viander M, Koivikko A. The seasonal symptoms of hyposensitized and untreated hay fever patients in relation to birch pollen counts: correlations with nasal sensitivity, prick tests and RAST. Clin Allergy 1978; 8: 387–96.
46. Ortolani C, Pastorello EA, Incorvaia C, Ispano M, Farioli L, Zara C, et al. A double-blind, placebo-controlled study of immunotherapy with an alginate-conjugated extract of *Parietaria judaica* in patients with *Parietaria* hay fever. Allergy 1994; 49: 13–21.
47. Bousquet J, Hejjaoui A, Skassa-Brociek W. Double-blind, placebo-controlled immunotherapy with mixed grass-pollen allergoids. 1. Rush immunotherapy with allergoids and standardized orchard grass-pollen extract. J Allergy Clin Immunol 1987; 80: 591a–98.
48. Bousquet J, Maasch HJ, Hejjaoui A, Skassa-Brociek W, Wahl R, Dhivert H, et al. Double-blind, placebo-controlled immunotherapy with mixed grass-pollen allergoids. 3. Efficacy and safety of unfractionated and high-molecular-weight preparations in rhinoconjunctivitis and asthma. J Allergy Clin Immunol 1989; 84: 546–56.
49. Frankland A, Augustin R. Prophylaxis of summer hay fever and asthma: a controlled trial comparing crude grass pollen extract with the isolated main protein components. Lancet 1954; 1: 1055–58.
50. Grammer LC; Shaughnessy MA, Suszko IM, Shaughnessy JJ, Patterson R. A double-blind histamine placebo-controlled trial of polymerized whole grass for immunotherapy of grass allergy. J Allergy Clin Immunol 1983; 72: 448–53.
51. Grammer LC, Shaughnessy MA, Finkle SM, Shaughnessy JJ, Patterson R. A double-blind placebo-controlled trial of polymerized whole grass administererd in an accelerated dosage schedule for immunotherapy of grass pollinosis. J Allergy Clin Immunol 1986; 78: 1180–84.
52. McAllen M. Hyposensitization in grass pollen hay fever. Acta Allergol 1969; 24: 421–31.
53. Machiels JJ, Buche M, Somville MA, Jacquemin MG, Saint-Remy JM. Complexes of grass pollen allergens and specific antibodies reduce allergic symptoms and inhibit the seasonal increase of IgE antibody. Clin Exp Allergy 1990; 20: 653–60.
54. Machiels JJ, Somville MA, Jacquemin MG, Saint-Remy JM. Allergen-antibody complexes can efficiently prevent seasonal rhinitis and asthma in grass pollen hypersensitive patients: allergen-antibody complex immunotherapy. Allergy 1991; 46: 335–48.
55. Ortolani C, Pastorello E, Moss RB, Hsu YP, Restuccia M, Joppolo G, et al. Grass pollen immunotherapy: a single year double-blind, placebo-controlled study in patients with grass pollen-induced asthma and rhinitis. J Allergy Clin Immunol 1984; 73: 283–90.
56. Starr M, Weinstock M. Studies in pollen allergy. 3. The relationship between blocking antibody levels, and symptomatic relief following hyposensitization with Allpyral in hay fever subjects. Int Arch Allergy 1970; 38: 514–21.
57. Varney VA, Gaga M, Frew AJ, Aber VR, Kay AB, Durham SR. Usefulness of immunotherapy in patients with severe summer hay fever uncontrolled by antiallergic drugs. Br Med J 1991; 302: 265–69.
58. Weyer A, Donat N, L'Heritier C, Juilliard F, Pauli G, Soufflet B, et al. Grass pollen hyposensitization versus placebo therapy. 1. Clinical effectiveness and methodological aspects of a pre-seasonal course of desensitization with a four-grass pollen extract. Allergy 1981; 36: 309–17.

59. Arbesman C, Reismann R. Hyposensitization therapy including repository: a double-blind study. J Allergy 1964; 35: 12–17.
60. Cockroft D, Cuff M, Tarlo S, Dolovich J, Hargreave F. Allergen-injection therapy with glutaraldehyde-modified-ragweed pollen-tyrosine adsorbate: a double-blind trial. J Allergy Clin Immunol 1977; 60: 56–62.
61. Grammer LC, Zeiss CR, Suszko IM, Shaughnessy MA, Patterson R. A double-blind, placebo-controlled trial of polymerized whole ragweed for immunotherapy of ragweed allergy. J Allergy Clin Immunol 1982; 69: 494–99.
62. Hirsch SR, Kalbfleisch JH, Cohen SH. Comparison of Rinkel injection therapy with standard immunotherapy. J Allergy Clin Immunol 1982; 70: 183–90.
63. Lichtenstein L, Norman P, Winkelwerder W. Clinical and *in vitro* studies on the role of immunotherapy in ragweed hay fever. Am J Med 1968; 44: 514–24.
64. Lichtenstein L, Norman P, Winkenwerder L. A single year of immunotherapy in ragweed hay fever. Am J Med 1971; 44: 514–24.
65. Lowell F, Franklin W. A double-blind study of the effectiveness and specificity of injection therapy in ragweed hay fever. N Engl J Med 1965; 273: 675–79.
66. Meriney DK, Kothari H, Chinoy P, Grieco MH. The clinical and immunologic efficacy of immunotherapy with modified ragweed extract (allergoid) for ragweed hay fever. Ann Allergy 1986; 56: 34–38.
67. Van MT Jr. Critique of controversial and unproven procedures for diagnosis and therapy of allergic disorders. Pediatr Clin North Am 1983; 30: 807–17.
68. Van-Metre TE, Adkinson N Jr, Amodio FJ, Lichtenstein LM, Mardiney MR, Norman PS, et al. A comparative study of the effectiveness of the Rinkel method and the current standard method of immunotherapy for ragweed pollen hay fever. J Allergy Clin Immunol 1980; 66: 500–13.
69. Van-Metre Te J, Adkinson N Jr, Lichtenstein LM, Mardiney MR, Rosenberg GL, Sobotka AK, et al. A controlled study of the effectiveness of the Rinkel method of immunotherapy for ragweed pollen hay fever. J Allergy Clin Immunol 1980; 65: 288–97.
70. Van-Metre T, Adkinson N, Amodio FJ, Kagey-Sobotka A, Lichtenstein LM, Mardiney MR, et al. A comparison of immunotherapy schedules for injection treatment of ragweed pollen hay fever. J Allergy Clin Immunol 1982; 69: 181–93.
71. Norman P, Winkelwerder W, Lichtenstein L. Immunotherapy of hay fever with ragweed antigen E: comparisons with whole extracts and placebo. J Allergy 1968; 42: 93–108.
72. Norman PS, Lichtenstein LM. Comparisons of alum-precipitated and unprecipitated aqueous ragweed pollen extracts in the treatment of hay fever. J Allergy Clin Immunol 1978; 61: 384–89.
73. Norman PS, Lichtenstein LM, Kagey-Sobotka A, Marsh DG. Controlled evaluation of allergoid in the immunotherapy of ragweed hay fever. J Allergy Clin Immunol 1982; 70: 248–60.
74. D'Amato G, Kordash TR, Liccardi G, Lobefalo G, Cazzola M, Freshwater LL. Immunotherapy with Alpare in patients with respiratory allergy to *Parietaria* pollen: a two year double-blind placebo-controlled study. Clin Exp Allergy 1995; 25: 149–58.
75. Pence H, Mitchell D, Greenly R, Updegraft B, Selfridge H. Immunotherarpy for mountain cedar pollinosis: double-blind controlled study. J Allergy Clin Immunol 1976; 58: 39–50.
76. Karmakar PR; Das A, Chatterjee BP. Placebo-controlled immunotherapy with *Cocos nucifera* pollen extract. Int. Arch Allergy Immunol 1994; 103: 194–201.
77. Juniper EF, Roberts RS, Kennedy LK, O'Connor J, Syty-Golda M, Dolovich J, et al. Polyethylene glycol-modified ragweed pollen extract in rhinoconjunctivitis. J Allergy Clin Immunol 1985; 75: 578–85.
78. Juniper EF, Kline PA, Ramsdale EH, Hargreave FE. Comparison of the efficacy and side effects of aqueous steroid nasal spray (budesonide) and allergen-injection therapy (Pollinex-R) in the treatment of seasonal allergic rhinoconjunctivitis. J Allergy Clin Immunol 1990; 85: 606–11.
79. Walker SM, Varney VA, Gaga M, Jacobson MR, Durham SR. Grass pollen immunotherapy: efficacy and safety during a 4-year follow-up study. Allergy 1995; 50: 405–13.
80. Current status of allergen immunotherapy: shortened version of a World Health Organisation/International Union of Immunological Societies Working Group Report. Lancet 1989; 1: 259–61.

81. Reed CE, Yunginger JW, Evans R. Quality assurance and standardization of allergy extracts in allergy practice. J Allergy Clin Immunol 1989; 84: 4–8
82. Marsh DG, Norman PS, Roebber M, Lichtensein LM. Studies on allergoids from naturally occurring allergens. 3. Preparation of ragweed pollen allergoids by aldehyde modification in two steps. J Allergy Clin Immunol 1981; 68: 449–59.
83. Grammer LC, Shaughnessy MA, Patterson R. Modified forms of allergen immunotherapy. J Allergy Clin Immunol 1985; 76: 397–401.
84. Dreborg S, Akerblom EB. Immunotherapy with monomethoxypolyethylene glycol modified allergens. Crit Rev Ther Drug Carrier Syst 1990; 6: 315–65.
85. Rinkel H. Inhalant allergy. 2. The co-seasonal application of serial dilutions. Ann Allergy 1949; 7: 639–45.
86. Hirsch SR, Kalbfleisch JH, Golbert TM, Josephson BM, McConnell LH, Scanlon R, et al. Rinkel injection therapy: a multicenter controlled study. J Allergy Clin Immunol 1981; 68: 133–55.
87. Norman PS. An overview of immunotherapy: implications for the future. J Allergy Clin Immunol 1980; 65: 87–96.
88. Creticos PS, Van-Metre TE, Mardiney MR, Rosenberg GL, Norman PS, Adkinson N Jr. Dose response of IgE and IgG antibodies during ragweed immunotherapy. J Allergy Clin Immunol 1984; 73: 94–104.
89. Hejjaoui A, Ferrando R, Dhivert H, Michel FB, Bousquet J. Systemic reactions occurring during immunotherapy with standardized pollen extracts. J Allergy Clin Immunol 1992; 89: 925–33.
90. Turkeltaub PC, Campbell G, Mosimann JE. Comparative safety and efficacy of short ragweed extracts differing in potency and composition in the treatment of fall hay fever. Use of allergenically bioequivalent doses by parallel line bioassay to evaluate comparative safety and efficacy. Allergy 1990; 45: 528–46.
91. Lowenstein H. Cross reactions among pollen antigens. Allergy 1980; 35: 198–200.
92. Lowenstein H, Sparholt SH, Klysner SS, Ipsen H, Larsen JN. The significance of isoallergenic variations in present and future specific immunotherapy. Int Arch Allergy Immunol 1995; 107: 285–89.
93. Lowenstein H, Wihl JA, Bache-Billesbolle K, Bowadt H. Rationale for specific immunotherapy of grass pollen allergy with extracts of rye pollen: skin test reactivity and immunochemical relationship between pollen allergens from rye and other common grasses. Allergy 1984; 39: 421–32.
94. Frostad AB, Grimmer O, Sandvik L, Moxnes A, Aas K. Clinical effects of hyposensitization using a purified allergen preparation from Timothy pollen as compared to crude aqueous extracts from Timothy pollen and a four-grass pollen mixture respectively. Clin Allergy 1983; 13: 337–57.
95. Moller C, Dreborg S. Cross-reactivity between deciduous trees during immunotherapy. 1. *In vivo* results. Clin Allergy 1986; 16: 135–43.
96. Petersen BN, Janniche H, Munch EP, Wihl JA, Bowadt H, Ipsen H, et al. Immunotherapy with partially purified and standardized tree pollen extracts. 1. Clinical results from a three-year double-blind study of patients treated with pollen extracts either of birch or combinations of alder, birch and hazel. Allergy 1988; 43: 353–62.
97. Moller C. Effect of pollen immunotherapy on food hypersensitivity in children with birch pollinosis. Ann Allergy 1989; 62: 343–45.
98. Kelso JM, Jones RT, Tellez R, Yunginger JW. Oral allergy syndrome successfully treated with pollen immunotherapy. Ann Allergy Asthma Immunol 1995; 74: 391–96.
99. Bousquet J, Hejjaoui A, Becker WM, Cour P, Chanal I, Lebel B, et al. Clinical and immunologic reactivity of patients allergic to grass pollens and to multiple pollen species. 1. Clinical and immunologic characteristics. J Allergy Clin Immunol 1991; 87: 737–46.
100. Pene J, Rivier A, Laier B, Becker WM, Michel FB, Bousquet J. Differences in IL-4 release by PBMC are related with heterogeneity of atopy. Immunology 1994; 81: 58–64.
101. Hedlin G, Silber G, Naclerio R, Proud D, Lamas AM, Eggleston P, et al. Comparison of the *in vivo* and *in vitro* response to ragweed immunotherapy in children and adults with ragweed-induced rhinitis. Clin Exp Allergy 1990; 20: 491–500.
102. Metzger WJ, Turner E, Patterson R. The safety of immunotherapy during pregnancy. J Allergy Clin Immunol 1978; 61: 268–72.

103. Lessof M, Chandler B. Experience with Spectralgen®/Pharmalgen®: a new kind of allergen preparation. Amsterdam: Excerpta Medica, 1983.
104. Osterballe O. Side effects during immunotherapy with purified grass pollen extracts. Allergy 1982; 37: 553–62.
105. Mosbech H, Osterballe O. Does the effect of immunotherapy last after termination of treatment? Follow-up study in patients with grass pollen rhinitis. Allergy 1988; 43: 523–29.
106. Grammer LC, Shaughnessy MA, Suszko IM, Shaughnessy JJ, Patterson R. Persistence of efficacy after a brief course of polymerized ragweed allergen: a controlled study. J Allergy Clin Immunol 1984; 73: 484–89.
107. Ariano R, Panzani RC, Chiapella M, Augeri G, Falagiani P. Local intranasal immunotherapy with allergen in powder in atopic patients sensitive to *Parietaria officinalis* pollen. J Investig Allergol Clin Immunol 1995; 5: 126–32.
108. D'Amato G, Lobefalo G, Liccardi G, Cazzola M. A double-blind, placebo-controlled trial of local nasal immunotherapy in allergic rhinitis to *Parietaria* pollen. Clin Exp Allergy 1995; 25: 141–48.
109. Georgitis JW, Reisman RE, Clayton WF, Mueller UR, Wypych JI, Arbesman CE. Local intranasal immunotherapy for grass-allergic rhinitis. J Allergy Clin Immunol 1983; 71: 71–76.
110. Georgitis JW, Clayton WF, Wypych JI, Barde SH, Reisman RE. Further evaluation of local intranasal immunotherapy with aqueous and allergoid grass extracts. J Allergy Clin Immunol 1984; 74: 694–700.
111. Georgitis JW, Nickelsen JA, Wypych JI, Kane JH, Reisman RE. Local nasal immunotherapy: efficacy of low-dose aqueous ragweed extract. J Allergy Clin Immunol 1985; 75: 496–500.
112. Georgitis JW, Nickelsen JA, Wypych JI, Barde SH, Clayton WF, Reisman RE. Local intranasal immunotherapy with high-dose polymerized ragweed extract. Int Arch Allergy Appl Immunol 1986; 81: 170–73.
113. Mathews KP, Bayne NK, Banas JM, McLean JA, Bacon J. Controlled studies of intranasal immunotherapy for ragweed pollenosis. Int Arch Allergy Appl Immunol 1981; 66: 218–24.
114. Nickelsen JA, Goldstein S, Mueller U, Wypych J, Reisman RE, Arbesman CE. Local intranasal immunotherapy for ragweed allergic rhinitis. 1. Clinical response. J Allergy Clin Immunol 1981; 68: 33–40.
115. Nickelsen JA, Goldstein S, Mueller U, Wypych J, Reisman RE, Arbesman CE. Local intranasal immunotherapy for ragweed allergic rhinitis. 2. Immunologic response. J Allergy Clin Immunol 1981; 68: 41–45.
116. Nickelsen JA, Georgitis JW, Mueller UR, Kane J, Wypych JI, Goldstein S, et al. Local nasal immunotherapy for ragweed-allergic rhinitis. 3. A second year of treatment. Clin Allergy 1983; 13: 509–19.
117. Passalacqua G, Albano M, Ruffoni S. Nasal immunotherapy to *Parietaria*: evidence of reduction of local allergic inflammation. Am J Respir Crit Care Med 1995; 152: 461–66.
118. Schumacher MJ, Mitchell GF. Inhibition of murine reaginic antibody responses by nasal immunotherapy with modified allergen. Int Arch Allergy Appl. Immunol 1980; 62: 382–88.
119. Schumacher MJ, Pain MC. Intranasal immunotherapy and polymerized grass pollen allergens. Allergy 1982; 37: 241–48.
120. Welsh PW, Zimmermann EM, Yunginger JW, Kern EB, Gleich GJ. Preseasonal intranasal immunotherapy with nebulized short ragweed extract. J Allergy Clin Immunol 1981; 67: 237–42.
121. Welsh PW, Butterfield JH, Yunginger JW, Agarwal MK, Gleich GJ. Allergen-controlled study of intranasal immunotherapy for ragweed hay fever. J Allergy Clin Immunol 1983; 71: 454–60.
122. Igea JM, Cuevas M, Lazaro M, Quirce S, Cuesta J. Susceptibility of a grass-pollen oral imunotherapy extract to the saliva and gastric fluid digestive process. Allergol Immunopathol Madrid 1994; 22: 55–59.
123. Bjorksten B, Moller C, Broberger U, Ahlstedt S, Dreborg S, Johansson SG, et al. Clinical and immunological effects of oral immunotherapy with a standardized birch pollen extract. Allergy 1986; 41: 290–95.

124. Moller C, Dreborg S, Lanner A, Bjorksten B. Oral immunotherapy of children with rhinoconjunctivitis due to birch pollen allergy: a double blind study. Allergy 1986; 41: 271–79.
125. Taudorf E, Laursen LC, Lanner A, Bjorksten B, Dreborg S, Soborg M, et al. Oral immunotherapy in birch pollen hay fever. J Allergy Clin Immunol 1987; 80: 153–61.
126. Taudorf E. Oral immunotherapy of adults with allergic rhinoconjunctivitis: clinical effects in birch and grass pollinosis. Dan Med Bull 1992; 39: 542–60.
127. Van-Niekerk CH, De-Wet JI. Efficacy of grass-maize pollen oral immunotherapy in patients with seasonal hay-fever: a double-blind study. Clin Allergy 1987; 17: 507–13.
128. Sabbah A, Hassoun S, Le-Sellin J, Andre C, Sicard H. A double-blind, placebo-controlled trial by the sublingual route of immunotherapy with a standardized grass pollen extract. Allergy 1994; 49: 309–13.
129. Troise C, Voltolini S, Canessa A, Pecora S, Negrini AC. Sublingual immunotherapy in *Parietaria* pollen-induced rhinitis: a double-blind study. J Investig Allergol Clin Immunol 1995; 5: 25–30.
130. Rebien W, Puttonen E, Maasch HJ, Stix E, Wahn U. Clinical and immunological response to oral and subcutaneous immunotherapy with grass pollen extracts: a prospective study. Eur J Pediatr 1982; 138: 341–44.
131. Horak F, Wheeler AW. Oral hyposensitisation with enteric-coated allergens as extension therapy following a basic subcutaneous course of injections. Int Arch Allergy Appl Immunol 1987; 84: 74–78.
132. Trede N, Urbanek R. Combination of parenteral and oral immunotherapy in grass pollen-allergic children. Allergy 1989; 44: 272–80.
133. D'Souza M, Pepys J, Wells I, Tai E, Palmer F, Overell BG, et al. Hyposensitization with *Dermatophagoides pteronyssinus* in house dust allergy; a controlled study of clinical and immunological effects. Clin Allergy 1973; 3: 177–93.
134. Amaral-Marques R, Avila R. Results of a clinical trial with a *Dermatophagoides pteronyssinus* tyrosine adsorbed vaccine. Allergol Immunopathol Madrid 1978; 6: 231–35.
135. McHugh SM, Lavelle B, Kemeny DM, Patel S, Ewan PW. A placebo-controlled trial of immunotherapy with two extracts of *Dermatophagoides pteronyssinus* in allergic rhinitis, comparing clinical outcome with changes in antigen-specific IgE, IgG and IgG subclasses. J Allergy Clin Immunol 1990; 86: 521–31.
136. Ewan PW, Alexander MM, Snape C, Ind PW, Agrell B, Dreborg S. Effective hyposensitization in allergic rhinitis using a potent partially purified extract of house dust mite. Clin Allergy 1988; 18: 501–8.
137. Gabriel M, Ng H, Allan W, Hill L, Nunn A. Study of prolonged hyposensitization with *D. pteronyssinus* extraxt in allergic rhinitis. Clin Allergy 1977; 7: 325–36.
138. Blainey A, Phillips M, Ollier S, Davies R. Hyposensitization with a tyrosine absorbed extract of *Dermatophagoides pteronyssinus* in adults with perennial allergic rhinitis. Allergy 1984; 39: 521–28.
139. Pastorello EA, Ortolani C, Incorvaia C, Farioli L, Italia M, Pravettoni V, et al. A double-blind study of hyposensitization with an alginate-conjugated extract of *Dermatophagoides pteronyssinus* (Conjuvac) in patients with perennial rhinitis. 2. Immunological aspects. Allergy 1990; 45: 505–14.
140. Corrado OJ, Pastorello E, Ollier S, Cresswell L, Zanussi C, Ortolani C, et al. A double-blind study of hyposensitization with an alginate conjugated extract of *D. pteronyssinus* (Conjuvac) in patients with perennial rhinitis. 1. Clinical aspects. Allergy 1989; 44: 108–15.
141. Lofkvist T, Agrell B, Dreborg S, Svensson G. Effects of immunotherapy with a purified standardized allergen preparation of *Dermatophagoides farinae* in adults with perennial allergic rhinoconjunctivitis. Allergy 1994; 49: 100–7.
142. Tari MG, Mancino M, Monti G. Efficacy of sublingual immunotherapy in patients with rhinitis and asthma due to house dust mite: a double-blind study. Allergol Immunopathol Madrid 1990; 18: 277–784.
143. Andri L, Senna G, Betteli C, Givanni S, Andri G, Falagiani P. Local nasal immunotherapy for *Dermatophagoides*-induced rhinitis: efficacy of a powder extract, J Allergy Clin Immunol 1993; 91: 987–96.

144. Scadding G, Brostoff J. Low dose sublingual therapy in patients with allergic rhinitis due to house dust mite. Clin Allergy 1986; 16: 493–99.
145. Reilly D, Taylor MA, Beattie NGM, Campbell JH, McSharry C, Aitchison TC, et al. Is evidence for homeopathy reproducible? Lancet 1994; 344: 1601–6.
146. Malling H, Weeke B. Immunotherapy. Position Paper of the European Academy of allergy and Clinical Immunology. Allergy 1993; 48 (suppl 14): 9–35.
147. The current status of allergen immunotherapy (hyposensitisation): report of a WHO/IUIS working group. Allergy 1989; 44: 469–79.
148. Bousquet J, Michel FB. Specific immunotherapy in asthma: is it effective? J Allergy Clin Immunol 1994; 94: 1–11.
149. Alvarez-Cuesta E, Cuesta-Herranz J, Puyana-Ruiz J, Cuesta-Herranz C, Blanco-Quiros A. Monoclonal antibody-standardized cat extract immunotherapy: risk-benefit effects from a double-blind placebo study. J Allergy Clin Immunol 1994; 93: 556–66.
150. Oppenheimer J, Areson JG, Nelson HS. Safety and efficacy of oral immunotherapy with standardized cat extract. J Allergy Clin Immunol 1994; 93: 61–67.
151. Nelson H, Oppenheimer J, Vatsia G, Buchmeier A. A double-blind, placebocontrolled evaluation of sublingual immunotherapy with standardized cat extract. J Allergy Clin Immunol 1993; 92: 229–36.
152. Bousquet J, Michel FB, Creticos PS. Sublingual Immunotherapy for cat allergy. J Allergy Clin Immunol 1995; 95: 920–21.
153. Bond JF, Brauer AW, Segal DB, Nault AK, Rogers BL, Kuo MC. Native and recombinant Fel dI as probes into the relationship of allergen structure to human IgE immunoreactivity. Mol Immunol 1993; 30: 1529–41.
154. Helm RM, Squillace DL, Yunginger JW. Production of a proposed international reference standard *Alternaria* extract. 2. Results of a collaborative trial. J Allergy Clin Immunol 1988; 81: 651–63.
155. Dreborg S, Agrell B, Foucard T, Kjellmann NI, Koivikko A, Nilsson S. A double-blind, multicenter immunotherapy trial in children, using a purified and standardized Cladosporium herbarum preparation. 1. Clinical results. Allergy 1986; 41: 131–40.
156. Karlsson R, Agarell B, Dreborg S. A double-blind, multicenter immunotherapy trial in children, using a purified and standardized *Cladosporium herbarum* preparation. 2. In vitro results. Allergy 1986; 41: 141–50.
157. Malling HJ, Dreborg S, Weeke B. Diagnosis and immunotherapy of mould allergy. 5. Clinical efficacy and side effects of immunotherapy with Cladosporium herbarum. Allergy 1986; 41: 507–19.
158. Horst M, Hejjaoui A, Horst V, Michel FB, Bousquet J. Double-blind, placebo-controlled rush immunotherapy with a standardized Alternaria extract. J Allergy Clin Immunol 1990; 85: 460–72.
159. Kaad PH, Ostergaard PA. The hazard of mould hyposensitization in children with asthma. Clin Allergy 1982; 12: 317–20.
160. International consensus Report on the Diagnosis and Management of Rhinitis. Allergy 1994; 49 (suppl 19): 1–33.
161. Frew AJ. Injection immunotherapy. British Society for Allergy and Clinical Immunology Working Party. Br Med J 1993; 307: 919–23.
162. Bush R, Huftel M, Busse W. Patient selection. In: Lockey R, Bukantz S, editors. Allergen immunotherapy. New York: Marcel Dekker, 1991: 25–49.
163. Cohn JR, Pizzi A. Determinants of patient compliance with allergen immunotherapy. J Allergy Clin Immunol 1993; 91: 734–73.
164. Position paper on allergen immunotherapy: report of a BSACI working party. January–October 1992. Clin Exp Allergy 1993; 3: 1–44.
165. Birkner T, Rumpold H, Jarolim E, Ebner H, Breitenbach M, Skvaril F, et al. Evaluation of immunotherapy-induced changes in specific IgE, IgG and IgG subclasses in birch pollen allergic patients by means of immunoblotting: correlation with clinical response. Allergy 1990; 45: 418–26.
166. Parker W Jr, Wishman BA, Apaliski SJ, Reid MJ. The relationships between late cutaneous responses and specific antibody responses with outcome of immunotherapy for seasonal allergic rhinitis. J Allergy Clin Immunol 1989; 84: 667–77.

Rhinitis: Immunopathology
and Pharmacotherapy
ed. by D. Raeburn and M.A. Giembycz

CHAPTER 9
Surgery of Rhinitis

James A. Cook

Department of Otolaryngology, Leicester Royal Infirmary, and University of Leicester, Leicester, UK

1. Introduction

Whilst the treatment of allergic and nonallergic rhinitis is primarily medical (as discussed in the accompanying chapters), a significant number of patients fail to obtain satisfactory relief from these measures, and surgical options may become of value.

Arguably, the principal symptom of rhinitis is obstruction to nasal airflow. The site of highest resistance of nasal airflow in the respiratory tract is found in the area of the anterior nasal valve and surgical strategies designed to relieve nasal airflow obstruction are usually targeted at this site and, in particular, at the inferior turbinate.

The inferior turbinate is composed of mucosa, cavernous tissue which possesses erectile properties [1, 2], periosteum and bone. Nasal obstruction may result as a consequence of engorgement of the erectile tissue, which is itself subject to autonomic neural influence. Parasympathetic stimulation leads to engorgement of the turbinate and rhinorrhoea, whereas sympathetic stimulation produces the converse. Surgery to control the influence of the inferior turbinates upon nasal airflow resistance may therefore be directed at both the turbinate itself and at its autonomic innervation. The chief purpose of this chapter is to evaluate these two approaches. A summary of the surgical options available for the treatment of atrophic rhinitis will also be given. For the surgical treatment of rhinosinusitis, the reader is referred to the milestone text on functional endoscopic sinus surgery by Stammberger [3].

1.1. Surgery of the Inferior Turbinate

A variety of procedures have been developed to reduce the bulk of the inferior turbinate or to reduce its ability to enlarge. These vary from attempts to induce scarring in the submucosal erectile tissue of the turbinate to radical amputation. Methods available to reduce the erectile capacity of the turbinate include injection of submucosal sclerosants [4], corticosteroids [5], cryosurgery [6] and various forms of cautery.

Surface cautery with a hot wire may be performed as an outpatient procedure but may result in crusting and incurs a risk of adhesion formation [7]. Submucosal diathermy (SMD) was initially performed using galvanic current [8] or hot wires [9]. Nagelschmidt [10] first described surgical diathermy in 1909, and later unipolar [11] and bipolar [12] techniques were developed. The beneficial effects of submucosal diathermy were subsequently described [13–15]. Von Haacke [16] described 204 cases of SMD to the inferior turbinate, performed over 6 years. Some of the cases also underwent antral lavage, but none underwent septal surgery. Symptomatic improvement was recorded in 72%, though the method of SMD was not recorded. Jones [17] has described a standardised method of performing SMD involving three passes of a unipolar electrode through the inferior turbinate. He also reported that it was possible to predict the outcome of SMD to the inferior turbinates by assessing the response to preoperative decongestion with xylometazoline. Unfortunately, the initial benefits of SMD do not seem to be maintained in the long term. Jones and Lancer [18] reported a series of 21 patients in whom a significant improvement in nasal airway resistance was obtained 2 months after the procedure, but at 15 months nasal airway resistance was not significantly different from the preoperative resistance. Nevertheless, these patients were still symptomatically better.

Talaat [19] studied 10 patients with nonallergic rhinitis and 10 patients with allergic rhinitis and described the mechanism by which SMD appears to work. At 1 month following SMD, punch biopsies were taken from the inferior turbinate and subjected to histological examination. Fibrosis was found which appeared to anchor the mucosa to the periosteum. A reduction in congestion and the number of tunical blood vessels was also found which could be expected to result in a reduction in oedema and cellular infiltration from blood. A reduction in the number of seromicinous glands was also noted, particularly in the nonallergic group. The latter also showed a significant improvement in the epithelial lining which returned to a pseudo-stratified type with reappearance of cilia and thinning of the basement membrane. Some cavernous sinusoids appeared to be destroyed. Histocytochemistry revealed no significant changes in the allergic group, indicating that the allergic process was still present.

1.2. Cryosurgery to the Inferior Turbinate

Cryosurgery as an effective treatment for rhinitis was first reported in 1970 [6]. Initially, freon was used as a coolant, but subsequently nitrous oxide was employed [20]. A cryoprobe was applied for 3–4 min at each of the sites indicated (Figure 1). Of 46 patients with nonallergic rhinitis undergoing this treatment, 100% were said to be relieved of their nasal obstructions and 92% of their rhinorrhoea. Although the maximum follow-up period was noted at 15 months, it is not certain how many patients were seen at this stage. Complications of the treatment included perforations of the nasal septum, serous otitis media (temporary), acute sinusitis and delayed healing. Modification of this technique was described in 1984 by Bumsted [21], who also emphasised the importance of careful patient selection: the sites of application of the cryoprobe are indicated in Figure 2. He reported that healing took place in 5–6 weeks and that nasal obstructions was eliminated in 46 (92%) of his 50 patients. His minimum follow-

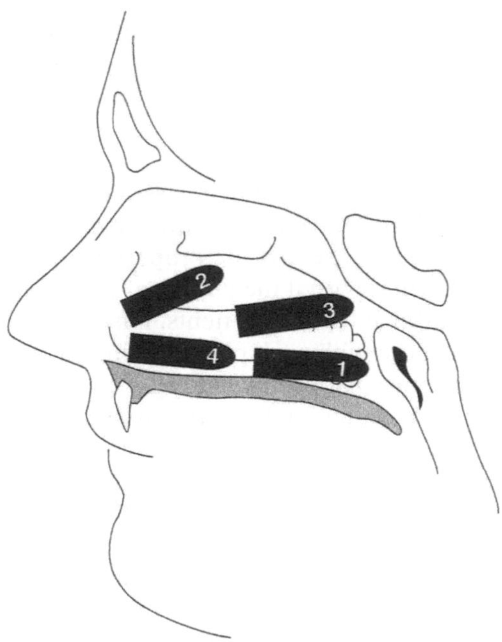

Figure 1. Four sites of application of the cryoprobe to the inferior and middle turbinates.

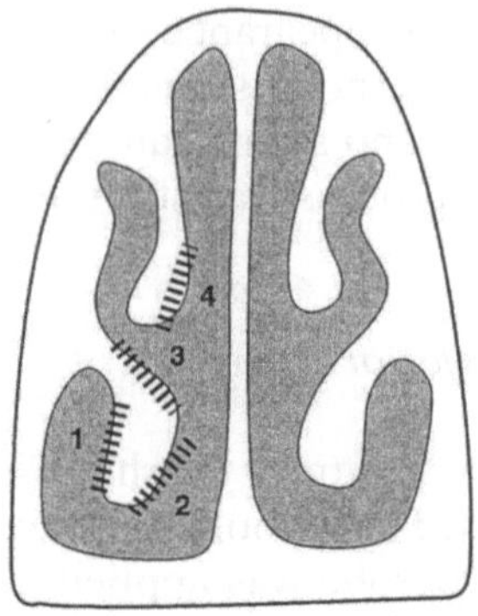

Figure 2. Modification of application of the cryoprobe to the inferior middle turbinates (adapted from Bumsted [21]).

up period was 2 years. Postoperative nasal airway obstruction usually lasted for up to 3 weeks, although Malony [22] reported nasal obstruction for only between 5 and 6 days. Principato [23] has emphasised the importance of removing slough from the nasal cavities at 5–7 days postoperatively. He also stated it was important to protect septal spurs and perform a septoplasty if necessary. Moore and Bicknell [24] compared the results obtained by cryosurgery with those obtained by SMD. There seemed to be no significant differences in effectiveness between the techniques at 2 months or at 6 months. Given that cryosurgery may be performed on an outpatients basis, it would seem to be a reasonable therapeutic option.

1.3. Laser Cautery of the Inferior Turbinate

As early as 1979 the use of a laser to decrease the bulk of the inferior turbinate was described [25]. The approach was later modified by Fukutake [26] in an attempt to reduce the erectile properties of the turbinate rather than decrease is bulk. He reported the effects of application of a CO_2 laser beam to the inferior turbinate on 140 patients. Laser surgery was performed as an outpatient procedure with each patient being treated once a week on five occasions. This somewhat protracted regimen was employed to avoid complications such as bleeding and reactive nasal obstruction. The entire surface of the inferior turbinate was subjected to vapourization by means of a defocused beam at 20–30 W for 1 min. Excellent or good results were achieved in 76% of patients at 1 month (from 140 cases) and 77% at 1 year (from 35 cases). However, selection criteria for the patients were not described. Kawamura [25] reported broadly similar results using a defocused CO_2 laser in patients with perennial allergic rhinitis caused by house dust. “Good or excellent” results were reported in 85% at 1 month, 76% at 2 years and 75% at 3 years in his cohort of 75 patients.

A comparison of CO_2 laser cautery of the inferior turbinate with submucosal diathermy [27] revealed that subjective nasal airway resistance was improved at 6 weeks in both groups but only in the laser group at 3 days postoperatively. Objective measurement by peak inspiratory nasal airflow revealed no significant differences. The follow-up of this cohort of 29 patients by the present author [28] revealed a significant improvement in subjective nasal airflow at 1 year, compared with the preoperative state in the laser group but not in the SMD group. This paper represented the first double-blind controlled trial examining the long-term effects of laser against SMD in the treatment of perennial rhinitis and confirmed that there was a long-term improvement in the nasal sensation of airflow following laser treatment. Laser cautery of the inferior turbinate would therefore appear to offer superior results to SMD, not least because it may be performed as an outpatient procedure. Mittelman [29] has also reported CO_2 laser turbinectomy to be superior to surgical reduction of the inferior turbinates since it may be performed on an outpatient basis using only topical anaesthesia and without the requirement for intranasal packing. It would also seem probable that the likelihood of postoperative haemorrhage would be reduced with the laser, though the incidence of postoperative haemorrhage was not compared with the incidence of bleeding after surgical turbinectomy.

1.4. Surgical Reduction of the Inferior Turbinates

Total turbinectomy was first described in the 19th century [30]. However, complications such as atrophic rhinitis and paradoxical nasal dyspnoea led to the procedure falling into disrepute. The development of less radical procedures led to a resurgence in the popularity of partial turbinectomy [31, 32] and submucosal resection of the inferior turbinate [33]. More recently, Mucci and Sismanis [34] reported a series of 54 patients in whom partial inferior turbinectomy had been performed with preservation of the inferior turbinate bone (Figure 3). In their series, 92% of the patients reported a decrease in nasal obstruction, 86% decrease in rhinorrhoea, 82% a decrease in snoring, 83% a decrease in headaches and 64% a decrease in "obstructive sleep apnoea". Average follow-up was for a period of 18 months (range 12–39 months). Bleeding was observed in 3.7%. Meredith [35] compared 100 patients who underwent electrocautery with 100 who underwent inferior partial turbinectomy. They stated 86% were improved following turbinectomy, but only 69% following electrocautery. However, there were no objective measurements and no statistical analyses. Bhargava [36] has recommended removal of the anterior one-third of each inferior turbinate under local anaesthesia. He performed this procedure on a series of 30 patients with allergic or nonallergic rhinitis and reported on 27 of them, though the duration of the follow-up was not mentioned. Eighty-

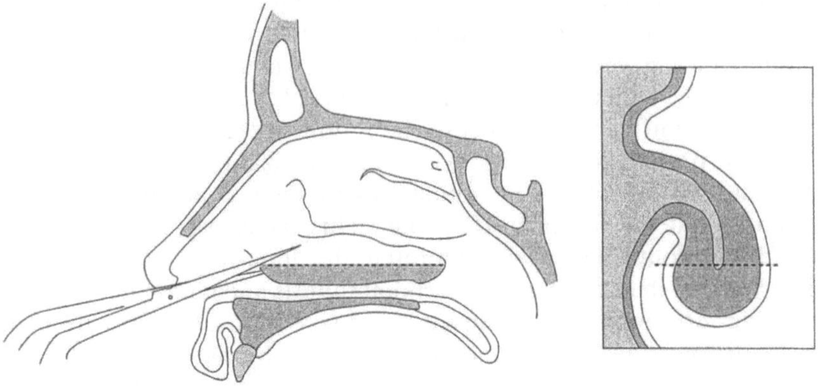

Figure 3. Inferior partial turbinectomy.

one percent an improvement in nasal obstruction, 80% in headaches, 78% in sneezing and 67% in rhinorrhoea. Whilst nothing that anterior turbinectomy should reduce nasal airflow resistance in the area of the anterior nasal valve, Jones found no evidence to support the subjective efficacy of this treatment [37]. The effectiveness and safety of reduction of the inferior turbinates has been assessed in children [38]. In a series of 22 children aged 15 years or younger, 68% reported a sustained improvement in the nasal airways with a period of follow-up ranging from 7 to 51 months. No serious cases of postoperative haemorrhage were encountered, although one child bled profusely following the removal of an intranasal pack but settled within a few minutes following the application of an ice-pack.

Whilst surgical reduction of the inferior turbinates is clearly likely to decrease nasal airway resistance due to purely mechanical factors, there may be other mechanisms involved. Shone [39] has studied the effect of reduction of the turbinates on mucociliary clearance and found no chance in saccharin transport time 3 weeks after turbinate reduction. However, the long-term effects were not evaluated. Cortes et al. [40] have postulated that autonomic microganglia in the inferior turbinates may be important in the pathophysiology of rhinitis. They suggested that vidian neurectomy, combined with reduction of the turbinates, may give a better result than either procedure performed in isolation, in that the cholinergic parasympathetic influence upon the nasal mucosa may be reduced at two anatomical sites by combining these procedures. They supported their data by simulating intrinsic rhinitis in cats by adminstering neostigmine. Three cats underwent inferior partial turbinectomy, another three Vidian neurectomy and a further three a combination of both these procedures. A combination of procedures was found to be more efficacious than either procedure performed alone in terms of reducing nasal hypersecretion. However, a change in nasal resistance to airflow was not reported.

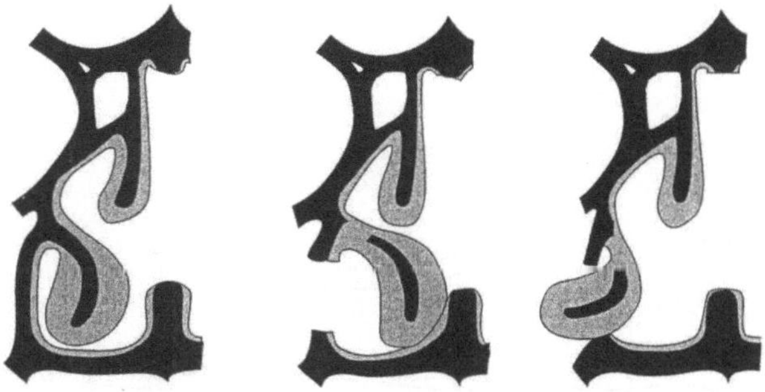

Figure 4. Antroconchopexy. The inferior turbinate is displaced via a large inferior meatal antrostomy into the maxillary antrum.

Antroconchopexy has been suggested as an alternative to turbinate reduction by reducing the impact of enlargement of the inferior turbinate on nasal airway resistance [41]. The procedure involves lateralicing the inferior turbinate through a large inferior meatal antrostomy into the maxillary antrum (Figure 4). The posterior end of the inferior turbinate extends beyond the limit of the antrostomy, and displacing this posterior end of the turbinate into the antrum to maintain the inferior turbinate in its lateralised position. The procedure was initially described by Fateen [42] and later Legler [43]. Lannigan [41] found significant reduction in nasal airway resistance as assessed by posterior active rhinomanometry 6 weeks after surgery. Reduction in the size of the inferior turbinate by application of silver nitrate has also been described [44], as has zinc intranasal ionisation [45].

2. Manipulation of Autonomic Innervation

The nasal mucosa receives three sources of innervation: (1) The maxillary division of the trigeminal nerve subserves sensation. (2) Vasoconstrictor influence is received from the sympathetic nervous system. Fibres from the superior cervical ganglion travel along the internal carotid artery, thence to the deep petrosal nerve where they travel with the parasympathetic fibres derived from the nervous intermedius. Sympathetic fibres from the deep petrosal nerve pass through the pterygopalatine ganglion without synapse. (3) Parasympathetic vasodilatatory and secretomotor influence is received from the superior salivatory nucleus via the nervus intermedius, thence to the greater superficial petrosal nerve, which travels with the deep petrosal nerve in the vidian canal. The parasympathetic fibres synapse in the pterygopalatine ganglion and are thence distributed to the nasal cavum. The innervation of the nasal mucosa is illustrated in Figure 5.

The predominant autonomic influence upon the nasal mucosa is parasympathetic. If both sympathetic and parasympathetic fibres to the nasal

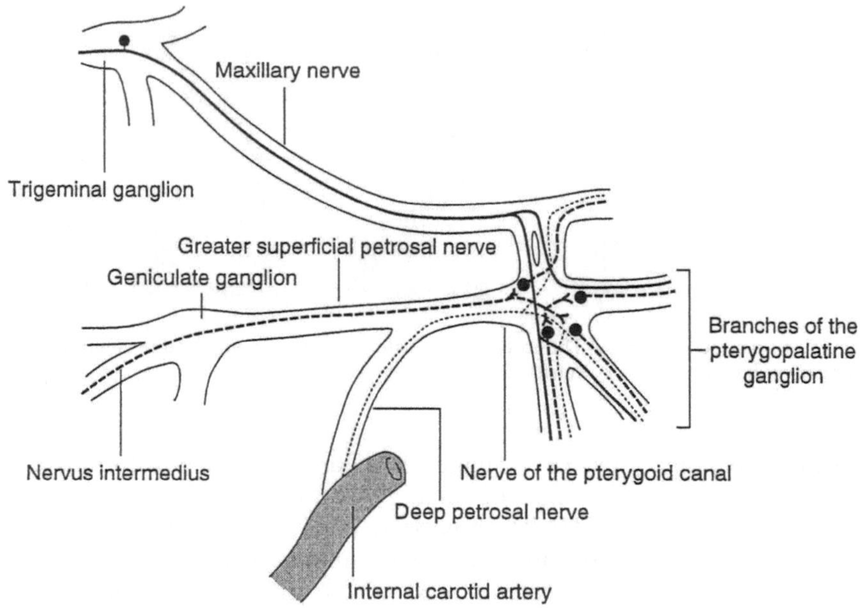

Figure 5. Sensory and autonomic innovation of the nasal mucosa.

mucosa are sectioned, the overall result is to decrease secretion and nasal airway resistance. The most common therapeutic methods used to achieve this are vidian neurectomy and pterygopalatine ganglionectomy.

2.1. Vidian Neurectomy

This procedure was first described by Golding-Wood in 1961 [46]. He employed a transantral (Cauldwell Luc) approach to the pterypopalatine fossa. After removal of the anterior bony wall of the pterygopalatine fossa, fat in the pterygopalatine fossa is dissected to expose the maxillary artery and its branches. These are clipped. The maxillary nerve is identified as it passes out of the foramen rotundum, and the vidian nerve sought more medially (Figure 6). Removal of bone on the medial wall of the antrum may be necessary to facilitate a view of the vidian nerve. The vidian nerve is then destroyed by diathermy. Initially, there were occasional cases of ophthalmoplegia produced by overinsertion of the diathermy probe into the vidian canal. Golding-Wood subsequently developed a unipolar diathermy electrode with shoulders such that penetration of the vidian canal beyond 2 mm was not possible (Figure 7). No cases of ophthalmoplegia have been reported using this modification. His approach allows preservation of the somatic fibres derived from the maxillary nerve and nasal mucosal

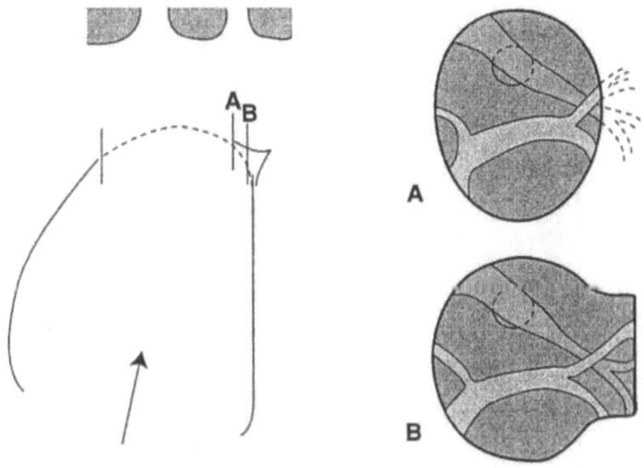

Figure 6. Transantral approach to the vidian canal. Bone between A and B requires removal to facilitate a view of the canal.

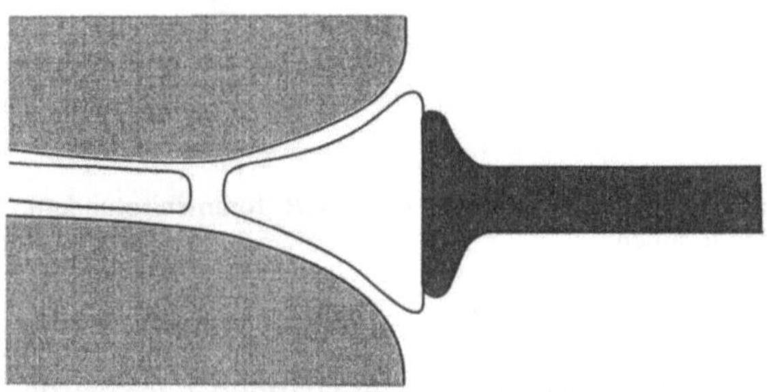

Figure 7. Unipolar diathermy electrode designed by Golding-Wood to limit penetration into the vidian canal.

sensation is preserved. Ablation of the pterygopalatine ganglion in contrast results in a loss of nasal mucosal sensation.

Largely due to the possibility of ophthalmoplegia and also the technical demands of the transantral route, various other approaches have been recommended. In 1975, Patel [47] pioneered a transantral approach to the vidian canal. This was further reported by Portman [48] and Kirtane [49, 50]. Fernandes [51] reported a series of 276 patients who had undergone transnasal vidian neurectomy. Eighty-two of these patients also underwent a septoplasty for reasons of access. One hundred and twenty patients also had a partial inferior turbinectomy. Fernandes performed the procedure under general anaesthesia. The middle turbinate was fractured medially and upwards, a long Killian's nasal speculum inserted and the posterior end of the middle meatus visualised by means of an operating microscope with a 300-mm objective lens. A small antrostomy was made into the maxillary at the posterior end of the middle meatus so that the posterosuperior margin of the maxillary antrum could be seen. The periosteum of the postero-

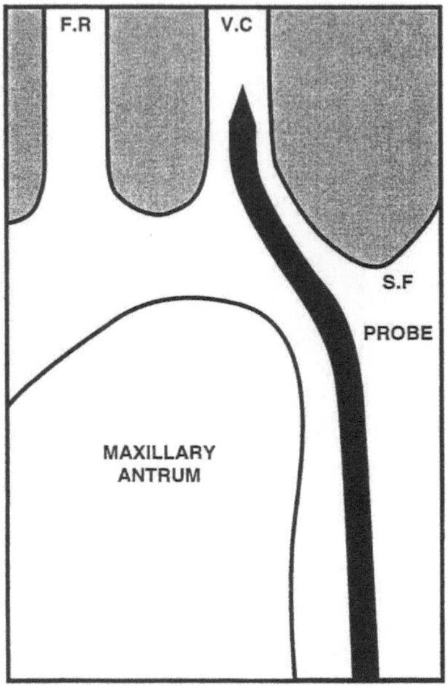

Figure 8. Transnasal approach to the vidian canal. F.R: foramen rotundum; V.C: vidian canal; S.F: sphenopalatine foramen.

medial margin of the antrostomy was stripped backwards off the lateral wall of the nose to reveal the sphenopalatine foramen (Figure 8). Bagatella [52] reported considerable variation in the location of the vidian nerve, and Fernandes' approach allows more certain identification of the vidian nerve and canal by identifying the landmark for the sphenopalatine foramen, the sphenopalatine artery, which exits from the foramen. The vidian canal has an anteroposterior orientation with its anterior opening in the posterior wall of the pterygopalatine fossa, level with the sphenopalatine foramen and 5–6 mm behind and lateral to it. A modified insulated bayonet electrode is introduced into the sphenopalatine foramen and into the vidian canal. The electrode is not inserted any further than 5 mm into the canal to avoid ophthalmoplegia. In Fernandes' series, 96% of patients with intrinsic rhinitis reported an improvement in the nasal obstruction, 88% of those with allergic rhinitis and 88% of those with nasal polyposis. Chandra [53] described a transpalatal approach which was subsequently improved by Mustafa [54], whilst Minnis and Morrison [55] described the trans-septal approach. El-Guindy developed the trans-septal approach using rigid 0° and 30° endoscopes [56] (Figure 9). The procedure is similar to the trans-nasal approach, but since the endoscope is passed into the contralateral nostril and through the nasal septum following a septoplasty, a more lateral view of the pterygopalatine fossa may be obtained. The procedure may be

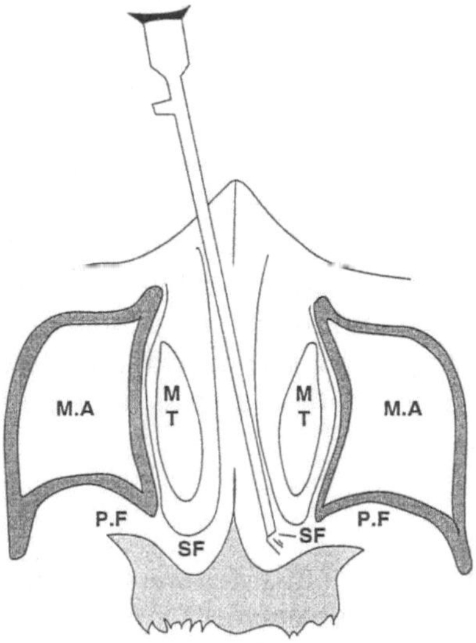

Figure 9. Transeptal approach to the sphenopalatine foramen. (MA: maxillary antrum; MT: middle turbinate; SF: sphenopalatine foramen; PF: pterygopalatine fossa).

performed endoscopically without septoplasty by insertion of the endoscope into the ipsilateral nostril [57]. Kamel [57] found an improvement in nasal rhinorrhoea and sneezing in 77 out of 102 patients, the minimum period of follow-up being 6 months.

The vidian nerve may also be ablated by means of the CO_2 laser [58]. Using the transantral approach, Williams [58] reported less pain and swelling than when performing a traditional transantral vidian neurectomy using chisels, rongers, diamond drills and electrocautery.

The biochemical and physical effects of vidian neurectomy have also been studied. Rucci [59, 60] looked at the nerve's influence on histamine turnover and mucosal mast cell function in nonallergic rhinitis. He reported a reduction in mucosal histamine and a reduction in the density and degranulation index of mast cells. He also found a reduction in histidine decarboxylase activity, which was interpreted as expressing parasympathetic involvement in the regulation of mast cell histamine.

Greenstone studied the effect of vidian neurectomy on nasal mucociliary clearance, assessed by saccarine transport time, but did not find any significant effect [61].

Vidian neurectomy is not commonly believed to provide long-term relief of nasal obstruction, rhinorrhoea or sneezing. Golding-Wood [62] has emphasised that patient selection needs to be rigorously maintained. Where watery rhinorrhoea is the principal complaint, symptoms seem to be best controlled. Nasal allergy also needs to be excluded. Only those patients resistant to medical treatment should be selected for surgery. He also states that nasal obstruction is best dealt with by means of linear cautery of the inferior turbinates, repeated three times at weekly intervals. Krant [63] assessed the amount of rhinorrhoea, nasal obstruction and sneezing following transantral vidian neurectomy and found that five out of seven patients with vasomotor rhinitis, symptoms returned within 4 to 12 months. This may serve to emphasise that patients with intractible watery rhinorrhoea may be the best candidates for this procedure. Conversely, Ogale [64] reported 208 cases undergoing transnasal vidian neurectomy by diathermy coagulation. One hundred and ninety-six patients had vasomotor rhinitis, and of these 184 were improved. The maximum follow-up was for a period of 5 years, but the minimum follow-up was not reported.

3. Atrophic Rhinitis

The aetiology of atrophic rhinitis remains an unsolved problem. The disease causes great embarrassment due to the formation of crusts and foul accompanying foetor. Fortunately, the incidence of atrophic rhinitis seems to be on the decline.

3.1. Surgery of Atrophic Rhinitis

A variety of surgical procedures have been developed. In 1873 Rouge (see [65]) curetted the whole of the nasal mucosa, hoping for healthy regeneration, but the results were disappointing and the procedure fell into disrepute. Extirpation of the sphenopalatine ganglion has been performed to reduce the sympathetic influence upon the nasal mucosa, but this procedure also results in disruption of the parasympathetic pathway, adding further to nasal dryness. A variety of procedures have been designed to reduce the size of the apparently large nasal cavity and to reduce nasal airflow. For a historical review the reader is referred to Girgis [65]. This section will concentrate on those procedures which still have their advocates.

3.1.1. Closure of the nostril: Young [66] described a procedure to obstruct the nostril completely by means of raising flaps from the nasal vestibular skin. An incision is made at the mucocutaneous junction inside the nostril and skin along with the joining mucosa reflected forwards by scissor dissection until adequate flaps are obtained for approximation without tension. The skin flaps are then sutured together and a small gauze wick, impregnated with antibiotics, is inserted and held in place with adhesive tapes over the suture line. The adhesive tapes help to counteract the tendency of the alar cartilage to spring the nostril open. Young subsequently performed a 5-year follow-up on his initial cohort of patients [67] and did not encounter a significant incidence of sponataneous reopening of the nostrils as long as the skin flaps were sufficiently undercut. Gadre [68] staged closures of the nostrils such that the second side was only closed following healing of the first side. Complete freedom from crusting was noticed within a month following bilateral closure but a dry mouth and snoring were occasional problems. In contrast to Young, Shah [69] found that complete nostril closure may not be necessary. He left a defect in the repair, approximately one-eighth the size of the nostril. The contralateral nostril was usually completely sealed, particularly in severe cases. Of his 97 cases, all reported an improvement at 1 year. Seventy-five per cent were free of nasal crusting when examined through the side of the partial closure. The nostrils of 11 patients were reopened at between 1.5 and 2 years after the initial procedure. In 10 these patients the nasal mucosa was reported to be clinically normal with no crusting. Histologically, there was persistence of squamous metaplasia in the reopened nostrils in some cases, with a return to respiratory ciliated epithelium in others. The inflammatory reaction was

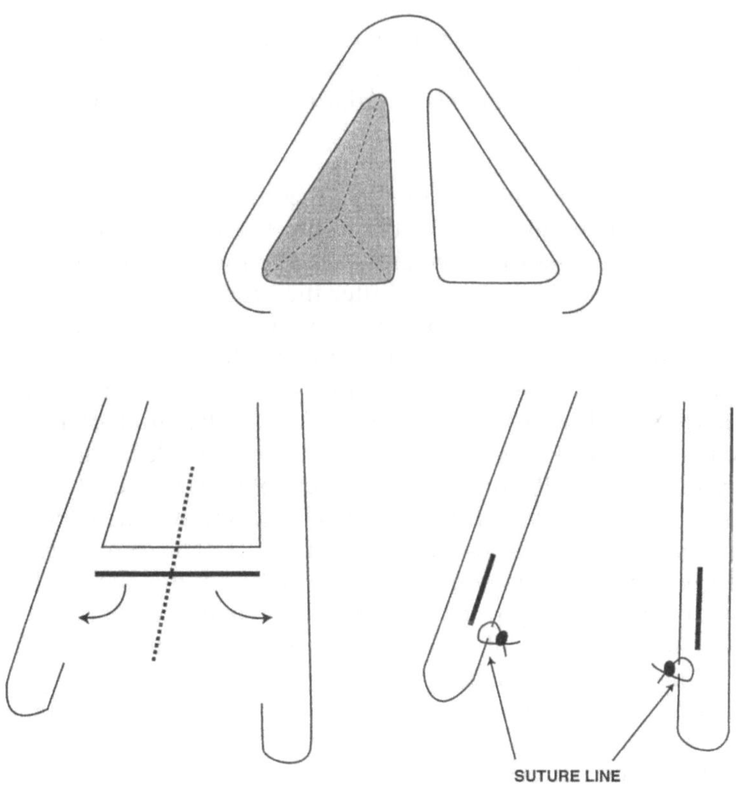

Figure 10. Method of reopening nostril after Young's procedure (Gadre). Three radial incisions are made into the occluded nostril. The rostrally based flaps are rotated caudally and sutured to the denuded nasal vestibule.

also reduced, and the number of mucous glands increased. Mustafa recommended complete closure of one nostril with partial closure of the other [70]. He also looked at when the nostril should be reopened. Ten cases underwent closure for 9 months, 10 for 12 months and 30 for 18 months. The cases were followed up for a year and half after reopening. The greatest improvement was obtained when the nostrils were closed for 18 months, with 24 of the 30 patients free of crusting on both sides of the nasal cavity. Reopening was performed by simple excision of the skin flaps but Gadre [71] reported a modification. Three radial incisions were made into the closure, and these rostrally based flaps were rotated caudally (Figure 10). This modification was reported to decrease the incidence of restenosis of the nostril.

3.1.2. Vestibulopexy: Ghosh [72] developed a modification of partial closure of the nostril. He suggested that if airflow could be directed away from the lateral wall of the nose, atrophic rhinitis would settle. To achieve this, he dissected a rostrally based skin flap from the lateral wall of the nasal vestibule and sutured this to itself to produce the narrowing of the nostril in the region of the mucocutaneous junction, leaving an airway approximately 6 mm × 12 mm (Figure 11). Satisfactory healing was obtained in 23 of his 25 patients, similar to that found following Young's procedure.

3.1.3. Insertion of implants: Girgis has recommended the insertion of a dermofat graft obtained from the thigh into the lateral wall of the nasal cavity [65]. In his series of 76 patients, 62 were found to be asymptomatic, 3 better and 3 the same at 1 month after the procedure. Forty-seven were followed up for 6 months, and the procedure was deemed successful in 36 with some improvement being obtained in a further 8. Chatterji implanted bone chips into the lateral wall of the nose under the mucoperiosteum but only reported good results in 12 patients [73]. Implantation of a fibromuscular temporalis graft was also reported by Papay [74], but this time into the floor of the nose. Rasmy [75] describes rotation of an osteoperiosteal flap from the anterior wall of the maxillary antrum into the lateral wall of the nose in the subperiosteal space (Figure 12). Thirteen patients were followed up for up to 18 months and improvement noticed in all though some shrinkage of the graft occured in two patients. Karnik [76] has recommended injection of placental extracts and Sinha [77] found it beneficial in 46 of a series of 60 patients.

Whitehead [78] reported the use of Proplast mixed with blood and Ampicillin. Shehata [79] suggested placing silastic implants into a subperichondreal and periosteal pocket developed in the nasal septum. In his 30 patients the implant was rejected in 9, and of these, 6 underwent reimplantation without further extrusion. Twenty-seven were found to be better at 1 year following surgery. Ward [80] injected Teflon into the floor of

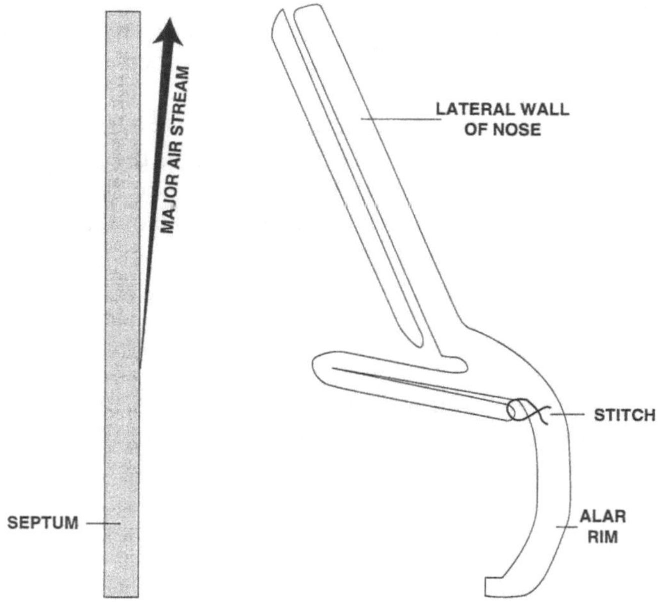

Figure 11. Vestibulopexy (Ghosh). A rostrally based lateral skin flap is sutured to itself to narrow the lateral portion of the nostril.

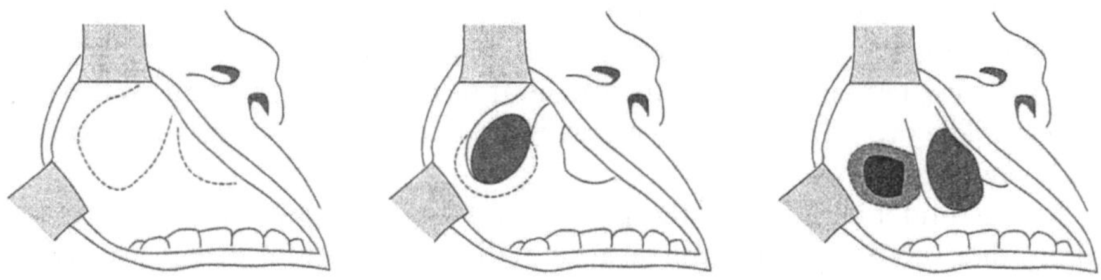

Figure 12. Rotation of an osteoperiosteal flap pedicled superiorly and taken from the anterior wall of the maxillary antrum. The flap is approached by means of a sublabial incision and is rotated into the lateral wall of the nose.

the nose of a patient with atrophic rhinitis, administering 19 cc into the floor of both nasal cavities, both under the inferior turbinate and into the angle between the floor of the nose and the nasal septum, apparently to good effect.

3.1.4. Other Methods: Ssali [81] suggested middle turbinectomy. He hypothesised that the middle turbinate would interfere with drainage of the ethmoids, resulting in stasis and infection of nasal secretions. This, he supposed, would lead to atrophic rhinitis. he treated 35 patients by middle turbinectomy and reported "reasonable success". Pharyngoplasty [82] has also been suggested, with elevation of a caudally based pharyngeal flap. The flap should be made as wide and as cranial as possible.

3.1.5. Surgical treatment of unilateral atrophic rhinitis: When atrophic rhinitis is combined with a deviated nasal septum, the procedure may be treated by means of a septoplasty [83]. This procedure has the advantage of improving the airway on the obstructed side and also reducing the size of the nasal cavum on the atrophic side.

3.2. Leprous Rhinitis

Leprous rhinitis results in atrophy of the nasal mucosa and crust formation, similar to that found in atrophic rhinitis. Partial closure of the nostrils may be of benefit [84].

4. Summary

The plethora of surgical options available to treat vasomotor, allergic and atrophic rhinitis would suggest that no single procedure can be recommended above all the others for each of these conditions. Factors which may come into the choice of procedure include the complexity of the technique and obviously the reported results. The possibility of performing a particular technique in the outpatient department may also be of benefit. Many procedures involve the insertion of nasal packs for haemostatic purposes; these are not popular with patients and have also been linked with toxic shock syndrome [85].

As our understanding of the pathophysiology of rhinitis improves, it is likely that medical treatment options will become more effective. Nevertheless, it is clear that surgery still has a major role to play.

References

1. Principato JJ. Chronic vasomotor rhinitis. cryogenic and other surgical modes of treatment. Laryngoscope 1979; 89: 619–38.
2. Abramson M, Harker LA. Physiology of the nose. Otolaryngol Clin N America 1973; 6: 623–35.
3. Stammberger H, editor. Functional endoscopic sinus surgery: the Messerklinger technique. Philadelphia: B.C. Decker, 1991.
4. Fishof FE. Treatment of vasomotor rhinitis and allied conditions with sodium morrhuate: preliminary report. Arch Otolaryngol 1938; 27: 413–19.
5. Simmons MW. Intranasal injection of corticosteroids in nasal disorders: further observations. Transactions Pacific Coast Oto-ophthalmological Society 1964; 45: 95–103.
6. Ozenberger JM. Cryosurgery in chronic rhinitis. Laryngoscope 1970; 80: 723–34.
7. Davison FW. Intranasal surgery. Transactions Pacific Coast Oto-opthalmological Society 1967; 51: 273–84.

8. Neres FE. Voltaic: turbinal puncture for the relief of intumescent and hypertrophic rhinitis. J Am Med Assoc 1907; 49: 1435–38.
9. Horn H. The treatment of intumescent rhinitis by a submucous method. Annals Otol Rhinol Laryngol 1908; 17: 490–94.
10. Nagelschmidt F, Uber Diathermie (Transthermie, thermopenetration). Munch Med Wschr 1909; 59: 2575.
11. Beck JC. Pathology and intramural electrode coagulation of inferior turbinate. Annals Otol Rhinol 1930; 39: 349–63.
12. Hurd LM. Bipolar electrode for electro-coagulation of inferior turbinate. Arch Otolaryngol 1931; 13: 442.
13. Richardson JR. Turbinate treatment in vasomotor rhinitis. Laryngoscope 1948; 58: 834–47.
14. Shahinian L. Chronic vasomotor rhinitis treatment by submucous diathermic coagulation. Arch Otolaryngol 1953; 57: 475–89.
15. Simpson JF, Groves J. Submucosal diathermy of the inferior turbinates. J Laryngol Otol 1958; 72: 292–301.
16. Von Haacke NP, Hardcastle PF. Submucosal diathermy of the inferior turbinates and the congested nose. J Otolaryngol 1985; 47: 189–93.
17. Jones AS, Wyght RG, Kabil Y, Beckingham E. Predicting the outcome of submucosal diathermy to the inferior turbinates. Clin Otolaryngol 1989; 14: 41–44.
18. Jones AS, Lancer JM. Does submucosal diathermy to the inferior turbinate reduce nasal resistance to airflow in the long term? J Laryngol 1987; 101: 448–51.
19. Talatt M, El-Sabawy E, Baky FA, Raheem AA. Submucous diathermy of the inferior turbinates in chronic hypertrophic rhinitis. J Laryngol Otol 1987; 101: 452–60.
20. Ozenberger JM. Cryosurgery for the treatment of chronic rhinitis. Laryngoscope 1973; 83: 508–16.
21. Bumsted RM. Cryotherapy for chronic vasomotor rhinitis: technique and patient selection for improved results. Laryngoscope 1984; 94: 539–44.
22. Molony TJ. Cryosurgery in chronic nasal obstruction. J Otolaryngol 1976; 5: 156–58.
23. Principato JJ. A fifteen year retrospective of chronic rhinitis and cryosurgery. ENT J 1986; 65: 558–63.
24. Moore JRM, Bicknell PG. A comparison of cryosurgery and submucous diathermy in vasomotor rhinitis. J Laryngol Otol 1980; 94: 1411–13.
25. Wang OI. Laser in otolaryngology. Chinese Med J 1979; 92: 857–61.
26. Fukutake T, Yamashita T, Tomoda K, Kumazawa T. Laser surgery for allergic rhinitis. Arch Otolaryngol Head Neck Surg 1986; 112: 1280–82.
27. McCombe AW, Cook JA, Jones AS. A comparison of laser cautery and submucosal diathermy for rhinitis. Clin Otolaryngol 1992; 17: 297–99.
28. Cook JA, McCombe AW, Jones AS. Laser treatment of rhinitis – one year follow-up. Clin Otolaryngol 1993; 18: 209–11.
29. Mittelman H. CO_2 laser turbinatectomies for chronic obstructive rhinitis. Lasers in Surgery and Medicine 1982; 2: 29–36.
30. Jones TC. Turbinotomy. Lancet 1895; 2: 496.
31. Courtiss EH, Goldwyn RM, O'Brien JJ. Resection of obstructing inferior nasal turbinates. Plastic Reconstr Surg 1978; 62: 249–56.
32. Pollock RA, Rohrich RJ. Inferior turbinate surgery. Plastic Reconstr Surg 1984; 74: 227–33.
33. Hause HP. Submucous resection of the inferior turbinal bone. Laryngoscope 1951; 61: 637.
34. Mucci S, Sismanis A. Inferior partial turbinectomy: an effective procedure for chronic rhinitis. ENT J 1994; 73: 405–7.
35. Meredith GM. Surgical reduction of hypertrophied inferior turbinates: a comparison of electrofulgeration and partial resection: Plastic Reconstr Surg 1988; 81: 892–7.
36. Bhargara KB, Shirali GN, Abhyankar US, Gadre KC. Turbinectomies for Allergic and Vasomotor Rhinitis. Ear Nose and Throat J 1987; 66(3): 125–127.
37. Jones AS, Wight RG, Stevens JC, Beckingham E. The nasal valve: a physiological and clinical study. J Laryngol Otol 1988; 102: 1089–94.
38. Thompson AC. Surgical reduction of the inferior turbinate in children: extended follow-up. J Laryngol Otol 1989; 103: 577–79.
39. Shone GR, Yardley MPJ, Knight LC. Mucociliary function in the early weeks after nasal surgery. Rhinology 1990; 28: 265–68.

40. Cortes JGG, Casas AP, Nieto CS. Autonomic microganglia of the nasal mucosa and their relation to vasomotor rhinitis. Clin Otolaryngol 1986; 11: 373–82.
41. Lannigan FJ, Gleeson MJ. Antroconchopexy for surgical treatment of perennial rhinitis. Rhinology 1992; 30: 183–86.
42. Fateen M. Concho-antropexy (CAP) in vasomotor rhinitis and chronic nasal obstruction. Rhinology 1967; 2: 20–24.
43. Legler U. Surgery of the turbinate bones and piriform crest. Rhinology 1976; 14: 65–71.
44. Bhargava KB, Abhyankar US, Shah TM. Treatment of allergic and vasomotor rhinitis by the local application of silver nitrate. J Laryngol Otol 1980; 94: 1025–36.
45. Weir CD. Intranasal ionization in the treatment of vasomotor nasal discorders. J Laryngol Otol 1967; 81: 1143–50.
46. Golding-Wood PH. Observations on petrosal and vidian neurectomy in chronic vasomotor rhinitis. J Laryngol Otol 1961; 75: 232–47.
47. Patel AH, Gaikward GA. Bilateral transnasal cauterisation of the vidian nerve in vasomotor rhinitis. J Laryngol Otol 1975; 89: 1291–96.
48. Portman M, Guillen G, Shabrol A. Electrocoagulation of the vidian nerve via the nasal passage. Laryngoscope 1982; 92: 453–55.
49. Kirtane MV, Prabhu VS, Karnik PP. Transnasal pre-ganglionic vidian nerve section. J Laryngol Otol 1984; 98: 481–87.
50. Kirtane MV, Rajaram D, Merchant SN. Transnasal approach to the vidian nerve: anatomical considerations. J Postgrad Med 1984; 30: 210–13.
51. Fernandes CMC. The management of intractible vasomotor rhinorrhoea by transanasal vidian neurectomy. South African Med J 1988; 74: 280–82.
52. Bagatella F. vidian nerve surgery revisited. Laryngoloscope 1986; 96: 194–97.
53. Chandra R. Transpalatal approach for vidian neurectomy. Arch Otolaryngol 1969; 89: 542–45.
54. Mustafa HM, Abdel Latif SM, Salah L, El-din SB. The transpalat approach for vidian neurectomy in allergic rhinitis. J Laryngol Otol 1973; 87: 773–80.
55. Minnis NC, Morrison AW. Transeptal approach for vidian neurectomy. J Laryngol Otol 1971; 85: 255–60.
56. El-Guindy A. Endoscopic transeptal vidian neurectomy. Arch Otolaryngol Head Neck Surg 1994; 120: 1347–51.
57. Kamel R, Zaher S. Endoscopie transnasal vidian neurectomy. Laryngoscope 1990; 101: 316–19.
58. Williams JD. Laser vidian neurectomy. Annals Otol Rhinol Laryngol 1983; 92: 281–83.
59. Rucci L, Borghi Cirri MB, Masini E, Fini Storchi O. Vidian nerve resection in chronic hypertrophic non-allergic rhinitis: the effects on histamine content, number and rate of degranulation processes of mast cells in nasal mucosa. Rhinology 1985; 23: 309–14.
60. Rucci L, Masini E, Arbiriccardi R, Giannella E, Fioretti C, Mannaioni PF, Borghi Cirri MB, Fini Storchi O. vidian nerve resection, histamine turnover and mucosal mast cell function in patients with chronic hypertrophic, non-allergic rhinitis. Agents Actions 1989; 28: 224–30.
61. Greenstone MA, Stanley PJ, Mackay IS, Cole PJ. The effect of vidian neurectomy on nasal mucociliary clearance. J Laryngol Otol 1988; 102: 894–95.
62. Golding-Wood PH. vidian neurectomy and other transantral surgery. Laryngoscope 1970; 80: 1179–89.
63. Krant JN, Wildervanck der Blecaurt P, Dieges PH, de Heer LJ. Long-term results of vidian neurectomy. Rhinology 1979; 17: 231–35.
64. Ogale SB, Shah A, Rao SE, Shah KL. Is vidian neurectomy worthwhile? J Laryngol Otol 1988; 102: 62–63.
65. Girgis IH. Surgical treatment of ozena by dermofat graft. J Laryngol 1966; 80: 615–27.
66. Young A. Closure of the nostrils in atrophic rhinitis. J Laryngol 1967; 81: 515–24.
67. Young A. Closure of the nostrils in atrophic rhinitis. J Laryngol 1971; 85: 715–18.
68. Gadre KC, Bhargava KB, Pradahan RY, Lodaya JD, Ingle MV. Closure of the nostrils (Young's operation) in atrophic rhinitis. J Laryngol 1971; 85: 711–14.
69. Shah JT, Karnik PP, Chitale AR, Nadkarni MS. Partial or total closure of the nostrils in atrophic rhinitis. Arch Otolaryngol 1974; 100: 196–98.
70. Mustafa H, Abdel-Latif S, El Fiky S, Hagras M. Surgical treatment of atrophic rhinitis by closure of the nostril. Otorhinolaryngology 1982; 44: 257–67.

71. Gadre AK, Savant R, Gadre KC, Bhargava KB, Juvekar RV. Re-opening of the close nostril in atrophic rhinitis. J Laryngol Otol 1988; 192: 411–13.
72. Ghosh P. Vestibuloplasty (a new one-stage operation for atrophic rhinitis). J Laryngol Otol 1987; 101: 905–9.
73. Chatterji P. Autogenous medullary (cancellous) bone graft in ozaena. J Laryngol Otol 1980; 94: 737–49.
74. Papay FA, Eliachari I, Rusica R, Fibro-muscular temporalis graft implantation for rhinitis sicca. Ent J 1991; 70: 381–83.
75. Rasmy E. Osteo-periosteal flap in the treatment of ozena: new technique. Annals Otol Rhinol Laryngol 1986; 95: 645–46.
76. Karnik PP. Placental extract therapy in atrophic rhinitis. The Eastern Pharmacist (India) 1971; 25: 113–114.
77. Sinha SN, Sardana DS, Rajbanshi VS. A nine years' review of 273 cases of atrophic rhinitis and its management. J Laryngol Otol 1977; 91: 591–600.
78. Whitehead E. Atrophic rhinitis: proplast as an implant material in surgical treatment. Can J Otolaryngol 1975; 4: 505–7.
79. Shehata M, Dohheim Y. Surgical treatment of primary chronic atrophic rhinitis (an evaluation of silastic implants). J Laryngol Otol 1986; 100: 803–7.
80. Ward PH. Uses of injectable Teflon in otolaryngology. Arch Otolarnygol 1968; 87: 91–97.
81. Ssali CL. Atrophic rhinitis: a new curative surgical treatment (middle turbinectomy). J Laryngol Otol 1973; 87: 397–403.
82. Huffstadt AJC, Hoeksema PE. Pharyngoplasty in atrophic rhinitis. Br J Plastic Surg 1976; 29: 132–33.
83. Gupta SE. Septoplasty in unilateral atrophic rhinitis with deviated nasal septum. J Laryngol Otol 1985; 99: 163–65.
84. Barton RPE. The management of leprous rhinitis. Leprosy Rev 1973; 44: 186–91.
85. Wilson JA, von Haacke NP, McAndrew PT, Murray JAM. Toxic shock syndrome after nasal surgery. Rhinology 1987; 25: 139–40.

Rhinitis: Immunopathology
and Pharmacotherapy
ed. by D. Raeburn and M.A. Giembycz

CHAPTER 10
Animal Models of Rhinitis

Ker-Sang Chen

Procter & Gamble Pharmaceutical Research Division, Health Care Research Center, Procter & Gamble Company, Mason, Ohio, USA

1. Introduction

The major clinical manifestations of rhinitis in the respiratory tract (nasal congestion, rhinorrhea) are the consequence of various aetiologies including infectious and allergic agents as well as the autonomic nervous system. However, the main pathogenic mechanisms of rhinitis differ with the causative agents. Many laboratory animals display pathologies and/or clinical signs in the upper respiratory tract following exposure to causative agents: many of the models show clinical symptoms resembling those observed in human subjects and are correspondingly responsive to human therapeutic agents; others only display limited rhinitic indications. This chapter provides a survey of published animal models that may serve as tools to aid the basic investigation of the pathogenesis of upper respiratory tract disorders and evaluate the efficacy of compounds for specific medial indications.

2. Types of Rhinitis

Rhinitis can be induced by infectious agents (viruses, bacteria, fungi, mycoplasma), allergens or have a noninfectious and nonallergic aetiology.

2.1. Infectious Rhinitis

2.1.1. Viral Rhinitis

2.1.1.1. Influenza virus-induced rhinitis.

Ferret model. Ferrets are highly susceptible to human influenza virus infection and display nasal congestion and rhinorrhea in the upper respiratory tract, in addition to systemic symptoms of febrile reaction and weight loss [1, 2]. These clinical symptoms are similar to those of human subjects with influenza virus infection. After infection, animals mount a protective immune response to the specific infectious agent. A subsequent infection with the homologous or a cross-reactive serotype of influenza virus undergoes a lower degree of clinical signs in animals pre-exposed to the virus. In order to stimulate maximum clinical manifestations, the use of ferrets seronegative to the challenge virus is a prerequisite.

Challenge virus. Influenza virus constantly undergoes minor antigenic modifications. The antigenicity of influenza virus presently in circulation in society is closely related to isolates in most recent years. The antigenic cross-reactivity is illustrated by the healthy adult ferret serum antibody reaction with influenza virus isolated in different years (Table 1). Every ferret serum specimen collected in 1990 reacts with the influenza A virus isolated in 1987 (A/Los Angeles/2/87), and the antibody titer, determined by hemagglutination inhibition (HI) assay, is at a high level (≥ 1280). This indicates that a great majority or all healthy ferrets have been naturally exposed to the circulating influenza virus in the environment, and the antigenicity of the infecting virus shares with that in the virus isolated only 3 years earlier. The degree of serum cross-reactivity diminishes with time: 97% of the same specimens react with the 1987 isolates (A/Mississippi/85 and A/Ann Arbor/3/85); 90% with a 1973 isolate (A/Port Chalmer/1/73); and 17% with a 1934 isolate (A/PR/8/34). Those seropositive specimens contain weak HI activity. It is therefore imperative to use a virulent influenza virus that is antigenically distinct (isolated as many years ago as

Table 1. HI reactivities of healthy adult ferret sera to influenza A viruses isolated in various years

	Percentage of serum samples with an HI titer of:				
Influenza A virus isolates	< 10	20	80	320	≥ 1280
Los Angeles/2/87	–	–	–	–	100
Mississippi/1/85	3	29	58	10	–
Ann Arbor/3/85	3	58	36	–	3
Port Chalmer/1/73	10	87	3	–	–
PR/8/34	83	14	3	–	–

possible) from the circulating virus so as to overcome the compromise by the seropositive status in ferrets that are exposed to current isolates. To assure susceptibility further, serum samples of ferrets prior to virus challenge are prescreened against the challenge virus by HI assay. Only those ferrets seronegative to the challenge virus are used in studies. The challenge virulent influenza virus (A/PR/8/34) pool was generated with a history of serial passages in mouse lungs and embryonated chicken eggs, in an alternate sequence, for a total of 902 times [2].

Virus secretion. Intranasal inoculation with influenza virus (A/PR/8/34) to seronegative ferrets produces a detectable level of infectious virus in the nasal secretion 1 day post challenge. The virus titer reaches a maximum 2 days post infection and declines gradually thereafter. Virus is undetectable in nasal lavages by 7 days post-infection (Figure 1).

Nasal inflammation. Leukocytes influx to the nasel lumen at an elevated level 1 day following the viral infection and reach a peak level 2 days after infection. The total cell count in nasal lavage fluids declines steadily and returns to the basal level 7 days after infection (Figure 1) [3, 4]. Among nasal leukocytes, polymorphonuclear neutrophils (PMN) are the predominant subpopulation that expands from a 15% level prior to infection to 75% at 2 days post-infection. At 1 week after infection, their prevalence rate is retained at an elevated (40%) level (Figure 2). Monocytes increase dramatically from a 4% basal level to 20 and 39% levels at 2 and 3 days post-infection, respectively, and the level reaches a plateau later (Figure 2). Lymphocytes constitute the smallest subset of leukocytes. Their presence is elevated from a preinfection basal level of 4% to a maximum level (15–20%) 2 days post-infection and remains at a low level thereafter (Figure 2). The onset of fever corresponds to the influx of inflammatory cells in the nasal lumen. Interaction of virus with phagocytes produces endogenous pyrogen. The intensity of febrile response correlates with the virulence degree of influenza virus [5]. The time course of febrile reaction, as indicated by rectal temperature, peaks 2 days after infection and returns to the normal level 7 days post-infection. Infected animals lose an ap-

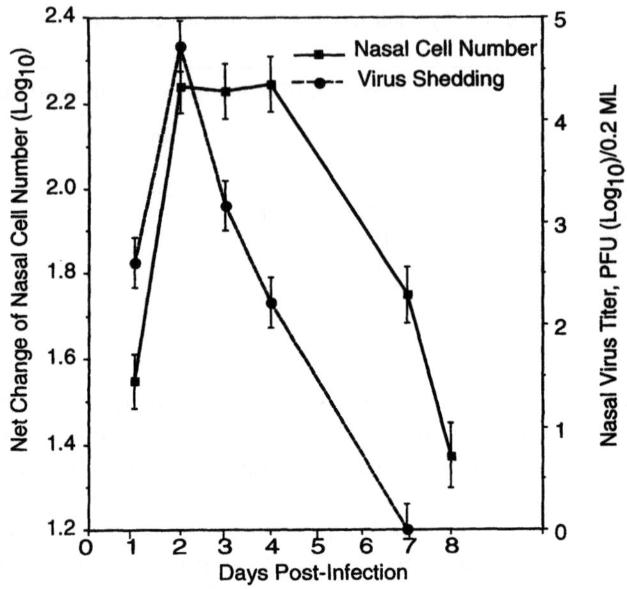

Figure 1. Kinetics of cellular influx and viral shedding in nasal lavages of influenza virus-infected ferrets.

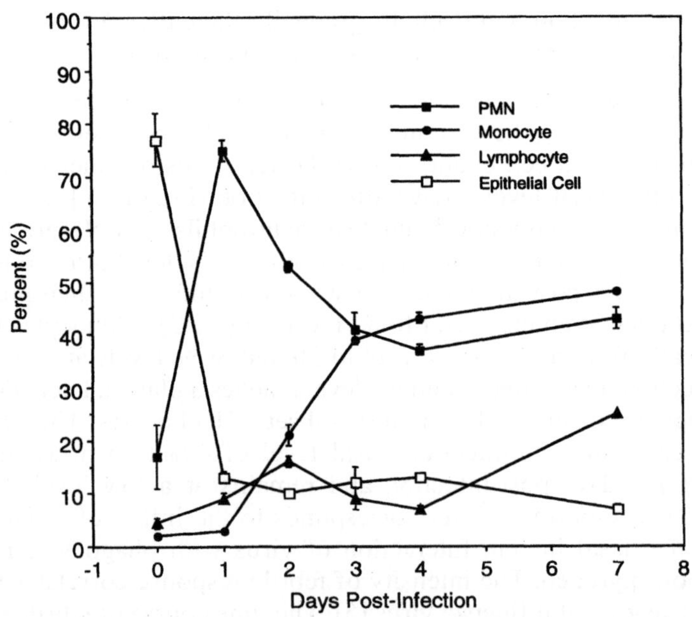

Figure 2. Kinetics of subpopulation change in nasal lavages of influenza virus-infected ferrets. PMN: polymorphonuclear neutrophil.

preciable amount of body weight 2 days after infection, which persists for an additional 5 days before they resume weight gain.

Histological sections of nasal turbinates in healthy ferrets show a clear outline of convoluted turbinates and a clean lumen space spotted with few leukocytes at low magnification (Figure 3 A). Cilia present on the epithelial layer of the nasal turbinate are well organized, and there are no or few leukocytes present in the interstitial space or venule (Figures 3 B and C). Virus infection greatly reduces the luminal space that is attributed by the swollen turbinate with an oedematous response in mucosal membrane and dilation of capacitance vessels. The luminal space is heavily filled with

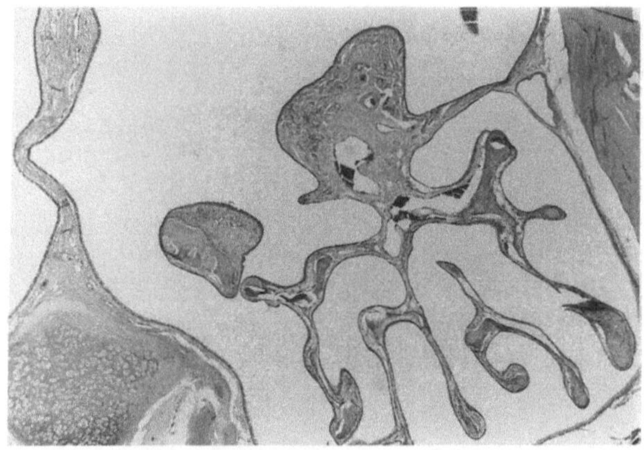

A

Figures 3 A–G. Histological changes of nasal turbinates before and after influenza virus infection in ferrets. 3 × magnification (uninfected).

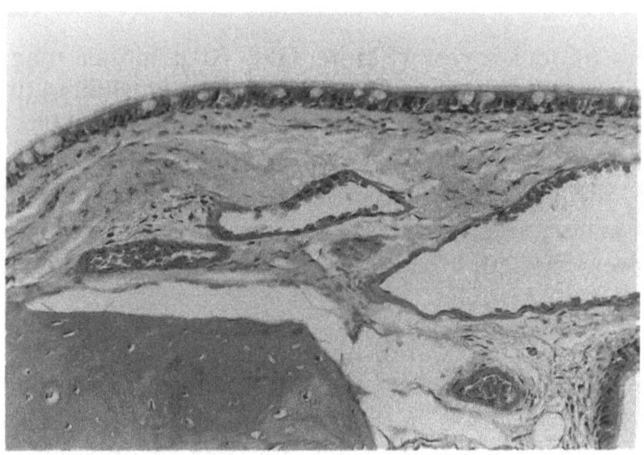

B

Figure 3 B. 25 × magnification (uninfected).

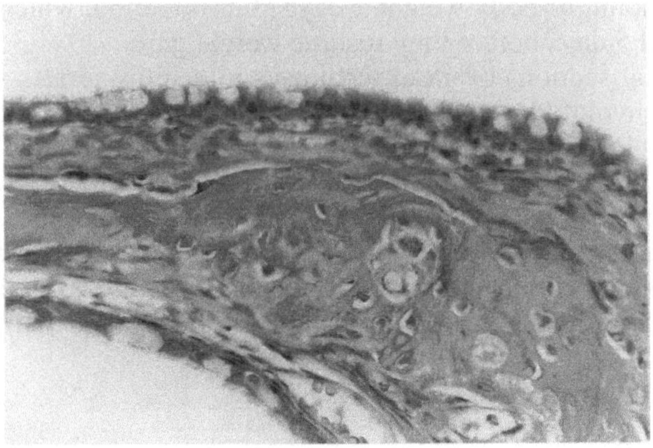

C

Figure 3 C. 40 × magnification (uninfected).

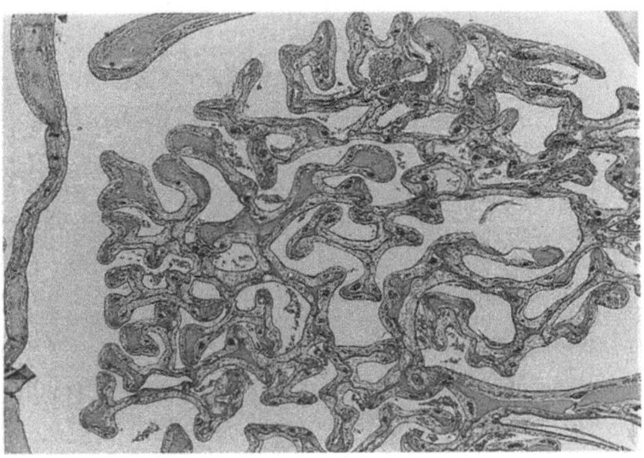

D

Figure 3 D. 3 × magnification (infected).

dense clusters of leukocytes (Figure 3 D). At a higher magnification, it clearly shows densely populated leukocytes are distributed throughout the swollen interstitial space in the turbinate tissue (Figure 3 E). The presence of leukocytes is greatly increased both in the venules and they massively transmigrate, through the distended interstitial space and the epithelial layer of turbinates, into the nasal lumen. The epithelial layer remains intact; however, the cilia become sparse in number and disorganized (Figures 3 F and G).

Nasal congestion. The level of nasal congestion, indicated by nasal airflow resistance (NAR), is measured by anterior active rhinomanometry (Figure 4). Mean resistance in healthy adult ferrets, under anaesthesia, is approximately 107 ± 24 cm H_2O per liter per second (cm l^{-1} s^{-1}). Upon influenza virus infection, the NAR is slightly elevated on day 1 post-infec-

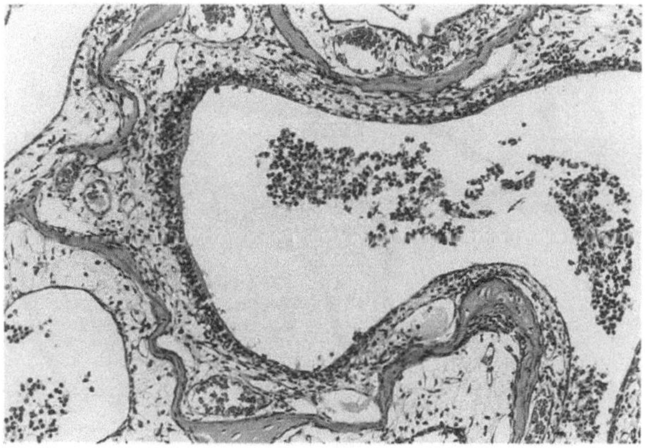

E

Figure 3 E. 20 × magnification (infected).

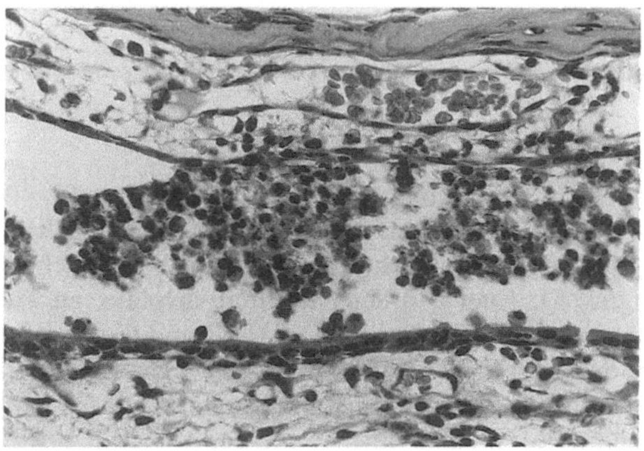

F

Figure 3 F. 60 × magnification (infected).

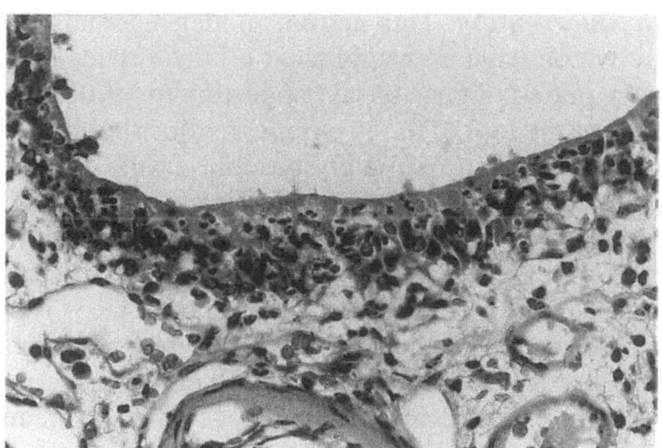

G

Figure 3 G. 60 × magnification (infected).

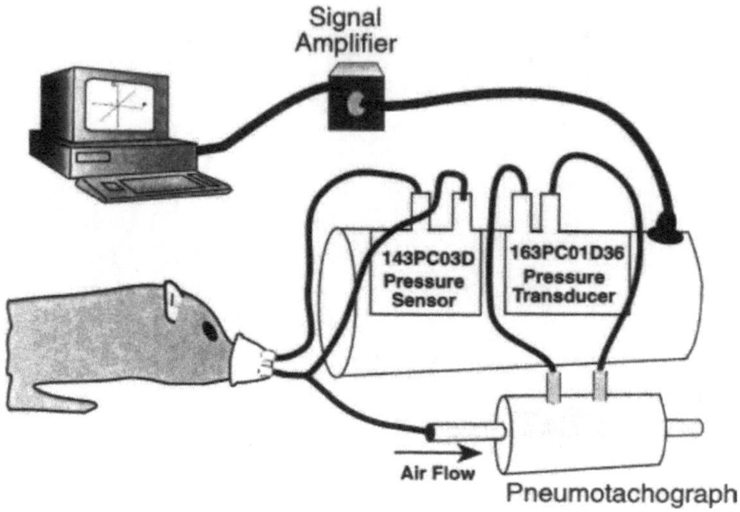

Figure 4. Diagram of active rhinomanometric system and its connection to anesthetized ferrets for measurement of nasal airflow resistance.

tion and reaches a maximum ranging between 4- and 40-fold higher than the baseline reading at 2 days post-infection. The NAR significantly declines the following day and returns to the baseline level by 7 days post-infection (Figure 5). Every infected animal displays an elevated NAR, although both the absolute magnitude of NAR and the exact occurrence in time can vary amongst individual animals. However, the kinetics profile of the mean NAR activity for a group of animals is highly reproducible. As stated previously, to enhance further the reproducibility in producing a consistent pattern of elevated NAR by virus infection, animals need to be preselected for their susceptibility to the challenge virus.

Therapeutic intervention. This animal model responds to several nasal decongestants which have an established clinical efficacy in human subjects. During the period of peak nasal congestion in influenza virus-infected ferrets, one intranasal dose of 0.1% oxymetazoline rapidly relieves congestion, reducing NAR to approximately baseline levels for hours within the study period (Figure 5). This provides an efficacy of 85% as determined by the area-under-the-curves method [2]. However, the next day, the treatment group experiences a greatly increased NAR as compared with nontreated animals (Figure 5). This exaggerated increase in NAR is reproducible and may be associated to a rebound phenomenon described by some human patients using topical nasal decongestants. Phenylephrine, another topical nasal decongestant, confers a similar efficacy (77%) in relieving nasal congestion in this infectious rhinitis model. An oral decongestant such as pseudoephedrine effectively relieves nasal congestion with an efficacy of

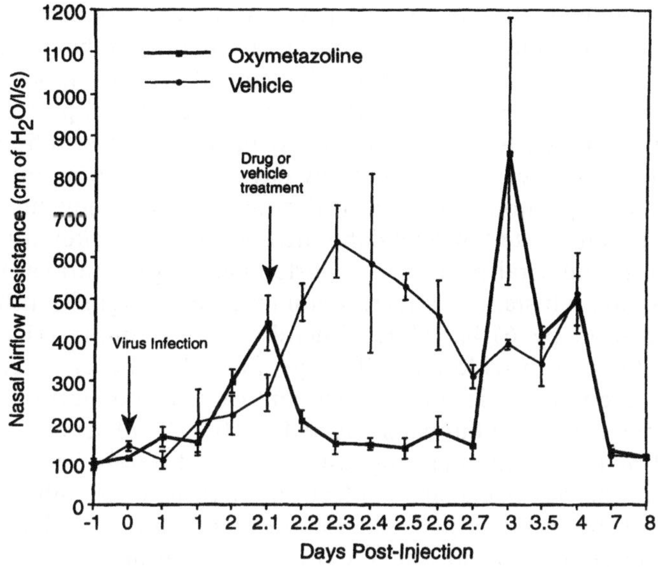

Figure 5. Patterns of nasal congestion and nasal decongestion by oxymetazoline in ferrets with influenza virus-induced rhinitis.

Table 2. Efficacy of nasal decongestants in influenza virus-induced rhinitis in ferrets

Test drug	Route of drug administration	Decongestion efficacy
0.1% Oxymetazoline	intranasal	85%
2% Phenylephrine	intranasal	77%
0.6% Pseudoephedrine	intragastric	84%
0.08% Ipratropium	intranasal	−35%
1% Pyrilamine	intranasal	61%
30% Cimetidine	intranasal	38%

* $P < 0.10$.

84%, when the medicine is administered once by the intragastric route (Table 2). Since the NAR response profile varies amongst individual animals, it is necessary to include a large number of test animals to represent the response activity of a study group, especially for evaluating the efficacy of therapeutic compounds quantitatively. Active anterior rhinomanometry enables easy and frequent NAR measurements to monitor the profile of kinetic changes in each animal. However, due to the length of time needed to take triplicate measurements for both nostrils and the intricate measuring procedures, this system limits the capacity to perform large population ferret studies and therefore limits its use in dose-response evaluation for rapid screening.

The pronounced efficacy of sympathomimetic decongestants clearly demonstrates the importance of the nasal vasculature in the production of congestion in this model and parallels the clinical manifestations in human subjects. Intranasal dosing with the muscarinic cholinoceptor antagonist ipratropium bromide to inhibit the parasympathetic drive inhibits virus-induced rhinorrhea seen in the first few days after infection, but does not reduce nasal congestion. The lack of decongestant efficacy suggests that nasal secretion mediated by acetylcholine does not play a key role in nasal congestion during viral rhinitis as reported earlier [6]. Intranasal therapy with pyrilamine, a histamine (H_1) receptor antagonist, significantly reduces nasal congestion by 61%, while cimetidine, a histamine (H_2) receptor antagonist fails to provide any efficacy (Table 2). The efficacy of antihistamines is controversial in the treatment of nasal congestion in rhinovirus-induced rhinitis in human subjects [7–10]. The observed efficacy in this model by pyrilamine may suggest a species difference for the role of histamine in the pathogenesis of infectious rhinitis, or a higher detection sensitivity of this study model under controlled conditions. The lack of a cimetidine effect may be attributed to the lack of histamine (H_2) receptors in the ferret nasal mucosa, the lack of a role for this receptor in nasal congestion or an insufficient drug concentration in the study. The influenza virus-induced rhinitis in ferrets corresponds to that in human subjects both in the clinical pathological profile and the therapeutic profiles by pharmacological agents. It reveals that activation of α-adrenoceptors and histamine (H_1) receptors modulates nasal patency. To the contrary, muscarinic cholinoceptors (secretory effects) and histamine (H_2) receptors appear to play a minor or no role in the pathogenesis of nasal congestion in viral rhinitis.

In conclusion, this animals model is useful for evaluating novel pharmacological agents to treat viral rhinitis-associated nasal symptoms. In view of the influx of inflammatory cells corresponding to the occurrence of nasal symptomatologies, this model also provides an excellent system to explore the potential roles of cellular components and soluble mediators involved in immunological and inflammatory responses in the pathogenesis of viral rhinitis.

Mouse model. The mouse-adapted PR8 strain of influenza A virus supports viral replication in albino Swiss mice when it is instilled into the nostrils of nonanaesthetized mice. A high level of virus titer is present in the nasal tissue 2–4 days after infection, depending on the titer of the virus inoculum. Virus is inconsistently found in the trachea, while non is detected in the lung. The pharyngeal ciliated epithelium is shown to be destroyed by viral infection [11]. While viral replication in the respiratory tract is demonstrated in mice, there is no information available on clinical signs in the upper respiratory tract.

2.1.1.2. Sendai virus-induced rhinitis

Rat model. Specific pathogen-free Sprague-Dawley rats (5–8 weeks old) infected with Sendai virus display severe, although temporary, rhinitis and pneumonia. Sendai virus antigen is detectable in the nasal mucosa 1 day after infection. Virus antigen intensity is most prominent at 3–4 days and becomes undetectable after 7 days post-infection [12]. The kinetics of antigen detection by immunohistochemical staining is similar to the infectious virus detected in the nasal secretion [13]. A marked infiltration of lymphocytes and some neutrophils into the nasal mucosal epithelium occurs at 1 day post-infection. Over the next 4 days post-infection, there is a progressive accumulation of inflammatory cells, chiefly lymphocytes, in the lamina propria that remains detectable 42 days later. Rhinitis with lesions most prominent in the respiratory epithelium of the naso- and maxilloturbinates occurs 4–6 days post-infection, and pneumonia persists to 21 days after infection [12].

2.1.1.3. Respiratory syncytial virus (RSV)-induced rhinitis

Ferret model. Ferrets are susceptible to RSV infection. Adult animals develop lesions limited to the nasal passage, but not lung, while infant ferrets (younger than 4 weeks of age) have viral replication in the lungs [14]. Intranasal infection of adult ferrets yields virus from their tracheas for 4 days and nasal turbinates for 1 week. RSV-infected adult ferrets shed the greatest amount of virus within 3–4 days, and no virus is detectable 8 days after infection. Epithelial destruction in the infected nasal turbinate begins on the third day of infection and is greatest 6 days after inoculation. It shows progressive changes: goblet cells are distended and increased in number; cilia are ragged and diminished in number; epithelial cells become desquamated so that the mucus sheet overlying the epithelium contains increasing amounts of cellular debris as the infection progresses. Later, binucleate epithelial cells and multinucleate cells containing eosinophilic intracytoplasmic inclusion bodies are observed. The epithelium becomes disorganized and heavily infiltrated by lymphocytes and PMNs. Inflammatory cells are present in the mucosa and submucosa regions 9 days after infection. These animals, however, do not show overt signs of illness [15]. Mink are also susceptible to RSV infection [15].

Primate model. At least five species of nonhuman primates are susceptible to RSV infection. Intranasal inoculation of adult squirrel monkeys and newborn rhesus monkeys leads to virus shedding in the nasal lumen, but no observable illness develops. Infant cebus monkeys also do not show illness, although virus shedding occurs in nasopharyngeal sites. Chimpanzees (15–18 months old) develop an upper respiratory illness characterized by profuse rhinorrhea, mild cough and sneezing 4 days after intranasal inoculation with RSV. The duration of illness lasts from 5 to 10 days. There is no evidence of lower respiratory tract illness [16]. The white lipped marmoset is also susceptible to RSV infection [15].

2.1.1.4. Sialodacryoadenitis virus infection

Rat model. Sialodacryoadenitis virus, a coronavirus, infects rats with a self-limiting necrosis and inflammation of mixed or serous salivary glands, lachrymal glands and upper airway epithelium [17]. Microscopic lesions begin in the nasal epithelium 2 days post-infection. Initial respiratory epithelial necrosis accompanied by congestion and oedema is rapidly followed by a mixed inflammatory cell infiltrate. Necrosis primarily occurs in the respiratory epithelium lining the ventral turbinate and lateral wall of the nasal cavity. The nasal meatuses may be filled with exudate composed of necrotic epithelial cells admixed with inflammatory cells and mucus [18].

2.1.2. Bacterial rhinitis

2.1.2.1. Atrophic rhinitis

Rat model. Newborn specific-pathogen-free rats are susceptible to infections with *Bordetella bronchiseptica* and *Pasteurella multocida*. Nasal turbinate atrophy is caused by colonization of *B. bronchiseptica* in the nasal cavity. Turbinate atrophy correlates with a severe inflammatory reaction, characterized by the infiltration of PMNs and mononuclear cells in the lamina propria and the epithelial layer. Oedema and exudation of PMNs into nasal cavity are evident. The inflammatory reaction, most severe at the tips of the conchae, is apparent 3 days after inoculation and is most severe between 9 and 16 days post-infection. Ciliated cells are lost 9 days after infection. The severity of the inflammatory reaction is dependent upon the size of bacterial inoculum and correlates with the degree of ventral turbinate atrophy [19].

Mouse model. Specific-pathogen-free newborn mice (5 days old or younger) of ddN strain are susceptible to *B. bronchiseptica* infection. Three weeks after intranasal inoculation, atrophy of nasal turbinates develops in 80% of infected mice [20]. The lesions are similar to those reported in swine (see below).

Rabbit model. Newborn rabbits free of antibody to *B. bronchiseptica* are susceptible to *B. bronchiseptica* infection. Intranasal inoculation with the pathogen develops ventral turbinate atrophy 10 days later. Catarrhal inflammation in the nasal and tracheal mucous membranes and bronchopneumonia with peribronchiolitis are evident [21].

Gnotobiotic pig model. Intranasal infection with *B. bronchiseptica* causes infectious atrophic rhinitis in swine [22]. Intranasal inoculation with a sterile sonicate of a toxigenic strain of *B. bronchiseptica* at 5 days of age, followed by intranasal infection with a live toxigenic strain of *P. multocida* at 7 days of age, results in nasal turbinate atrophy. Although turbinates are atrophied, there is no significant infiltration of inflammatory cells histologically. The experimental regimen is a useful model for testing vaccine strategies [23].

Pig model. Intranasal infection with *P. multocida* toxin in 4-week-old pigs causes development of subclinical signs of atrophic rhinitis [24].

2.1.3. Fungal rhinitis

A high incidence of fungal rhinitis is described in male Wistar CRI: (WI)BR rats. *Aspergillus* rhinitis is generally limited to the naso- and maxilloturbinates. Hyphal conglomerates are usually associated with foreign bodies and are surrounded by PMNs, bacteria, debris, and nasal secretions. The underlying respiratory epithelium is usually hyperplastic, hypertrophic or shows evidence of squamous metaplasia. Subepithelial connective tissue and submucosal glands often are infiltrated by aggregates of lymphocytes, plasma cells and neutrophils. It is hypothesized that Sendai and Sialodacryoadenitis viral infections predispose the rats to the fungal infection [25].

2.1.4. Macoplasma rhinitis

Mycoplasma pulmonis infection in rats causes rhinitis, otidis media, laryngitis and tracheitis [26]. Gross lesions in the upper respiratory tract are generally not discernible, although rats may occasionally show mucopurulent nasal exudate and/or discharge. The microscopic pathology is characterized by epithelial changes, including cellular hypertrophy as well as metaplastic changes. Neutrophilic exudation and lymphoplasmacytic infiltrates are common throughout the upper airway. Subepithelial lymphoid accumulations can occur. Ciliary loss and epithelial hyperplasias can be severe and quite extensive [27]. Certain chemical agents, including ammonia, can exacerbate the infection. Inhalation of the important industrial compound hexamethylphosphoramide can cause a synergistic enhancement of the progression and severity of the infection [28, 29].

2.2. Allergic Rhinitis

Allergic rhinitis is the consequence of immunological responses. The mast cell is the principal cell that secretes inflammatory mediators (histamine, prostanoids, leukotrienes (LT)), in the presence of immunoglobulin (Ig)E complexes with allergen, and culminates in nasal symptoms (nasal congestion, rhinorrhea, itching sensation). A variety of agents are capable of inducing allergic reactions in the upper respiratory tract of experimental animals. Upon nasal challenge with the homologous allergen, an early-phase reaction (mostly histamine production) in the nasal cavity occurs rapidly within minutes and subsequently subsides. After a lag period of several hours, an inflammatory late-phase reaction ensues.

2.2.1. Antigen (ovalbumin)-induced allergic rhinitis

Guinea pig model. Adult guinea pigs can be actively sensitized to ovalbumin (OV) by an intraperitoneal injection containing OV and $Al(OH)_3$ as an adjuvant. Booster injections with the same preparation are repeated intraperitoneally on days 7 and 14. Four to 5 weeks after the first vaccination, sensitized animals are anaesthetized and two polyethylene cannulae inserted into the trachea for the measurement of nasal congestion. One is inserted caudally to permit spontaneous (or mechanical) ventilation, the other cephalically through which air supplied from a compressed air tank is directed retrograde through the nasal cavities and nose. The oesophagus is ligated and the mouth sealed by filling the oral cavity with pliable modeling plastic material. The pressure in the nasal cavities is visualized by a water manometer and recorded via a pressure transducer and electronic amplifier [30]. Sensitized guinea pigs challenged intranasally with OV develop allergic rhinitis and nasal congestion. Intranasal treatment with fenspiride or mepyramine effectively reduces allergen-induced nasal airflow resistance [30]. The release of chemical mediators (kinins and LTC_4) in the nasal lavage fluid is augmented not only immediately after the antigenic challenge, but also during 60–90 min after the stimulation. Release of histamine into the nasal lavage fluid is observed only immediately after the antigenic stimulation. Release of histamine into the nasal lavage fluid is observed only immediately after the antigenic stimulation. In nonsensitized guinea pigs, nasal stimulation with bradykinin accelerates nasal vascular permeability, while histamine or LTC_4 results in an increase of nasal vascular permeability and of kinins concentration in the nasal lavage fluid. Therefore, kinins might be associated with immediate and later vascular permeability during the allergic response [31]. Similarly, guinea pigs actively sensitized with the DNP-*Ascaris* conjugate as an antigen also develop allergic rhinitis when the homologous antigen solution is perfused into the nasal cavities. The antigen-induced release of histamine and dye leakage into the nasal cavity is significantly increased 0–15 min following antigen administration and decreases thereafter [32].

Rat model. Brown Norway rats, a high IgE responder strain, sensitized with OV develop allergic rhinitis following the OV challenge to the nasal cavity. Chlorpheniramine maleate inhibits the release of Evans blue and elevates that of histamine without affecting the level of *N*-acetyl-*β*-D-glucosaminidase. Halopredone acetate inhibits the releases of all the three markers (Evans blue, histamine and *N*-acetyl-*β*-D-glucosaminidase). This model is therefore a potentially useful experimental system for evaluating the effect of drugs on allergic rhinitis [33].

2.2.2. Fungus-induced allergic rhinitis

Guinea pig model. Tricoloured adult guinea pigs are immunized three times with a fungal extract of *Cladosporium cladosporioides* or *Alternaria alternata* by the subcutaneous route at 4-day intervals. Nasal instillation (three drops in each nostril) is further carried out twice a day for a period of 10 days. Seven days and 1 month later, animals are boosted with two subcutaneous injections. This immunization protocol induces the production of allergen-specific IgG and IgE antibodies and rhinitis. Nasal challenge with the homologous soluble allergen causes degranulation of mast cells at the nasal mucosa. The ciliated epithelium remains unchanged after the allergen challenge [34]. This model makes it possible to monitor the intervention of chemicals or immunological factors other than IgE in the degranulation process in nasal mucosa.

2.2.3. Chemical conjugate-induced allergic rhinitis:

Guinea pig model. Nasal allergy in guinea pigs can be developed by painting a 2,4-toluene diisocyanate (TDI) 10% solution onto the nasal vestibule once a day for 5–10 days. Both rhinorrhea and sneezing are apparent upon nasal challenge with the inducer and indicate a nasal hypersensitive reaction [35, 36]. A marked eosinophil infiltration, rhinorrhea and other changes indicative of acute inflammation are evident in the nasal mucosa. Furthermore, mast cells are found not only in the epithelial and subepithelial layers of the nasal mucosa but also in the enlarged venous vessels. A significantly higher level of histamine release in the mucosa from TDI-treated animals is present [35]. This model displays of close resemblance to human nasal allergy in both symptomatologies and pathogenesis (morphological changes in nasal mucosa and mucus). Hence, this animal model not only provides a convenient tool for studying nasal allergic rhinitis but also may be useful for understanding the pathogenesis of TDI-induced physical disorders.

2.2.4. House dust mite extract-induced allergic rhinitis

Guinea pig model. Guinea pigs actively sensitized by parenteral injection of house dust mite extract (HD) for 3 weeks. Aerosol challenge of HD does not induce bronchoconstriction but does induce intense lacrimation and rhinorrhea. This model has possible utility as a model of allergic rhinitis [37].

2.2.5. Passive sensitization-induced rhinitis

Guinea pig model. Guinea pigs are passively sensitized by an intravenous injection of anti-DNP (dinitrophenol) guinea pig IgE antibody. One week later, animals are challenged by nasal application of DNP-BSA (DNP modified bovine serum albumin). The passive cutaneous anaphylaxis antibody-dependent nasal allergic rhinitis reveals that eosinophils transmigrate into the nasal lumen through the tight junctions of epithelial lining cells [38]. Similarly, guinea pigs can be passively sensitized with an intraperitoneal injection of OV antiserum and display allergic rhinitis following intranasal challenge with OV [39, 40].

To evaluate the efficacy of therapeutic agents in relieving nasal congestion, 48 h after antiserum sensitization animals are anaesthetized and respired spontaneously through a cannula inserted into the trachea while the oesophagus is ligated with a thread to interrupt perfusate flow across the cavities. Test compounds such as flutropium bromide, diphenhydramine hydrochloride, atropine sulfate, cimetidine etc. are introduced into test animals 1 min prior to antigen challenge through the intravenous route. Their effects on intranasal pressure change are monitored with passive posterior rhinomanometry [39, 40].

Rat model. Rats can also be sensitized with a hyperimmune serum to OV and develop allergic rhinitis upon intranasal challenge with the allergen. The induced nasal congestion can be modulated by a variety of decongestants or antihistamines in this model and is detectable by passive posterior rhinomanometry [39].

2.2.6. Chemical mediator-induced rhinitis

Rat model. Nasal cavities of anaesthetized male Wistar rats are ventilated between cannulae inserted into the nasopharynx and bilateral nostril, with an artificial respirator. Intranasal resistance can be recorded with a modification of a Konzett-Rossler apparatus as a change in ventilation overflow. To provoke rhinitis, some mediators are inhaled into the nasal cavities with an ultrasonic nebulizer for 5 min. To assess the capillary permeability of the nasal mucosa, exudation of Evans blue is determined by injecting the dye before inhalations of mediators (histamine, bradykinin, acetylcholine, serotonin) [41]. The histamine-induced nasal congestion in anaesthetized rats is inhibited by methoxyphenamine in IgE-dependent allergic rhinitis [42]. Salem and Clemente [39] reported a similar system that evaluates decongestant activity of known standards at clinically effective concentrations and can differentiate decongestant drugs by durations of action.

Guinea pig model. Inhalation of histamine in healthy nonsensitized guinea pigs causes a concentration-related increase in intranasal pressure and secretion and a reduction in mucosal volume. Flutropium, atropine and diphenhydramine effectively inhibit intranasal pressure in this model [40, 43].

2.3. Noninfectious, Nonallergic Vasomotor Rhinitis

Vasomotor rhinitis is a clinical manifestation with an aetiology that is independent of an infectious or allergic origin. Vasomotor rhinitis may be the consequence of the combined effects of an imbalanced autonomic nervous system with an overreactive parasympathetic nerve and modulated immune competence [44]. Stimulation of parasympathetic nerves activates nasal secretion. An attempt has been made to develop an animal model with vasomotor rhinitis. In sympathectomized dogs, a majority of them have oedema as well as a greater proportion of lymphocyte infiltration in the nasal mucosa, determined histologically, 1 month after surgery; these signs disappear 3 months later, and the rhinitis is thus transient. In addition, IgG and IgA levels in serum, but not in nasal secretions, of sympathectomized dogs are reduced significantly [44]. It is with reservation that this sympathectomized model completely reflects parasympathetic nerve overreactivity.

3. Methods for Quantitative Measurement of Nasal Congestion

In rhinitis, open space in the nasal lumen can be reduced due to one or combined factors: oedema vasodilatation, inflammatory reactions. The typical key clinical signs are manifested by nasal congestion and rhinorrhea that can be objectively quantified by several means: rhinomanometry, rhinometry and magnetic resonance imaging (MRI) for the measurement of nasal congestion, and nasal fluid weight or absorption distance on absorbing materials for rhinorrhea.

3.1. Rhinomanometry

The rhinomanometric technique to measure nasal congestion relies on resistance to airflow across the nasal turbinate and therefore assesses the change in nasal patency. The principle involves a laminar-type flow passing through a tube that generates a differential flow rate at two separate locations that in turn generates a pressure drop. The magnitude of pressure drop is proportional to the airflow rate. Therefore, a resistance (R) is reflected by the ratio of pressure (P) and flow rate (V) ($R = P/V$). In the nasal cavity, the pressure drop across the nasal airway during airflow (transnasal pressure) is detected by a pneumotachograph, and is in turn monitored by a pressure transducer to generate a flow signal. The airflow rate can be expressed in liters per second, and the transnasal pressure can be expressed in centimeters of H_2O. Both pressure and flow signals are amplified and recorded concurrently. Measurements are made in the range that the $V–P$ curves are essentially linear to assure laminar-type airflow and eliminate turbulence.

Active rhinomanometric measurement relies on the air supply originated from the active respiration of the test animal [2]. To the contrary, passive rhinomanometric measurement involves the external supply of airflow at a constant rate to the naris [45].

3.1.1. Active rhinomanometry

3.1.1.1. Active anterior rhinomanometry. The anaesthetized animal's nose area is shaved to minimize obstruction for the mask fitting over the nose. A silicon rubber mask moulded from a cast of the nose is mounted to the nose with a nontoxic reusable adhesive dough. The left and right nostrils are separated by a strip of the adhesive dough inside the mask. To measure the NAR of each nostril, animals breath only through one nostril (the test nostril); no airflow is allowed to pass through the other nostril or the mouth during the measurement. The test nostril is connected to a pneumotachograph. Airflow across the test nostril is measured by the pressure drop across the pneumotachograph using a pressure sensor. The transnasal pressure is obtained by measuring the pressure gradient at the front of the test nostril and the pressure in the second nostril using a second pressure sensor. The signals from the pressure sensors are amplified and are converted in a computer in which NAR is calculated. Each NAR reading can be expressed as cm of H_2O per liter per second (cm l^{-1} s^{-1}). Each NAR reading takes 10 s to complete, and a total of three readings for each nostril for each time point are taken. From each of the three replicate measurements, the higher reading from either nostril is determined and chosen for the calculation of the geometric mean NAR for the specific time point of each animal.

Test compounds can be administered intranasally, intravenously, or intragastrically to animals, and the NAR measurements performed as above. The effect of a nasal decongestant (see Figure 5) is expressed as a function of the area under the curve (AUC) above basal state for responses over time. The net change in NAR from the basal state (i.e. the mean of the two NAR readings obtained prior to viral infection) is calculated for each animal. AUC for each animal for the 5- to 6-h time course following drug or vehicle intervention is calculated. The efficacy of a drug is assessed by comparing AUC for all animals treated with the drug ($AUC_{\text{drug-treated group}}$) to those treated with a vehicle ($AUC_{\text{vehicle-treated group}}$). In addition, the percent change from vehicle was calculated for each drug as: $(AUC_{\text{vehicle-treated group}} - AUC_{\text{drug-treated group}})/(AUC_{\text{vehicle-treated group}}) \times 100\%$.

The system has several advantages in that it is noninvasive; it allows a repetitive monitor of NAR activity in a living animal over a period of days or longer term, and the same animal serves as its own control to provide the baseline value for subsequent data comparison; the data acquisition time is short, thus allowing frequent measurements to generate a more representative drug efficacy; it is more sensitive in detecting the change in NAR than previously reported in a passive posterior rhinomanometric measurement; the system provides reproducible data that consistently measure an NAR baseline level of 107 ± 24 cm l^{-1} s^{-1} in healthy adult ferrets and detect an elevated NAR ranging between 4- and 40-fold increase during the viral rhinitic processes; and it allows easy measurement that enables monitoring the profile of kinetic changes in each animal during progression of a disease. However, there are certain limitations. The animals must be anaesthetized; the nostrils must be measured one at a time; the nasal cycling can obscure drug response or change the response of the primary nostril during testing; and, due to the length of time required to take triplicate measurements for both nostrils and the intricacy of the measuring procedures, the system limits the capacity to perform large-population ferret studies and thus limits its use for dose-response drug evaluation. To derive a representative efficacy value of a test drug, it is necessary to include a large population of study animals.

3.1.2. Passive rhinomanometry

3.1.2.1. Passive posterior rhinomanometry. The trachea of an anaesthetized animal is surgically exposed, and two polyethylene cannulae are inserted into the trachea. One cannula is inserted caudally to allow spontaneous ventilation, the other via the cephalad to permit a humidified air supply, directed retrograde through the nasal cavities and naris, from a compressed air tank (Figure 6) [39]. The oesophagus is ligated and the mouth sealed. The pressure in the nasal cavities is detected from the airflow line and is recorded from a water manometer or through a pressure transducer coupled with an electronic recorder. After a period of equilibrium, airflow rate is adjusted for each animal to between 235 and 425 ml/min, for example for rats, so that the resultant pressure is within a limited physiological range. The flow rate (F) is held constant throughout the study. The pressure (P) in the nasal passage is converted to air flow resistance (R) by

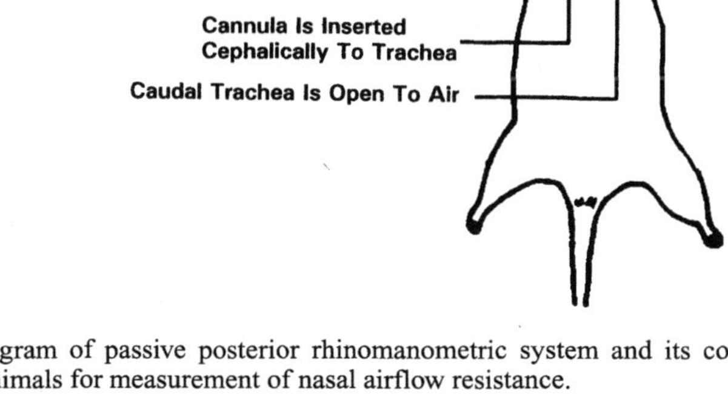

Figure 6. Diagram of passive posterior rhinomanometric system and its connection to anaesthetized animals for measurement of nasal airflow resistance.

the equation: $(R) = P/F$. Nasal resistance is recorded every minute for 10 min and the mean of these 10 values represents the degree of nasal air flow resistance. Prior to introduction of the test drug, the baseline level of nasal resistance is monitored. Test compounds or saline can then be administered intravenously, intraduodenally or through rubber tubing connected to the cephalad tracheal cannula and flushed through the nasal cavities by the air stream. Nasal resistance is then measured every minute for 30 min and is averaged for 10-min periods [39].

This method has the advantages that direct deposition of test compound on the nasal cavity can occur and thus exert therapeutic effects directly on the target tissue, it requires no specialized mask, and it is highly reproducible. At the same time it has the drawbacks that it is an invasive method; the terminal state of the study animal does not allow a kinetic study of a drug repetitively on the same animal for a long term (over a period of days); it does not permit a dynamic assessment of a drug's efficacy in infectious diseases that undergo a constant change in disease progression, which limits assessment of its therapeutic efficacy to modulate the disease in its entirety; it is labour-intensive, and requires a large number of study animals to obtain representative data. The model is thus not ideally suited for rapid-screening, a limitation that is especially apparent in disease models.

Similar set-ups, using the same principles, have been reported by others using guinea pigs [40], rats [41, 42] pigs [46] and miniature pigs [47].

3.1.2.2. Passive anterior rhinomanometry. Following the same principles described above this system supplies moist air to the anterior nares of the anaesthetized animal. Between the air supply and the nares, a pressure transducer is situated after a pneumotachograph to measure airflow change (Figure 7). The animal breathes through its mouth, instead of its nose, and care should be taken that the posterior nares are unobstructed and open to the atmosphere [45].

The advantages of this system are that it is nonterminal and noninvasive, allowing drug efficacy testing in ferrets [45, 48]. Associated disadvantages are that it takes a long time, 10 min in the case of ferrets [45], to monitor the effect of the drug, which limits acquisition of data and thus provides weaker sensitivity in detecting drug efficacy; it is labour-intensive, it requires a large number of study animals to obtain representative data, and it is difficult to perform a kinetic study over a long period of time. Thus this system also has limited applicability for rapid-screening purposes, and the limitation is especially apparent in disease models.

3.1.3. Acoustic rhinometry

Acoustic rhinometric measurements relies on the principle of an ultrasound wave from the emitting source bouncing back when it comes in contact

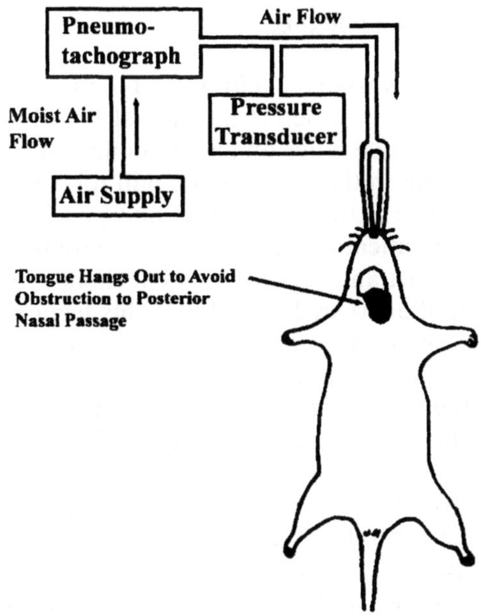

Figure 7. Diagram of passive anterior rhinomanometry and its connection to anaesthetized animals for measurement of nasal airflow resistance.

with a barrier surface. The time interval between the emission and the receipt of the return wave is dependent upon the distance it travels. It is affected by the distance, area and shape of the lumen in the nasal cavity. From the composite sound wave, the cross-sectional area at any given distance from the naris is calculated and thus provides a continuous distance-cross-section area as a representation of the nasal cavity. This technique has been used in minipigs to measure the degree of nasal congestion and the efficacy of nasal decongestants. A comparative study indicates that acoustic rhinomanometry generates results comparable to those of passive posterior rhinomanometry in miniature pigs [47].

Again the technique has several advantages in that it is very easy to operate, with a high degree of data reproducibility; it requires a very short time (seconds) to obtain one data point, and is thus able to perform frequent assessments to derive a kinetic profile; it is a noninvasive technique, it has the potential to use conscious animals for long-term studies and it depends less on the sophisticated skill of an operator to generate reliable data. While the technique is user-friendly, the system is difficult to apply for small animals (rats, mice) due to the very small apertures present in these animals.

3.2. Magnetic Resonance Imaging

MRI is a powerful noninvasive technique used to visualize soft tissues and fluids. It is primarily used to detect the spatial distribution of water and lipid protons. The technique relies on the principle that activated protons of water and lipids present in the target tissue will relax and return to equilibrium. The consequence is the emission of energy which can be detected, digitized and mathematically transformed to produce an image. This results in image contrast and produces an excellent differentiation of the mucosa surrounding the airway lumen [49]. This technique has been used evaluate the effects of histamine and methacholine in the upper airways of ferrets [50, 51]; to visualize the changes in the nasal turbinates of sensitized guinea pigs following an antigenic challenge (Figure 8, [52]); and to demonstrate histamine-induced change in the upper airway in guinea pigs [43].

By employing MRI, the drug efficacy of the histamine (H_1) receptor antagonists loratadine in relieving antigen-induced changes in the nasopharyngeal airway and in mucosal volumes is demonstrated [43]. Similarly, the methodology shows that the nasal decongestant oxymetazoline also has a partial therapeutic effect in guinea pigs after allergen challenge [52]. This technique offers an alternative measurement of rhinitis status with the following advantages. It provides a visual illustration of localized morphological changes in target tissues, and minimal animal preparation is required. It also has some limitations in that it is difficult to perform continuous measurements over a period of hours or days on the same animal; once the animal is removed from the chamber, it is difficult reproducibly to reposition the animal at the same place; and it can take up to several minutes to obtain images with the quality and spatial resolution required to visualize the nasal structures. Additionally, the congestion state could change during image acquisition, and it is difficult to distinguish luminal from interstitial fluid. However, a recent approach developed by Reo et al. [51] allowed distinction between challenges which produced the two types of fluids. The usefulness of MRI is further limited because image analysis procedures to identify the open airway objectively have not been developed, and the convolutions in their airway makes quantification a technical challenge.

4. Methods for Quantitative Measurement of Nasal Secretions

One of the typical signs of rhinitis is nasal secretions, which might be caused by stimulation of sensory nerves or vasculature. Secretions can be objectively measured by several methods in the following examples.

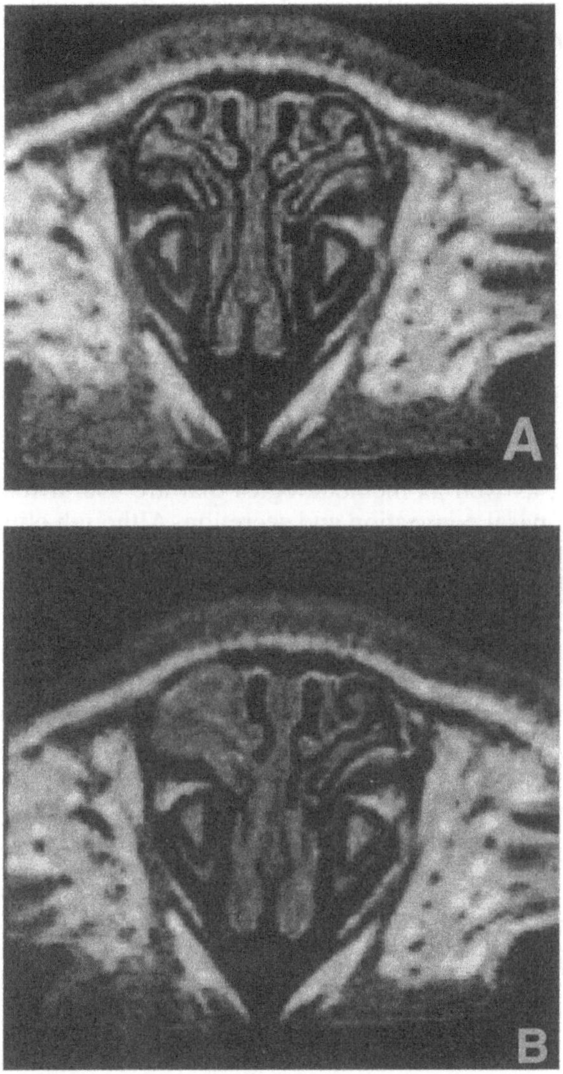

Figure. 8. MRI photographs of nasal turbinates of ovalbumin-sensitized guinea pigs (A) prior to and (B) post intranasal challenge with the homologous allergen. (A) Prior to nasal challenge. (B) Post nasal challenge. Swelling is evident at the lower portion of the septum and the turbinate at the upper left section. Reproduced with permission from [55].

4.1. Guinea Pigs

Defatted cotton threads are dyed with 10% fluorescein sodium in saline at one end and cut to yield pieces 100 mm in length; 10 mm from one end is coloured. Ten minutes after nasal provocation, the nasal secretion is measured with the dyed thread. One end of the thread is inserted into the unilateral anterior naris and retained for 60 s. The length of the colour revealed on the thread is indicative of the quantity of nasal secretion produced [53].

4.2. Ferrets

The content of nasal secretion can be collected over a 10 min period with a pipette [54]. Glandular fluid output is obtained via the cannula inserted at the opening of the gland duct as free-flowing fluid [55], and the quantity is expressed as weight (mg) per 10 min.

5. Conclusion

This review introduces various animal models of rhinitis induced by diverse causes, as well as methodologies that are useful for an objective quantitation of nasal congestion and secretion. Although clinical manifestations of rhinitis may be similar and overlap, their pathogenic mechanisms are different. Every model offers a potentially useful preclinical tool, but they all have inherent advantages and disadvantages. Although clinical symptoms in many animal models resemble human clinical symptoms, the underlying pathogenic mechanisms may not be fully identical to those in human subjects, thus, careful interpretation and extrapolation of findings from experimental models for application in developing human therapeutic agents is warranted.

Acknowledgements

Permission to reproduce MRI photographs of guinea pig nasal turbinate from Dr M.K. Robinson and the critical review of the manuscript by Drs M.K. Robinson, R. Henry and M.D. Cockman are greatly appreciated.

References

1. Kingsman SM, Toms GL, Smith H. The localization of influenza virus in the respiratory tract of ferrets: the importance of early replication events in determining tissue specificity. J Gen Virol 1977; 37: 259–70.
2. Chen K-S, Bharaj SS, King EC. Induction and relief of nasal congestion in ferrets infected with influenza virus. Int J Exp Path 1995; 76: 55–64.
3. Toms GL, Bird RA, Kingsman SM, Sweet C, Smith H. The behaviour in ferrets of two closely related clones of influenza virus of differing virulence for man. Br J Exp Path 1976; 57: 37–48.
4. Toms GL, Davies JA, Woodward CG, Sweet C, Smith H. The relation of pyrexia and nasal inflammatory response to virus levels in nasal washings of ferrets infected with influenza viruses of differing virulence. Br J Exp Path 1977; 58: 444–58.
5. Tinsley CM, Sweet C, Coates DM, Smith H. The local origin of fever in influenza; differential production of endogenous pyrogen by nasal inflammatory cells of ferrets exhibiting different levels of fever. FEMS Microbiol Lett 1987; 42: 103–8.

6. Gaffey MJ, Hayden FD, Boyd JC, Gwaltney MJ Jr. Ipratropium bromide treatment of experimental rhinovirus infection. Antimicrob Agent Chemother 1988; 32: 1644–47.
7. Howard JC Jr, Kantner TR, Lilienfield LS, Princiotto JV, Krum RE, Crutcher JE, Belman MA, Danzig MR. Effectiveness of antihistamines in the symptomatic management of the common cold. J Am Med Assoc 1979; 242: 2414–17.
8. Crutcher JE, Kantner TR. The effectiveness of antihistamines in the common colds. Pharmacology 1981; 21: 945–52.
9. Gaffey MJ, Gwaltney JM Jr, Sastre A, Dressler WE, Sorrentino JV, Hayden FG. Intranasal and oral antihistamine treatment of experimental rhinovirus colds. Am Rev Respir Dis 1987; 136: 556–60.
10. Gaffey MJ, Kaiser DL, Hayden FD. Ineffectiveness of oral terfenadine in natural colds: evidence against histamine as a mediator of common cold symptoms. Ped Infect 1988; 7: 223–28.
11. Iida T, Bang FB. Infection of the upper respiratory tract of mice with influenza A virus. Am J Hyg 1963; 77: 169–76.
12. Giddens WE Jr, Van Hoosier GL Jr, Garlinghouse LE Jr. Experimental Sendai virus infection in laboratory rats. 2. Pathology and immunohistochemistry. Lab Anim Sci 1987; 37: 442–448.
13. Garlinghouse LE Jr, Van Hoosier GL Jr, Giddens WE Jr. Experimental Sendai virus infection in laboratory rats. 1. Virus replication and immune response. Lab Anim Sci 1987; 37: 437–41.
14. Prince GA, Porter DD. The pathogenesis of respiratory syncytial virus infection in infant ferrets. Am J Pathol 1976; 82: 339–52.
15. Coates HV, Chanock RM. Experimental infection with respiratory syncytial virus in several species of animals. Am J Hyg 1962; 76: 302–12.
16. Belshe RB, Richardson LS, London WT, Sly DL, Lorfeld JH, Camargo E et al. Experimental respiratory syncytial virus infection of four species of primates. J Med Virol 1977; 1: 157–62.
17. Jacoby RO, Bhatt PN, Jonas AM. Pathogenesis of sialodacryoadenitis in gnotobiotic rats. Vet Pathol 1975; 12: 196–209.
18. Brownstein DG. Sialodacryoadenitis virus infection, upper respiratory tract, rat. In: Jones TC, Mohr U, Hunt RD, editors. Monographs on pathology of laboratory animals: respiratory system. Berlin: Springer-Verlag 1985: 84–87.
19. Kimman TG, Kamp EM. Induced atrophic rhinitis in rats. Am J Vet Res 1986; 47: 2426–30.
20. Sawata A, Kume K. Nasal turbinate atrophy in young mice inoculated with *Bordetella bronchiseptica* of pig origin. Am J Vet Res 1982; 43: 1845–47.
21. Maeda M, Shimizu T. Nasal infection of *Alcaligenes bronchisepticus* (*Bordetella bronchiseptica*) and lesions in newborn rabbits. Natl Inst Anim Hlth Quart 1975; 15: 29–37.
22. Duberstein LE, Hessler JR. Porcine atrophic rhinitis: a model for studying nasal physiology and pathophysiology. Rhinology 1978; 16: 31–39.
23. Ackermann MR, Rimler RB, Thurston JR. Experimental model of atrophic rhinitis in gnotobiotic pigs. Infect Immun 1991; 59: 3626–29.
24. van Diemen PM, de Jong MF, Reilingh GV, van der Hel P, Schrama JW. Intranasal administration of *Pasteurella multocida* toxin in a challenge-exposure model used to induce subclinical signs of atrophic rhinitis in pigs. Am J Vet Res 1994; 55: 49–54.
25. Rehm S, Waalkes MP, Ward JM. *Aspergillus* rhinitis in Wistar (Crl:(WI)BR) rats. Lab Anim Sci 1988; 38: 162–66.
26. Schoeb TR, Lindsey JR. Murine respiratory mycoplasmosis, upper respiratory tract, rat. In: Jones TE, Mohr U, Hunt RD, editors. Monographs on pathology of laboratory animals: respiratory system. Berlin: Springer-Verlag 1985: 78–84.
27. Everitt JI, Richter CB. Infectious diseases of the upper respiratory tract: implications for toxicology studies. Environmental Health Perspectives 1990; 85: 239–47.
28. Overcash RG, Lindsey JR, Cassell GH, Baker HJ. Enhancement of natural and experimental respiratory mycoplasmosis in rats by hexamethylphosphoramide. Am J Pathol 1976; 82: 171–90.
29. Lee KP, Trochimowicz HJ. Pulmonary response to inhaled hexamethylphosphoramide in rats. Toxicol Appl Pharmacol 1982; 62: 90–103.

30. Broillet A, White R, Ventrone R, Giessinger N. Efficacy of fenspiride in alleviating SO_2 induced chronic bronchitis in rats and allergic rhinitis in guinea pigs. Rhinology 1988; 4 (suppl): 75–83.
31. Shirasaki H, Kojima T, Asakura K, Kataura A, Shimamoto K, Iimura O. The pathophysiological role of kinin and chemical mediators on experimental allergic rhinitis. Adv Exp Med Biol 1989; 247A: 375–78.
32. Ishida M, Amesara R, Ukai K, Sakakura Y. Antigen (DNP-AS)-induced allergic rhinitis model in guinea pigs. Ann Allergy 1994; 72: 240–44.
33. Takahashi N, Aramaki Y, Tsuchiya S. Allergic rhinitis model with Brown Norway rat and evaluation of antiallergic drugs. J Pharmacobiodyn 1990; 13: 414–20.
34. Bouziane H, Latgé JP, Prévost MC, Chevance LG, Paris S. Nasal allergy to fungi in guinea pigs. Mycopathologia 1988; 101: 181–86.
35. Tanaka K, Okamoto Y, Nagaya Y, Nishimura F, Takeoka A, Hanada S, et al. A nasal allergy model developed in the guinea pig by intranasal application of 2,4-toluene diisocyanate. Int Arch Allergy Appl Immunol 1988; 85: 392–97.
36. Zhao XJ, Experimental models of nasal hypersensitive reaction. Chung Hua Erh Pi Hou Ko Tsa Chih 1993; 28: 17–18, 58–59.
37. Underwood DC, Osborn RR, Hand JM. Lack of late-phase airway responses in conscious guinea pigs after a variety of antigen challenges. Agents Actions 1992; 37: 191–94.
38. Samejima Y, Masuyama K, Ishikawa T. Transepithelial migration of eosinophils in experimental nasal allergy in guinea pigs. Auris Nasus Larynx (Tokyo) 1988; 15: 33–42.
39. Salem H, Clemente E. A new experimental method for evaluating drugs in the nasal cavity. Acta Otolaryngol 1972; 96: 524–29.
40. Mizuno H, Kawamura Y, Iwase N, Ohno H. Effects of flutropium on experimental models of drug- and allergy-induced rhinitis in guinea pigs. Jpn J Pharmacol 1991; 55: 321–28.
41. Misawa M. A new rhinitis model using chemical mediators in rats. Jpn J Pharmacol 1988; 48: 15–22.
42. Lau WAK, King RG, Boura ALA. Methoxyphenamine inhibits basal and histamine-induced nasal congestion in anesthetized rats. Br J Pharmacol 1990; 101: 394–98.
43. Sherwood JE, Hutt DA, Kreutner W, Morton JB, Chapman RW. A magnetic resonance imaging evaluation of histamine-mediated allergic response in the guinea pig nasopharynx. J Allergy Clin Immunol 1993; 92: 435–41.
44. Whicker JH, Neel, HB III, Kern EB, Reynolds HY. A model for experimental vasomotor rhinitis. Laryngoscope 1973; 83: 915–22.
45. Wardell JR Jr, Familiar RG, Haff RF. A technique for measuring nasal airway resistance in ferrets. J Allergy 1967; 40: 100–6.
46. Eccles R. The domestic pig as an experimental animal for studies on the nasal cycle. Acta Otolaryngol 1978; 85: 431–36.
47. Mack CE, Henry RT. Comparison of acoustic rhinometry with rhinomanometry in assessing nasal patency in anesthetized minipigs. A Folha Medical (suppl 1): 18.
48. Haff RF. Symptomatic therapy of influenza rhinitis in ferrets by topical application of compounds. J Allergy 1970; 45: 163–77.
49. James TL, Margulis AR, editors. Biomedical magnetic resonance. San Francisco, CA: Radiology Research and Education Foundation 1984.
50. Reo NV, Barnett JKC, Neubecker TA, Alexander ME, Goecke CM. A nuclear magnetic resonance investigation of the upper airways in ferrets. 1. Effects of histamine and methacholine. Magn Reson Med 1992; 27: 21–33.
51. Reo NV, Alexander ME, Goel R. A nuclear magnetic resonance investigation of the upper airways in ferrets. 2. Contrast-enhanced imaging to distinguish vascular from other nasal fluids. Magn Reson Med 1992; 27: 34–43.
52. Robinson MK, Schrotel KR, Neubecker TA. Use of magnetic resonance imaging (MRI) to study allergic rhinitis responses in the guinea pig. J Allergy Clin Immunol 1992; 89: 302.
53. Namimatsu A, Go K, Tanimoto H, Okuda M. Mechanism of nasal secretion mediated via nerve reflex in guinea pigs and evaluation of antiallergic drugs. Int Arch Allergy Immunol 1992; 97: 139–45.
54. Mizoguchi H, Bergeron ML. Effect of capsaicin on nasal secretion in anesthetized ferrets. J Appl. Physiol 1991; 70: 282–86.
55. Mizoguchi H, Widdicombe JG. Lateral nasal gland secretion in the anesthetized ferrets. J Appl. Physiol 1989; 67: 2553–55.

Index

PHYSIOLOGY • PHARMACOLOGY

D. Raeburn, *Rhône-Poulenc Rorer Ltd, Dagenham, UK*
M.A. Giembycz, *Royal Brompton National Heart and Lung Institute, London, UK (Eds)*

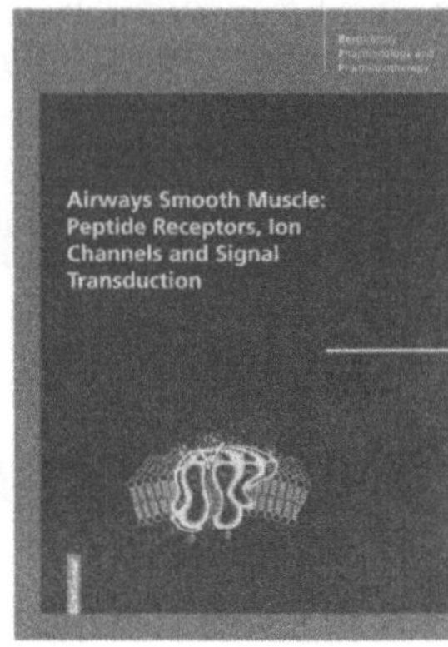

Airways Smooth Muscle: Peptide Receptors, Ion Channels and Signal Transduction

1995. 288 pages. Hardcover • ISBN 3-7643-5140-3

This is the second volume of the Airways Smooth Muscle series to focus on the pharmacological control of airways smooth muscle tone. Each monograph concentrates on the expression and distribution of peptide receptors and describes how their activation may modulate airways calibre at the biochemical level.

In addition, specific chapters are presented on those ion channels and transporter proteins that are currently believed to play major roles in regulating contractility. Current theories regarding signalling at steroid receptors are also considered.

Containing reviews of the latest research developments in the field, this book will prove an invaluable source of reference for pharmacologists, biochemists, clinicians and other biological scientists interested in drug-receptor interactions.

Contents:

Birkhäuser Verlag • Basel • Boston • Berlin

MIX
Papier aus verantwortungsvollen Quellen
Paper from responsible sources
FSC® C105338

If you have any concerns about our products,
you can contact us on
ProductSafety@springernature.com

In case Publisher is established outside the EU,
the EU authorized representative is:
Springer Nature Customer Service Center GmbH
Europaplatz 3, 69115 Heidelberg, Germany

Printed by Libri Plureos GmbH
in Hamburg, Germany